The

PARENT'S

Guide to

HOMEOPATHY

The
PARENT'S
Guide to
HOMEOPATHY

SAFE, NATURAL REMEDIES FOR CHILDREN,
FROM NEWBORNS THROUGH TEENS

SHELLEY KENEIPP
MH, DiHOM

Foreword by Colin Griffith, MCH, MHMA

North Atlantic Books
Berkeley, California

Homeopathic Educational Services
Berkeley, California

Published by   Homeopathic Educational Services
North Atlantic Books   and   812 Camelia Street
Berkeley, California   Berkeley, California 94710

Cover and book design by Jasmine Hromjak
Printed in the United States of America

The Parent's Guide to Homeopathy: Safe, Natural Remedies for Children, from Newborns through Teens is sponsored and published by The Society for the Study of Native Arts and Sciences (dba North Atlantic Books), an educational nonprofit based in Berkeley, California, that collaborates with partners to develop cross-cultural perspectives, nurture holistic views of art, science, the humanities, and healing, and seed personal and global transformation by publishing work on the relationship of body, spirit, and nature.

North Atlantic Books' publications are available through most bookstores. For further information, visit our website at www.northatlanticbooks.com or call 800-733-3000.

MEDICAL DISCLAIMER: The following information is intended for general information purposes only. Individuals should always see their health care provider before administering any suggestions made in this book. Any application of the material set forth in the following pages is at the reader's discretion and is his or her sole responsibility.

Library of Congress Cataloging-in-Publication Data
Keneipp, Shelley.
  The parent's guide to homeopathy: safe, natural remedies for children, from newborns through teens / Shelley Keneipp, M.H., DiHom; foreword by Colin Griffith.
     pages cm
  Includes bibliographical references.
  Summary: "A practical, concise, comprehensive and easy-to-use guide for parents who want to use homeopathy to treat their children's illnesses, with remedies for more than 150 acute conditions that arise in the everyday lives of their children, from annoying to threatening. Includes instructions on how to observe physical and emotional symptoms in children from newborns to teens"—Provided by publisher.
  ISBN 978-1-58394-905-4 (trade pbk.)—ISBN 978-1-58394-906-1 (e-book)
  1. Homeopathy—Popular works. 2. Children—Diseases—Alternative treatment—Popular works. I. Title.
  RX76.K46 2015
  615.5ʲ32—dc23
                              2014021829

              1 2 3 4 5 6 7 8 SHERIDAN 20 19 18 17 16 15

                     Printed on recycled paper

To
My daughters, Michelle and Julia
My grandsons, Zachary, Eli, and Henry Scott
All the children of the world, in hopes that homeopathy
will alleviate much suffering

Acknowledgments

I would like to thank my husband, Marshall, for always supporting my endeavor of studying homeopathy, mostly in England. Thank you for the financial support and your willingness to allow my absence for such long periods of time. Thank you for patiently enduring the long hours I have been unavailable while writing this book.

I would also like to thank all the parents who have given me feedback on how to make this a user-friendly book. It has been invaluable. Parents are the best healers!

Special thanks to my teachers:
Jody Shevins, ND
Colin Griffith, MCH, MHMA

In memory of my teacher:
Martin Miles, FSHom

Contents

Foreword

How often have you wished you knew more about medical matters so that you could ease or heal a problem without having to call or visit the doctor? Have you regretted that you were not able to take responsibility for minor and acute conditions? In these days when medical technology rules, we have all but lost a valuable heritage of knowing what to do in a crisis beyond handing over the problem to an "expert."

In this practical guide, we have a means of taking back some of that responsibility for ourselves and our families. Shelley's book admirably covers just about anything acute witnessed in an average household. Within these covers you'll find out how to deal with conditions that range from annoying to threatening. You'll find out why using homoeopathy is gentler, safer, and more satisfactory than relying on drugs. You'll get to know what remedies are the most useful to keep in your first-aid kit—essential remedies for any household where accidents, trauma, bugs, and other crises happen with any regularity.

Shelley has written a book for everyone. It is user-friendly. It explains just what you need to know and adds no complication. Behind Shelley's wise words is the intention of offering an alternative and complementary way of thinking about health in the home. There is encouragement here for those who might feel reluctant to break the habit of relying exclusively on medical expertise. There is a wealth of experience too; for many years Shelley has lived, breathed, studied, and practiced homoeopathy in just the way she is advocating that you try. She has seen for herself within her own family and among her patients the beauty of homoeopathy at work.

I have known Shelley for many years and can honestly say that in my forty years of involvement in homoeopathy I have not met another person more devoted to or more passionate about its benefits. Though homoeopathy may go in and out of fashion, it remains always true to itself—the gentlest possible cure in the shortest possible time, with the fewest reasons for intervention. It is a system used across the world; it is known in every continent of the globe; and it has advocates in almost every country, even in the jungles of South America and the islands of the South Pacific.

If you are new to homoeopathy, then you hold in your hands a book of discovery. If you already know something about it and want to learn more, then I can't imagine a better way than to refer to these pages whenever the need arises.

I wish you all the very best of health!

—Colin Griffith, MCH, MHMA

A Note about Homeopathy in the United States

In 1862 Congress passed the first Homestead Act, which granted the head of a family 160 acres of land if they cultivated it for five years.

The year is 1863. In the city of Saint Louis, Missouri, people wanting to take advantage of the Homestead Act are preparing their wagons for the adventure west. Most wagon trains did not have a doctor for the journey, and the doctors in the West were few and far between, especially in the Plains states. There is a pharmacy by the name of Luties, where the pioneers can buy a homeopathic kit and a book, *The Domestic Physician* by Constantine Hering, MD (the father of United States homeopathy). Pioneers used this book and remedy kit to treat any illnesses that might arise on their journey. Settling on a ranch—say out in the middle of Wyoming—would mean a total reliance on the homeopathic kit and the knowledge put forth in Dr. Hering's book. To this day, homeopathy is still used to treat people and animals on ranches in Wyoming, where I was raised.

Homeopathy was very helpful and an invaluable modality for the pioneers who settled the western part of the United States. It has been used for generations to treat families in an effective and safe way, with no toxic or harmful side effects.

Introduction

Important! Please read:

Any information contained in this book is not intended to diagnose, treat, cure, or prevent any chronic disease or emergency condition. Information in this book is not intended as a substitute for advice from your physician or other healthcare professional. You should consult with your physician or healthcare professional before taking any medication yourself, or giving a medication to your infant, child, or other members of your family. You should always consult with your physician or healthcare professional and carefully read all information provided by the manufacturer, including the label, of any homeopathic remedy.

What is homeopathy?

The word homeopathy comes from the Greek words *homoios* and *patheia,* which translate into "similar suffering." Hippocrates, a Greek physician born around 460 BC, is considered the father of medicine. Hippocrates stated that there are two ways of treating ill health—the Law of Opposites and the Law of Similars. In 1796, a German doctor named Samuel Hahnemann based his approach to healing on the principles of the Law of Similars originally set forth by Hippocrates. Thus homeopathy was born.

Homeopathy is based on the principle that "like cures like." Suppose a child has a cold with watery eyes and a burning nasal discharge. According to the principles of homeopathy, these symptoms represent the body's attempt to restore itself to health. If a substance can cause symptoms in a healthy person, then it can stimulate self-healing of similar symptoms in a sick person. The remedy **Allium Cepa** (Latin for "onion") might be given because onion is known to cause watery eyes and a burning nasal discharge. This is how homeopathy utilizes the Law of Similars. Practicing the Law of Opposites, a cold would be treated by giving a drug to dry mucus in the nose, a different drug to bring down the fever, a cough syrup to suppress the cough, and/or something to get rid of the headache.

Homeopathy is effective because it evaluates the whole person, taking into account the physical, emotional, and mental symptoms. Homeopathic case-taking looks at each person individually, as each person suffers from health conditions in his or her own unique way. Observing four different children suffering from the same cold virus, we see that one child will develop a horrible sore throat, another a deep cough, another an ear infection, etc. Homeopathy looks at each person's unique symptoms: Is the person chilly or hot? Is the nose running or stuffed up? What color is the discharge? Did the cold come on after stress, anger, or loss of sleep? Does the person want sympathy, or to be left alone? A complete picture of the whole person is looked at from a truly holistic perspective. Therefore, the homeopathic remedy is chosen based on the best match of the person's own unique set of symptoms. Once the remedy is taken, it restores the body and mind into a complete biological and psychological balance.

Homeopathy is a science of healing that stimulates and strengthens the vital force by the use of a minute dose of a substance. In the case of homeopathy, "less is better and more powerful." The message from the chosen remedy is sent through the central nervous system, which pervades all systems in the entire body. The body receives the message from the similar energy pattern being presented by the remedy, which stimulates the self-healing process into action.

This is a very simple explanation of homeopathy. If you wish to learn more about homeopathy, you can go to www.homeopathic.com, the site for Homeopathic Educational Services. If you would like a more in-depth study of homeopathic knowledge and philosophy, they have a good selection of beginner, intermediate, and advanced books available for purchase. This book will only provide a simple explanation of how homeopathy works.

Where else is homeopathy used— and why isn't it more common in the U.S.?

Over 200 years of clinical experience, along with modern research published in *The Lancet, Pediatrics, Pediatric Infectious Disease Journal, The British Medical Journal, The British Journal of Clinical Pharmacology, Journal of Head Trauma Rehabilitation,* and *Clinical Journal of Pain* have all confirmed homeopathy's effectiveness. Included in some of the research are double-blind clinical trials, especially from the German homeopathic community.

The use of homeopathy is advocated by the World Health Organization. Its use is commonplace in Germany, the United Kingdom, France, India, Israel, Brazil, Mexico, Canada, the Netherlands, Greece, Australia, New Zealand, and Russia. There are homeopathic hospitals, not to mention scores of homeopathic clinics, in Moscow, France, India, Denmark, Shanghai, and the United Kingdom. The royal family of the United Kingdom has been using homeopathy as its main healthcare modality since the 1840s and has its own homeopathic physician for consultations. As evidenced by the royal family's longevity, homeopathy shines forth.

Sadly, it is only used by two percent of the population in the U.S. today. There is a statue of Samuel Hahnemann in Washington, DC. In 1900 there were twenty-two homeopathic medical schools, more than one hundred homeopathic hospitals, and over 1,000 homeopathic pharmacies in the U.S. It is estimated that there were approximately 15,000 homeopathic practitioners. What happened to the hospitals and homeopathic medical schools?

In 1850, the American Medical Association (AMA) stated that orthodox physicians would lose their membership in the AMA if they even consulted a homeopath. In 1866, the AMA banned any discussion of homeopathic medical theory in their journals and expelled any doctors caught consulting a homeopath or using homeopathy for their patients. They even went so far as to say that any doctor married to a homeopath would be expelled. Because of heavy lobbying and scare tactics, people were frightened into thinking that everyone in the healthcare field needed licensing. Licensing measures, heavily weighted by AMA standards and beliefs, were adopted by Congress and state legislatures between 1900 and 1920. The U.S. government was even giving subsidies to the AMA. By 1930, the AMA had almost entirely eroded the influence of homeopathy and other natural healing arts in the U.S. Homeopathic hospitals and the majority of homeopathic teaching schools were closed down.

In the book *Patient Power: Solving America's Health Care Crisis* (Cato Institute, 1992), John C. Goodman and Gerald L. Musgrave wrote, "Virtually every law restricting the practice of medicine in America has been enacted not on the crest of public demand, but due to intense pressure from the political representatives of physicians."[1]

Fortunately for children in the United States, homeopathy is making a comeback. Every year, more and more medical doctors are studying homeopathy and incorporating it into their practices. The September 2003 edition of *Plastic and Reconstructive Surgery* reported on two studies that supported the safety and efficacy of the homeopathic remedy **Arnica**. Following this article, thirty doctors who are certified by the American Society of Aesthetic Plastic Surgeons have come forward endorsing its usefulness in their surgical practices.

How safe is homeopathy?

Homeopathy is one of the safest modalities of healing. The majority of homeopathic remedies are taken from plants. Some other remedies are taken from minerals, elements of the periodic table, and animal sources. These remedies assist the body to restore its healthy balance. Homeopathic remedies are free of any harmful or toxic side effects. They are safe and gentle enough for infants and children. Homeopathic remedies have never had to be taken off the market because of damaging or dangerous side effects. Homeopathic remedies are not addictive. Many of the same remedies being used today were used two

[1]John C. Goodman and Gerald L. Musgrave, *Patient Power: Solving America's Health Care Crisis* (Washington, DC: Cato Institute, 1992).

hundred years ago, and new ones are being proven all the time to broaden the scope of treatment. If a remedy is not appropriate, there will be no response and nothing will happen.

It is, however, important to keep all homeopathic remedies out of the reach of children. The small vials can present a choking hazard—and no parent wants their child to consume their store of remedies! If your child does ingest an entire vial, in most instances there is nothing to worry about. Homeopathic remedies do not pose a threat of poisoning. Except for a few instances in this book, all remedies you will be using are of a 30C potency. This potency will not cause any harm to your child even if they ingest the whole vial.

Homeopathic remedies are not tested on animals. They are only given to healthy humans in order to understand the unique healing properties of each particular remedy.

What does this book address?

This book gives detailed information about how to use homeopathy to treat acute and first-aid conditions for infants, children, teens, and the whole family. Explanations are geared toward infants and children. A screaming baby cannot tell you what is happening. "It hurts," from a toddler, does not give you enough information to choose the appropriate remedy. No chronic illnesses will be addressed in these pages.

In this book, there are explanations of what each acute condition is, and guiding principles for observing them. Also provided is a precise thumbnail sketch of the most common remedies as they pertain to each particular condition. There are exact dosage directions. Supplemental practical tips are given to facilitate a safe and complete recovery. Clear guidelines are presented where the development of certain symptoms would require a call to your healthcare practitioner or a visit to an emergency room.

Only the most common remedies for each condition are addressed. You will have a very high likelihood of successfully choosing the correct remedy given the choices in this book. Tables are provided at the end of major sections for quick reference on each major condition and how to identify the most commonly used remedies for it.

Acute illness produces symptoms that appear very quickly, are relatively short in duration, and go through a typical progression of changes. This includes injuries, fevers, colds, cuts, bruising, teething, stomach upsets, etc. Normally, the body has its own self-healing resources and can find its own resolution. Homeopathy sets the body right again through its gentle powerful action, much more quickly than doing nothing. Given the correct remedy, your child will have less suffering with no repression of symptoms.

Chronic illness is a long-term condition for which the body has no ultimate internal solution; the self-healing mechanism has somehow been compromised. A chronic condition tends to get progressively worse over many months or years. A recurring acute illness is not actually acute—if someone suffers repeated colds over a long period of time, the real problem lies in the dysfunction of the immune system, nutritional deficiencies, and/or environmental toxins. These chronic conditions require a constitutional treatment, with an assessment of family history, history since birth, psychological makeup, and every system of the body as well as current symptoms. If you choose to treat homeopathically, an experienced homeopath is needed to deal with chronic conditions.

Do I need to consult a professional homeopath in order to use homeopathy at home?

No, but it's much easier if you do. There are times when we all need guidance. If you do not have a homeopath, you may log on to www.homeopathic.org/resources/practitioners to find a homeopathic practitioner in your area.

Are there any warning signs that tell me when to seek professional advice?

This is mostly a question of common sense, prudent judgment, and parental intuition. Nevertheless, there are a number of symptoms that should never be ignored. There is a section entitled "Call your healthcare practitioner if" at the end of almost every condition section, which lists conditions requiring immediate medical attention or a call to your healthcare practitioner. When in doubt, do not hesitate to call your healthcare practitioner for confirmation.

How should I store remedies?

Remedies should be stored in a cool, dry place away from excessive heat, strong sunlight, and electrical equipment. Do not let your remedies stay within ten feet of a cellphone, cordless digital phones, microwave ovens, computers, or stereo equipment. There are homeopaths who do not believe that remedies can be affected by any of what has been mentioned, but it is my recommendation to be safe rather than sorry, especially if you have invested in a homeopathic kit. The best protection from microwave radiation or x-rays is aluminum foil, or a lead-lined photographer's bag, available from photography shops.

If you are traveling, you need to protect your remedies from the x-ray machines at the airport. Carry-on and checked bags are x-rayed. Wrap all remedies, or your whole kit, in aluminum foil. Some place their remedies in a lead-lined photographer's bag. Do not carry remedies on your body if you go into the full-body scanner at the airport. You can, however, put remedies or small kits in your pocket if you simply walk through the metal detector. This will not hurt the remedies because it does not use x-rays.

Note: Some pharmacies are now putting remedies in plastic instead of the traditional colored glass. Plastic outgasses petroleum products into the remedies, so it is best to obtain remedies in glass containers. You can link onto a reputable pharmacy using glass vials from my website, www.hchild.com. There is also a resource section in the back of this book that will give you further information on homeopathic pharmacies that do not package their products in plastic.

What is the shelf life of a remedy?

Remedies made in the traditional way by reputable homeopathic pharmacies will keep their potency for years. If you store the remedies properly, they can last a lifetime. There are cases of remedies being 100 years old and still working just fine. These remedies have been prepared by a process called "succussing." Many health-food stores now carry remedies from pharmacies that take the shortcut of shaking their remedies rather than succussing them, and then package them in plastic, in order to increase their profit margin. Homeopaths have found that shaken remedies will lose their potency over time.

How do I select the indicated remedy?

- Address the condition sooner rather than later! If you try to treat a cold three days after it began, the cold has already set in. You can still treat any new symptoms that arise, such as a cough. If a child has been in a cold north wind and the cold symptoms came on quickly, **Aconitum** will usually clear the cold in twenty-four hours with supportive measures employed.
- Choose three important symptoms in order to identify the correct remedy. No child will have all of the symptoms. If a child is hacking away and you think they have three strong symptoms that indicate **Cuprum Metallicum,** but there is no metallic taste, give the remedy anyway. Or if there are three strong symptoms for **Belladonna,** but the child is not craving lemonade, give the remedy. See below for choosing the most important symptoms.
- Stop the remedy once there is improvement, unless otherwise indicated. Your child should steadily improve over minutes, hours, or days, depending on the condition. Repeat *only* if there is a return of symptoms.

To read symptoms in a child is rather like learning a foreign language—the language of the body. Symptoms are the way that the body and mind communicate that the vital force is not in balance. When you analyze your child's symptoms, this is called "taking a case." After observing the symptoms, you will be able to choose the correct remedy.

The first step is to look at the child to see if there is any obvious change in the mood, the coloring, the expression, energy, temperature, sensitivity (or not) to the environment, thirst, appetite, or changes in sleep patterns. Moods and temperament are very important because they are related to the emotional state. Emotional symptoms can sometimes eliminate your consideration of a whole range of remedies. Temperature is important because each fever is very different. Some remedies will deal with very high fevers, while others will deal with fevers where the child is playing as if nothing is amiss. Coloring can be useful; for instance, observing whether a boil is very red or purple. Energy is important; a child whose energy is lively will need a different remedy from a child who is trashed on the sofa, or from another who is weak but restless. Sensitivity to the environment is important because it can give a clue as to how the child reacts to drafts, heat, cold, sunlight, or noise. Thirst and appetite can also be helpful in guiding you to the correct remedy; however, these tend to be less important guiding symptoms. If your child is waking at 4 AM, this can also point to a specific remedy.

Symptoms can be qualified by what are known as "modalities." These are symptoms that tell us what makes the child feel better or worse. For example, the child may feel worse from being in a hot, stuffy atmosphere, and better from being in the fresh air. Or a child may feel better from sitting than lying down. Some conditions are better from motion and worse from rest.

Besides helping you to choose the correct remedy, the "Worse from" sections will give you an indication of how to eliminate further suffering of the child, while "Better from" will give you an indication of how to make your child more comfortable. *Please be sure to use these modalities in caring for your sick child; they will help to alleviate their suffering and make them feel more comfortable.*

Pain and other sensations are good guides as well. Pains can be achy, sharp, shooting, burning, cramping, pinching, erratic, steady, or throbbing. Sensations can be numbness, trembling, weakness, cold, heat, heaviness, or pressure. It can be very difficult for a child to describe pain. Babies and sometimes your child cannot give you specific answers. Don't worry; there will be other symptoms to look at in order to choose the best remedy. There is a "What to observe" guide in the Newborn section that will help you to choose the remedies needed for babies and young toddlers.

The symptoms that can be the most valuable of all are known as "strange, rare, or peculiar" symptoms. The more strange, rare, or peculiar they are, the more likely you will be led to the correct remedy. This is because those strange symptoms may indicate only one remedy, or just a few. For example, it is very strange for a child to have a dry mouth but no thirst, thus indicating **Pulsatilla**. Or the child may have burning pains in the stomach but wants a heating pad, thus indicating **Arsenicum**. If a child gets a cold after having their hair cut, this can indicate **Belladonna**. This being said, most of the symptom picture must fit. Do not prescribe based on only one strange, rare, or peculiar symptom.

Note: There may be times when you are exhausted or losing sleep from taking care of a sick child. If this is the case, it is advisable to use **Bach Flower Essence Rescue Remedy.** Put three drops in a small glass of spring water, and drink it. Sit quietly for a few moments and then go back to analyzing the case.

Rescue Remedy is found in health-food stores and natural pharmacies. It is a liquid made up of five different flower essences preserved in an alcohol-water solution. This flower essence was invented by an English homeopath by the name of Dr. Edward Bach. It has calming and comforting properties to reduce stress and shock when there has been a crisis, emergency, or accident. The Bach Flower Essences are usually next to the homeopathic remedies in the health-food store or natural pharmacy. They are completely safe. If your child or any member of your family is experiencing any of the above conditions, you can administer it in the following way: Add three drops to a glass of water, and have the child sip it frequently until you see progress; repeat as long as needed. Stop when emotional stability has returned.

How do I administer remedies?

You will give 2 pellets of the remedy at a time. **Two pellets are considered to be one homeopathic dose.** Do not open the remedy vial in a room where strong odors are present. Carefully and slowly put 2 pellets into the lid of the vial. Do not touch the pellets. If more than 2 pellets come out, *do not* put excess pellets back into the vial, as they can contaminate what remains in the vial. Have the child tip their head back and lift their tongue; then administer 2 pellets under the tongue. Be careful not to touch the lid to the child's lips, tongue, or mouth. If you are using tiny pellets, you only need two of them, but do not worry if the child gets even seven or eight.

Do not wake a baby or child to give them a remedy. If they go to sleep after taking a remedy, this is a good sign. Allow the remedy to take action.

How to administer remedies to a baby: If the pellets are large, you can crush one pellet between two spoons, add a drop of spring water, swish it around, wait a few seconds, and then administer the water onto the baby's lips. Once you put a pellet into water, you are causing the water to become "medicated."

If you do not have any spring water, just crush 2 pellets on a clean spoon. Gently pull back the baby's lower lip, and let the remedy slide off of the spoon so that it goes between the lip and gum. The pellets in the kits from my website, Homeopathy for the Child (www.hchild.com), are so small that you do not need to crush them into a powder and choking is not a hazard.

Frequency of the dose is actually the most important thing. Each dose, separated by a period of time, is a fresh input of the energy of the remedy for the vital force. Sometimes it is necessary to repeat a dose because the vital force has used up the energy of a previous dose. So a child that has begun to respond to **Belladonna** for a fever, or **Podophyllum** for diarrhea, might need a repeat dose after two hours if the symptoms begin to return. It is not unusual for remedies to be repeated quite a few times.

- If the condition is **life-threatening**, give the remedy *every 5–15 minutes.*
- If a condition **comes on fast and furious**, give the remedy *every 15 minutes.*
- If the onset is **slower and less intense**, give the remedy *every 2–4 hours.*
- If the onset is **mild**, give the remedy *every 4–6 hours.*
- If the condition is **quite slow to heal**, as with a muscle strain, give the remedy *2–3 times per day for a few days.*
- *Stop repeating the remedy* as soon as there is improvement of symptoms. Repeat *only* if there is a return of symptoms.

Sometimes you are getting good results from a remedy, but then it fails to hold. At this point, you will need to administer the same remedy with more frequency. If there is still no holding power, you need to reassess the case and look to another remedy. It might be that your choice was not quite similar enough to the symptoms of your child. Or the first remedy was needed but now the child has moved on, and requires another remedy to complement the first remedy you gave. In this case, the second remedy will then finish the cure. This can be common if a child was chilled in a north wind and goes down fast, indicating **Aconitum.** Twenty-four hours later, they are coughing and have different symptoms. At that point you need to reassess, and look to a cough remedy.

Note: A common mistake that parents make is not giving enough doses of the remedy. If you follow the instructions in the **Dosage** section under each remedy, you do not need to worry about giving your child too much medication. You do, however, need to make sure that enough of the selected remedy has been given before ever moving on to another remedy.

It is common to give remedies to animals in their food, so don't worry about giving a remedy before or after meals or drinks. If the child has eaten something with a strong flavor, though, wait ten minutes before giving the remedy.

Should I avoid touching the remedies?

Yes, because if you are either sensitive to or need the same remedy yourself, then your body will take up the remedy through the skin. Because the skin is so rich in nerve endings, it is quite capable of transferring the remedy's energy to the central nervous system. Another reason is that the remedy might be tainted if your hands have been in contact with something heavily scented such as perfumed hand lotion. Also, the normal oils on your hands are not good for the remedies.

What potency should I give?

Ninety-nine percent of the conditions in this book are set for 30C potency. This is the most commonly recommended potency for acute conditions. This potency will act for a good amount of time, and also act on the child's temperament, and the organs and tissues of the body. If you have a baby or child with low vitality, please consult a homeopath. A baby who is failing to thrive will need a lower potency, and professional help. A child who is extremely weak will have the same remedy picture, but will need a lower potency. Call your homeopath.

Are there any substances that will antidote the remedies?

Yes, there are. The main ones are *strong peppermints* (such as Altoids® breath mints), *camphor, eucalyptus, menthol,* and *tea tree oil.* Always avoid these substances. These are very powerful essential oils with medicinal potentials of their own, and they can completely negate the action of a remedy given. Do not use decongestants such as mentholated lozenges or vapor rubs. Avoid inhalations of things like Vicks VapoRub® or Tiger Balm, because these can also antidote a remedy. Be sure to check your toothpaste, shampoos, conditioners, and soaps for such aromatic products. Most health-food stores will carry alternative toothpastes without the above ingredients. Although I do not recommend that children drink coffee, your teenager might be indulging in it. Do not allow them to drink coffee *two hours before or after* taking a homeopathic remedy. Some children are so sensitive that coffee or even dental work can undo a remedy. If your child or a family member is particularly sensitive, you will need to adhere strictly to this protocol.

If you suspect that the remedy has been compromised or nullified and the condition has returned, repeat the remedy. An example of this might be that you gave a remedy for a cough, and the cough went away. Then your child was exposed to someone using Tiger Balm, and the child started coughing again.

Many parents have become disenchanted with the failures of antibiotic use for ear infections. Others have put their children through operations to place tubes in their ears, only to find that they didn't work or ended up falling out and starting another round of infections. By using the tools in this book you are helping to revive a modality that works! I applaud your courage to take back the responsibility of caring for your children's good health using a gentle, efficient, non-invasive, and effective system. Please spread the word of your successes among your family, friends, and neighbors. As always, I encourage feedback and new ideas. You may contact me on my website, www.hchild.com.

Good luck to you and your family on your journey using homeopathy!

Caring for a Sick Child

If you are a first-time parent and your baby becomes ill, it can be scary because you do not know what to do or how to help your child who is suffering. All children are going to get sick from time to time; it is part of life. The immune system is like any other muscle in the body—using it on a consistent basis keeps it strong and vital. This does not mean that a child should be contracting illness after illness, which would put too much stress on the immune system. The child's constitutional state must be evaluated if they are always getting sick.

There may come a time when a child needs urgent medical attention. Most parents know instinctively when something is not right with their child; I encourage you to listen to your intuition and use prudent judgment. Better to be safe than sorry! A call to your healthcare practitioner can help calm many fears.

In our modern-day life of frantic hustle, it may be overwhelming for a parent when a child falls ill, especially for working parents. "Who can cover for me at work?" "I can't take off any more time at work; I've used all my vacation time!" "I have a deadline to finish this project!" "How can I get my child over this quickly?" These are just a few of the unfortunate questions or realities of modern life that arise when our children are ill.

If you are a working parent, you might want to put in place ahead of time some help to call upon when your child falls ill. Utilizing the help of neighbors, friends, or family ahead of time can ease the pressure and stress on yourself and your partner. It is always best if children can stay at home when they are sick. You will also need to get as much rest as possible, and be sure to eat well.

When a child becomes ill, it is imperative that the child slow down and rest. Healing and repair takes place faster and more completely if the body is allowed to rest. The atmosphere needs to be low-stress, with few comings and goings of outside people, and with only quiet activities. These may consist of soothing music, reading or being told stories, playing board games, or drawing. A little TV or a movie may help with boredom, but too much is overstimulating and can keep the child from deeply resting.

A sick child needs extra nurturing, comforting, and reassurance in order to get better. They need to be encouraged to drink plenty of water, diluted juices, and herbal teas. If they do not want to drink, they can suck on ice cubes, frozen juice bars with no sugar added, or even a clean natural sponge dipped in water. Do not force a child to eat if they are not hungry. Offer nutritious light snacks, soups, or pureed vegetables and fruits.

A sick, demanding child can be very trying and tiring. The potty-trained toddler may have an accident. A child may ask for something and then throw it down. They may have no patience, and be impossible to please. Your child needs to hear, in a reassuring and comforting voice, that everything is going to be all right. Share with the child what is wrong, why you are doing certain things, and how soon they can look forward to feeling better. Please keep your child at home until there is no fever, their appetite has returned, and they are sleeping normally.

Don't forget to use **Bach Flower Essence Rescue Remedy** yourself if you are frustrated or exhausted. Refer back to the Introduction of the book and look at the "How do I select the indicated remedy?" section.

Note: When children are under stress, their bodies begin producing symptoms of illness. If your child is unhappy at school, he or she can develop headaches, stomachaches, anxiety, or sleep difficulties. It is important to not let this become a chronic situation. Encourage the child to talk to you about it. Listen carefully, and address their fears and frustrations. If necessary, intervene by speaking with teachers, coaches, or school counselors. Children can be the victims of bullying; do not hesitate to speak with other parents to remedy this kind of situation. You are your child's only advocate.

Teens of today have many more temptations to deal with than their parents' generation did. In this sometimes frantic-paced world, it is easy for a teen to feel lots of pressure to perform, and they can easily become overwhelmed. Again, keep the lines of communication open. In our society, there are some children who have no downtime, or are being forced to participate in sports. Your son may not want to play football. Your daughter may not want to play basketball.

Make sure your child is not eating junk food, playing too many video games, or watching too much TV, and that they are getting adequate hours of sleep. Studies have shown that it is optimal for a teenager to get at least nine and a quarter hours of sleep a night. If your child is not responding to remedies, stress could be an obstacle. Any child or teen who has suffered a great emotional shock, e.g., divorce or death, will more than likely need professional psychological help and a professional homeopath for support.

How To Use This Book

Only acute conditions or acute phases of conditions are addressed in this book. You will need to address any chronic conditions with a professional homeopath.

The full Latin names of remedies are not spelled out in the text. Abbreviations will be obvious.

The following sections are included for all or most conditions:

The condition: Each condition is explained in detail, with information about how it manifests generally in the body. There may also be information on when to call your healthcare provider, or other cautions.

What to observe: This section under each condition will aid you in how to read symptoms and detect what is happening to your baby or child. There is a checklist in the "Newborn Discomforts" section on how to observe infants and young toddlers. Some but not all condition sections also include this.

The most common remedies for each condition: Each child manifests symptoms differently. Each remedy section provides a description of the unique set of symptoms for that particular remedy. Most descriptions will also tell you what the mood of the child is like when the remedy is indicated. Again, remember that we are taking a look at the whole picture. *Please remember* that your child is unlikely to have every symptom described. If the description says "the child *may have*" or "*sometimes* the child is," this indicates a minor symptom that may or may not be present. You will be choosing the remedy that most closely matches *most* of your child's symptoms.

At the end of most remedy descriptions, you will see what makes the child feel worse or better. This is a further indication for choosing the correct remedy. These modalities can also help you care for the sick baby or child. **"Worse from"** actions tell you how to reduce the child's suffering. In other words, this is what the child's body does *not* want or need for the present condition. **"Better from"** actions tell you how to make your child more comfortable. In the "Colic in Babies" section, for instance, a nursing mother will be given an indication of what to eliminate from her diet so it does not aggravate the baby's colic. Paying close attention to these details will help you and your child.

Dosage: This section will tell you how often to give a remedy, or when to change a remedy if it was not the best match.

Supportive measures: This section will give you tips for dealing with the particular condition, and ways of further comforting your baby or child.

Call your healthcare practitioner if: These sections will give clear parameters about when to seek emergency care or call your child's healthcare practitioner. *Please pay particular attention to this section, and use your good judgment.* If in doubt, do not hesitate to call your healthcare practitioner, or seek urgent or emergency care. It is very important to familiarize yourself with any complications that may arise. Please always read this section, to become familiar with any complications associated with the condition your child has. Then take any necessary actions.

Remedy tables: These tables at the end of some sections provide a thumbnail sketch of only the most common remedies. Tables are provided for the most commonly used remedies for some but not all conditions. The tables can be helpful if your child is exhibiting symptoms indicating two closely related remedies. They will provide you a quick reference guide, but please always read the more in-depth description about each remedy when you are assessing your child's condition.

PART ONE

Common Childhood Ailments,
from Newborns to Teens

ANXIETY ABOUT GOING TO PRESCHOOL, KINDERGARTEN, SCHOOL, OR COLLEGE

A preschool or elementary school child may exhibit such behaviors as crying, screaming, clinging to you, and/or throwing a tantrum. They can become so upset that they may hyperventilate. A middle or high school-age child may withdraw, experience a drop in academic grades, or suffer panic attacks.

Certain things need to be eliminated as possible causes of your child's anxiety. Please listen to your child and explore their resistance to attending school. You are your child's only advocate. Some children may be the victims of merciless teasing, demeaning name-calling, bullying, a mean teacher, a teacher exhibiting inappropriate behaviors, breaking up with a girl/boyfriend, or being excluded from a clique. Also, get feedback from your child's teacher about classroom dynamics, and make sure your child does not have a learning disability.

The following are the most commonly indicated remedies for anxiety:

Arsenicum: The whole body, and/or different body parts, tremble. The child is irritable, restless, oversensitive, anxious, impatient, demanding, critical, and forgetful. The toddler will want to be carried briskly. They may want mom, then dad, then to go back to mom again. The older child may have a fear of dying or catching a serious disease. They get upset about any disorder, wanting to have their bedroom or surroundings orderly and neat. They have a strong need for order and consistent routines. They may pace back and forth. They worry a lot about what may or may not happen. They are usually chilly, and thirsty for sips of water. This anxiety can manifest with heartburn or burning stomachaches, diarrhea, and/or rashes.

Baryta Carb: This is for a very shy child who hesitates to speak in a group or raise their hand in class. They have anxiety about being made fun of or laughed at. This is a child that may be more immature both physically and mentally compared to others in

3

their age group. They usually learn to walk and talk late. They may also lack reading skills; their development seems delayed. They generally lack confidence, and may say they are stupid. They sit in the corner at school by themselves. This anxiety can manifest in a sore stomach, weakness, sleepiness, chilliness, and cold, clammy feet.

Calc Carb: This remedy is especially helpful for a child entering preschool or kindergarten. They are very dependent. They dread new situations because they need stability and protection from the unknown.

Calc Phos: These children are fretful, dissatisfied, easily frustrated, forgetful, and easily fatigued from mental strain. School may just be too academically overwhelming and exhausting. Their memories are very weak. You many notice involuntary sighing. They can have a hard time waking up in the morning. Their anxiety manifests with headaches, stomachaches, and sometimes trembling.

Ignatia: This remedy is indicated for the child who is very sensitive, especially to pain; who is nervous, excitable, introspective, easily frustrated, moody, or weepy, sighs a lot, yawns, grieves quietly, does not want sympathy, and may become antisocial. This child will complain of a lump in the throat, a sore throat, tightness in the chest, cramping of muscles, numbness or tingling of the nerves, spasms, or a stomachache. They may have strange sensations anywhere in the body. This is a good remedy for a child starting preschool, for separation anxiety and homesickness. They may bite their lips or cheeks. They may say, "I can't believe it," over and over again. They can have unpredictable reactions—hysterically crying one moment, laughing the next, furious the next, distant the next, anxious and restless the next. They may try to hold the tears back, but end up sobbing. There is often a loss of appetite.

Natrum Mur: This is for the child who is irritable, angry, serious, abrupt, absent-minded, confused, and likely to cry at the least little thing. They get their feelings hurt easily. However, they absolutely do not want consolation, and desire to be alone. They tend to hold grudges. They have a fear of being rejected, humiliated, or hurt emotionally. Because of this, they may not want to return to school if they have lost a close friendship. A middle-school youngster will be depressed, discontented with life, withdrawn, irritable, and inclined to listen to melancholic music. They are emotionally sensitive, but find it hard to cry in front of others. The anxiety is manifested with achy sore throats with pain extending into the ears, or throbbing, bursting, blinding headaches, or tingling in the extremities, or palpitations with a faint feeling.

Pulsatilla: The child is mild, timid, clingy, tearful, whiny, weepy, and fretful—but affectionate, and craves attention. The younger child will be quite pouty if they feel others are not paying enough attention to them. They are very dependent on others for reassurance. This child needs attention, reassurance, and gentleness. They may tend to feel sorry for themselves, and need to be gently encouraged out of their self-pity and not allowed to wallow in it for too long. They may state, "It is not fair." They will feel better after a good cry. They have very changeable moods, like being on an emotional roller coaster, especially at the middle-school level. This anxiety manifests with stomachaches, symptoms that come and go, discharges from the eyes, one-sided headaches, shortness of breath, or a dry mouth without thirst.

Stramonium: This child exhibits hysteria, ceaseless talking, rage, loud laughter, or a fear that they are going to die. They can be terrified. Look for a red, flushed face with an expression of intense anxiety or terror. The pupils can be widely dilated. There is often much tension in the abdomen. The child needing this remedy may become afraid of the dark, need to have a light on, and may not want to sleep alone. They can also wake screaming from nightmares. They cannot bear solitude or darkness. They have a feeling that they have been forsaken, or are all alone in the wilderness. Your teen may exhibit anxiety by wearing all black and becoming isolated. This anxiety manifests with headaches, difficulty swallowing along with intense thirst, or constriction in the chest.

Dosage: Give 2 pellets every day for up to 3 days. If there is improvement after the first dose, you can stop. If there is no response after the third dose, try a different remedy. Repeat the remedy only if there is a return of any symptom.

Call your healthcare practitioner if:

- Your child is lacking in social skills for maintaining good relationships.
- Your child develops a phobia about going to school.

BOILS

A boil is a skin abscess in which pus accumulates just beneath the surface of an oil gland or hair follicle. Boils develop because of an internal process in which the body needs to rid itself of toxicity. The boil will start out as a small, hard, red bump. As days go by, it becomes more tender, fills with pus, forms a head, bursts open, and then drains. The pus consists of dead white blood cells that have died after killing bacteria. If a boil comes to a head and bursts, it expels the dead bacteria.

Sometimes the boil will not burst, and the body will absorb the pus into the system. However, it is best to pop the core out so the boil will fully discharge all the material and resolve itself. If the boils are large, they are called carbuncles, which can leave scars. If there is a lot of toxicity to expel, your child may develop a low-grade fever. If your child develops a boil, you should regard it as the immune system working to cleanse the body of unwanted toxins.

The following are the most commonly indicated remedies for boils:

Apis: This is for a boil in the beginning stages. The swelling is red, shiny, and puffy. The boil stings, prickles, and burns. It feels terribly hot. It may or may not come to a head. Cold compresses make the child feel better. The child is irritable and wants to be left alone to rest or sleep. If there is any sign of redness or heat, look to **Hepar Sulph**, because **Apis** will not resolve a boil in the later stages.

Belladonna: For a hot, hard, red swelling that may or may not have a head. There is burning heat with dry, swollen, red skin. The onset is rapid and violent. The pains are throbbing and cutting. This remedy dries up the pus. There may be a fever of up to 102 degrees. Usually the boils are on the right side. There may be swelling of glands under the arms or in the groin. The child is sensitive to noise, light, touch, or being jarred.

Echinacea: This is a remedy for boils or carbuncles that are bluish-red. The pains are intense, sharp, darting, and shifting. The boil progresses and then stops, with no more growth or discharge. This remedy will allow the boil to start draining again. The child's face is usually red and flushed, with a sensation of fullness in the head. Many times there is a tingling sensation in the tongue and lips. This is a good remedy for recurring boils and carbuncles. The child feels quite weak, drowsy, and tired, with achy muscles. The child is confused, slow to react, or walks slowly. They become angry if contradicted.

Hepar Sulph: These boils are hard, hot, very painful, and sometimes throbbing. The surrounding skin is very tender to the touch. This remedy can help the boil come to a head and burst, which gives relief. There is usually a lot of pus that is thick, acidic, and may contain blood. This remedy will help dry up the pus. The discharge may smell like old rotten cheese. Local glands may be swollen. The child is irritable and quite sensitive, especially to touch, pain, or cold.

Mercurius Viv (also known as **Mercurius Sol**): For slow-forming boils with lots of thin, yellow-green, foul-smelling pus. The pains are burning and stinging. There may also be oozing ulcers around the boil. The breath, pus, and sweat smell foul. The child will drool excessively, and may have a metallic taste in the mouth.

Silicea (also known as **Silica Terra**): This is a slow-forming boil with thick or thin, foul-smelling, yellow or green pus. This is a good remedy to give if the boil is not discharging, the pus is continuing to ooze, or the wound is not healing. These boils tend to be hard. There may be swelling of nearby glands. The child is very sensitive and withdrawn.

Sulphur: For boils that are stinging, burning, with flushes of heat, and may be itchy. They ooze foul-smelling, thin, yellow, and bloody pus. There may be a group of boils. These boils are slow to heal, remaining red and sore. This is a good remedy for recurring boils.

Dosage: Give 2 pellets every 2–4 hours, depending on the severity. If there is no response after twenty-four hours, try a different remedy. As soon as there is improvement, repeat the remedy only if there is a return of any symptoms.

Supportive Measures:

Do not squeeze boils unless they have come to a white head. You can aid this process by applying a hot compress, which will bring it to a head. Boils are best left uncovered where practical. Never cover a boil so that the air cannot reach it. Use gauze coverings while the boil is discharging, and then leave it to open air. To relieve pain, you may use one drop of Hypericum Tincture in 25 drops of spring water. This tincture can be found in health-food stores or natural pharmacies. Apply topically every 4–6 hours until healed.

Call your healthcare practitioner if:

- Your baby is under three months old and has any rise in temperature.
- Your child is over three months old and has a temperature over 103 degrees.
- Your child is under two years of age and has had a fever for more than twenty-four hours.
- Your child is over two years of age and has had a fever for more than three days.
- The boil is draining foul-smelling pus, or has not improved after coming to a head.
- The boil does not drain after ten days.
- A group of boils develop near the original one.
- There are recurring boils.

COLD SORES

Cold sores are caused by a virus in the Herpes Simplex One group. They are also known as fever blisters. After the virus enters the body, it lies dormant in a local nerve ganglia. A cold sore erupts if the body's resistance is lowered from emotional stress, fatigue, illness, hormone imbalances, or drugs. They can also erupt due to environmental changes such as strong sunlight or bitter cold. The first symptoms start with tingling, burning, itching, or numbness. A blister or several small blisters then form, which can become quite tender. At this stage, the fluid in the blister is infectious. The child may develop a mild fever.

Cold sores commonly manifest around the lips, below or in the nose, or on the chin. After about two weeks, the blisters start to dry out and form a yellowish, grey, or black scab that is flaky or crusty. Cold sores are actually a sign of a chronic state that requires homeopathic treatment. However, the following remedies can help acute symptoms so that the child may be more comfortable. Call your homeopath before giving a remedy. Try to keep the child from scratching, so that the sores do not become infected.

The following are the most commonly indicated remedies for cold sores:

Arsenicum: Skin is dry and tingling, with much burning. The blister is red and itchy as it erupts out of the swollen area. A crust usually forms over an ulcerous-looking blister. The child is nervous, anxious, and restless. Even though there is burning, warm compresses feel good.

Dulcamara: Red blisters with much stinging and prickling. The blister forms a thick, brown-yellow crust that will bleed if scratched. They are worse before a teen girl's period, or exposure to cold, wet weather, and better with cool applications. The child is confused, quarrelsome, impatient, and rejects what has been asked for.

Graphites: Skin is dry and rough, with a burning sensation. The blister oozes a sticky, honey-colored fluid, and forms a thick crust that may be itchy. The skin feels drawn and tight, and may even crack open. The breath tends to be foul. Cool applications feel best. The child is sad, weepy, miserable, and unhappy.

Hepar Sulph: The skin is extremely sensitive, with prickly and stinging pains. The blisters bleed easily, and ooze a foul-smelling fluid that smells like old, rotten cheese. The blisters tend to be itchy, red at the base, and surrounded by groups of small pimples. They feel better with warm applications. The child is sweaty, irritable, and extremely sensitive, especially to pain and cold.

Mercurius Viv (also known as **Mercurius Sol**): The skin tends to be moist and tender, with burning and stinging pains. The blisters ooze a thin, foul-smelling, greenish-yellow fluid that may be streaked with blood. A yellow-brown crust forms that is itchy and feels worse from warmth. The child usually has bad-smelling breath and drools. The child is likely to be restless, and is easily chilled or overheated.

Natrum Mur: The skin is raw, inflamed, stinging, and dry to the point of cracking. Circular blisters form a red crust, usually on the lips, and feel numb, tingly, and itchy. There may be a crack in the middle of the lip. Blisters occur from exposure to sun, emotional shock, or during a fever. The child is thirsty, but craves salty things. Cool applications feel best. The child's feelings are hurt easily, and they are withdrawn.

Rhus Tox: The skin tingles, burns, stings, and violently itches. Prior to the eruption, there often is aching in the muscles on arising. Several small red, intensely itching blisters may form that ooze a watery, yellowish fluid. Later, a moist crust forms over a swollen blister, which can be scaly. Warm applications feel best. The child is restless and wants to stretch.

Sepia: The skin is sore and dry, with a sensation of burning. The circles of blisters are red, very itchy, stinging, and form thick crusts that can be scaly. They ooze a clear, watery, or slightly milky fluid. In teen girls, it is worse before and during the period, or in spring. Warm applications feel best. The child is weak, tired, sad, and indifferent to family.

Dosage: Give 2 pellets 3–4 times a day during the outbreak, depending on the discomfort of the child. Then reduce to two times a day, and then once daily. If there is no response after forty-eight hours, try a different remedy.

Supportive Measures:

Keep the area dry. Keep a hat on the child that covers the face if they are out in the sun. Keep the child out of extreme cold. Do not let the child kiss anyone.

Call your healthcare practitioner if:

- The sores become red and swollen, and form foul-smelling pus.
- The child has a temperature over 103 degrees, or a fever that persists for more than three days.
- The cold sore is near the eye.
- There is no improvement after a week.

COLIC IN BABIES

Colic is spasmodic abdominal pain in infants, usually in the first three to four months of life. Trapped gas in the large intestine is the most frequent reason for colic in babies. The pains become sharp, making the infant cry, double up, and pass gas, which only temporarily helps. Colic usually makes the infant irritable and/or restless. In newborns, the gas may be from an immature digestive system, eating too quickly, intolerance or aversion to the mother's milk or formula, the mother's diet, or a first-time mom who may be nervous and worried about doing it right.

In an older baby, the gas can be caused by eating unsuitable solids. Soymilk can cause constipation and colic. Cow's milk can be hard for babies to digest because of a high level of salt and grease, or there may be a lactose intolerance, causing curd-like stools and abdominal pains. If the baby does not respond to the remedies, consult your healthcare practitioner to make sure nothing else is occurring. Teething can cause colic problems, especially with the eruption of molars. If your baby seems extremely anxious, it can be related to birth trauma, for which you should seek help from your healthcare practitioner and a cranial-sacral osteopath. If the anxiety has to do with family dynamics, call your healthcare practitioner.

Note: *Do not give honey to a baby under one year old. Honey may be contaminated with bacteria that may be harmful to babies.*

What to observe:

Does the baby double up, curl up, or throw themselves backward? What position do they sleep in? Do they like to be held, carried, or left alone? Can they be satisfied if they are given attention? What color is the baby's face? If they have diarrhea, what color and consistency is it? If they spit up or vomit, what does it look like?

Note: The nursing mother should avoid foods listed in the "Worse from" category after each remedy description. *Avoidance of listed foods can go a long way in preventing colic.*

The following are the most commonly indicated remedies for colic:

Aethusa: The baby has cold hands and feet. The face is pale and sometimes puffy. The baby is unable to digest breast milk or formula, spits up after every feeding, or may projectile-vomit within an hour. The vomit contains curds (white, yellow, or green). Infant is sweaty, restless, anxious, and weepy, and weak to the point of not being able to hold their head up; there is a lot of limpness. They can have yellow or green slimy diarrhea of undigested milk, or lack of thirst. The baby cries all the time—which may make the mother anxious so that she constantly feeds the infant, making colic worse. The baby is restless, and may have an anxious expression.

Note: If you suspect this remedy is indicated, consult your healthcare practitioner, because sometimes these babies may be failing to thrive.

Worse from: Evening time and around 3–4 AM, frequent feeding, summer heat, and a nursing mom drinking wine. **Better from:** Open air.

Antimonium Crud: This remedy tends to be for plump babies. After nursing, the baby vomits curds of milk, refuses to nurse anymore, and is very irritable. Later the baby has a great desire to nurse, but not enough strength. Constant burping. Bloated abdomen after nursing. Baby has thick white coating on tongue, but edges can be red. Baby does not like to be carried and cannot stand to be touched or looked at. They are fretful, temperamental, and weepy, sometimes shrieking.

Worse from: Evening hours, heat, cold dampness, overfeeding, and nursing moms eating pork, vinegar, or wine, or overeating. **Better from:** Open air, rest, moist warmth, and lying down.

Belladonna: Intense, violent, sharps pains that come and go suddenly. Baby screams and involuntarily bends forward or arches the back. Abdomen will stick out and feel hot to the touch, and you may see it throbbing. Face is red, hot, and dry. Hands and feet are cool. Pupils of eyes may be dilated. Restless sleep—tired but cannot sleep. They startle easily, and are excitable because their senses become acute. Infant sometimes moans. May have fever, be constipated, or bite at the nipple. May have a look of anger on their face.

Worse from: Noise, light, jarring, touch, lying on stomach, around 3 PM, or from nursing mom eating meat, acidic foods, coffee, milk, or beer. **Better from:** Bending backward, a darkened room, quiet, and light covers.

Borax: This is useful for babies who have ulcers in their mouths that bleed and cause excess saliva. The infant's mouth feels hot on the mother's nipple. They may even refuse the breast. The baby will cry while nursing and when having a bowel movement. This condition may become worse during teething. The baby dislikes strangers. Easily startled, nervous, and sensitive to noise. Will jump at sudden loud noises. Very upset when put down in the crib. They can wake screaming and grasping the sides of the crib.

Worse from: Downward motion, touch, and breastfeeding. **Better from:** Quiet, and after a bowel movement.

Calc Carb: Frequent burping and vomiting of sour, curdled milk. Abdomen bloated and hard. Milk upsets the stomach. Hands and feet tend to be cold and clammy. They sweat easily, especially on the head while sleeping. All discharges smell sour. Feel better if constipated. Stool is hard at first, followed by diarrhea full of undigested food. Infant usually has large head, and may have enlarged glands. This baby is fearful, restless, and cries out at night. Slow, easygoing baby, usually obstinate. Likes affection.

Worse from: Cold damp, movement, full moon, and nursing mom eating beans, peas, eggs, smoked food, and wine. **Better from:** Dry warmth, drawing legs up, and lying on back.

Calc Phos: Brought on by any feeding. Squirms around trying to get comfortable. Slow teething and poor growth rate. The baby will refuse the breast. Vomits because of possible intolerance to milk. May want to be fed constantly, because of great hunger. Tends to be pale, thin, and can have large head. May have a hard time gaining weight. Sleeps on knees and elbows. Cranky, discontent, irritable, fretful, always restless, and dissatisfied.

Worse from: Wet cold, cold air, and nursing mom eating too much fruit. **Better from:** Riding in the car, passing gas, and lying down.

Chamomilla: Terrible, writhing pains. Has gas, but passing it does not relieve the pain. Abdomen is bloated and sensitive to the touch. Can have greenish diarrhea that may smell sulphurous, like bad eggs. Starts to nurse, then turns away. May bite at the nipple. Is overtired, but cannot sleep. One cheek may be red and hot, and the other pale; this symptom may be subtle or quite obvious. May arch the back. Severe, piercing screams and shrieks. Wants to be held, but is only comforted for a short time. After being put down, they want to be held again. Hard to please, angry, impatient (especially when hungry), irritable, cranky, and oversensitive to pain.

Worse from: Evening, cold, touch, anger, and nursing mom drinking coffee or alcohol. **Better from:** Warmth on abdomen, being carried or rocked, and patience.

Colocynthis: Pains come on suddenly, are violent, severe, and cutting, usually moving from left to right. They may have watery, sour, yellowish diarrhea with gas and pain. Passing gas will give only temporary relief. Twists and doubles up. Wants to lie on abdomen, and will scream if moved. Infant sometimes moans. Agonized expression on the face. Extreme restlessness; oversensitive and easily irritated.

Worse from: Nighttime, after eating, overexcitement, anger, and nursing mom eating cheese or unripe, rotten, or large quantities of fruit. **Better from:** Warmth and firm pressure in the abdominal area—put the infant over the top of your shoulder, or lie the baby on its back and draw their knees up to their chest.

Dioscorea: Pains from going too long between feedings, or not getting enough to eat. They have cramping and cutting pains around the navel. These babies scream, writhe about, and twist in agony. They arch their back and extend their legs. Abdominal area rumbles and is full of gas. They are restless and want quiet.

Worse from: Around 2 AM, onward through early morning, bending forward, lying down, or nursing mom eating old cheese, raw fruit, pastry, and tea. **Better from:** Being held upright, stretching out, bending backwards, and burping.

Lycopodium: There is much loud gas and belching, even after the slightest amount of milk. Abdomen bloated. Very hungry, but is satisfied quickly and doesn't nurse for long. It is a good idea to feed this baby just before sleep. This remedy is usually for infants who are lean and long, especially in the trunk. They can sleep well at night but cry all day long. They have a look of anxiety or worry, with a wrinkled brow. This is a good remedy if there is anxiety in the baby, mom, or family. They can scream out suddenly from sleep, and cannot be pacified. They are irritable, serious, and wake up irritable and angry.

Worse from: Either 4 AM or 4 PM–8 PM, after eating, warm rooms, diapers or clothes that are too tight, strangers, on the right side, and nursing mom eating oysters, too much bread or pasta, milk, peas, beans, broccoli, cauliflower, Brussels sprouts, or raw cabbage. **Better from:** Warm applications on the abdomen, which will aid in the release of gas.

Mag Phos: Cramping pain from lots of trapped gas. Pains come and go suddenly. Abdomen is very bloated. Burps and passes gas; however, the burping does not help to get rid of the gas. May draw all limbs into body because of the pain. The baby may also have hiccups. Irritable, and whimpering with the pain. Wants to be nurtured and lie in a fetal position, with knees drawn to the chest. The baby is nervous, intense, and restless.

This remedy is best given in hot (not boiling) water. Put 2 pellets in one ounce of water and carefully spoon it into baby's mouth. Test the water to make sure it is not too hot.

Worse from: Cold drafts, possibly with constipation, evening time, and nursing mom eating acidic foods or coffee. **Better from:** Knees to chest, with warm baths, being comforted, gentle pressure and rubbing, a warm blanket, and warm drinks.

Nux Moschata: *This is a baby that may be in shock from birth trauma.* Please consult the section on "Newborn Discomforts" and look under "Birth or Circumcision Trauma." These babies are so sleepy that they cannot latch onto the breast. They nurse for a few minutes and then fall back asleep, because they are so exhausted and in shock from the birthing process. The abdomen is excessively bloated. All food turns to gas. They may get hiccups easily. The baby has cold hands and feet; the face is pale, and the skin is dry. Heavy, droopy eyelids may make the baby look drunk. Baby may have bright yellow diarrhea with cramping. May have sore ulcerated navel. If you have given this remedy a few times and there has been no response, *consult your healthcare practitioner,* because sometimes these babies are failing to thrive.

Worse from: Cold, dampness, cold wind, jarring, shock, excitement, and nursing mom consuming dairy products, alcohol, or overeating. **Better from:** Warmth, moist heat, warm rooms, calm, and quiet. Keep this baby warm at all times.

Nux Vomica: Stuck gas with constipation. Infant strains and grunts, but there is no movement in the bowels, even though the stool may be soft. Colic may be caused by overfeeding. The baby may have hiccups and belching. Pain comes in waves, and they may arch their back. Fitful, intermittent crying. May retch without vomiting, or vomit violently, which will make them feel better. Face is pinched. Infant is tense, angry, easily frustrated, sensitive, and irritable. Tends to be chilly.

Worse from: Morning hours, 3 AM, noise, odors, light, touch, diaper or clothes that are too tight, and nursing mom ingesting spicy rich food, too much bread or pasta, stimulants, coffee, or alcohol. **Better from:** Warmth, moist air, covering up, and after bowel movements.

Pulsatilla: Gas with vomiting. Develops hiccups soon after eating. Loud rumbling and gurgling noises in the abdomen, with bloating, usually about one hour after feeding. Wants to nurse or be fed constantly, not from hunger but because they are craving comfort. May be a plump infant. Face may have visible small veins. May have diarrhea that alternates with constipation, with no two stools alike. May vomit long after eating. For infants who cry a lot and who are clingy, weepy, whiny, and tearful. They stop crying when picked up, feeling best in mother's arms. Moods change often. A good remedy if there is anxiety in the baby, mom, or family.

Worse from: Warm and stuffy indoors, evenings, and nursing mom ingesting fatty, rich food, e.g., ice cream, too much pasta or bread, cabbage, or large quantities of fruit. **Better from:** Fresh air, after crying, gentle motion, and a soothing voice.

Rheum: Colic preceding sour-smelling diarrhea. The whole child smells sour, as well as their sweat, breath, vomit, and stools. Diarrhea is brown, green, and slimy. They may change their routine completely. They eat and sleep very little. They scream and cry a lot, and their crying turns into screams at night. Scalp and hair become sopping wet with sweat. They get into strange positions in order to rest for a while. They tend to frown. The child either dislikes their favorite things, or only wants particular ones. Very irritable, restless, and sleeps little. This remedy will really help to improve the infant's digestion and appetite.

Worse from: Uncovering any part of the body, eating, nighttime, mornings after sleeping, and a nursing mom eating too much fruit, especially plums or unripe fruit, and milk. **Better from:** Warmth, wrapping up, and bending double.

Silicea (also known as **Silica Terra**): Infant has large head with fine features, and looks emaciated. Head tends to be sweaty. This baby has a tendency toward constipation, and may only have a stool every two or three days. Stool is hard, dry, and light-colored. They are chilly and thirsty. There will be constant spitting up, but rarely do they vomit. They may have an aversion to mother's milk. These infants do not have the intense reactions to pain as with the other types; however they are sensitive and easily startled.

Worse from: Cold damp, uncovering, bathing, and nursing mom drinking wine or milk. **Better from:** Warmth; this infant will do well to always wear a hat if it is even a little cool.

Sulphur: Bloated abdomen, with rumbling and gas in the lower intestines after eating. Abdomen is sore, tender to the touch, and sensitive to pressure. Belches smell sour, or sulphurous, like rotten eggs. There will be redness of the eyelids, and maybe of the lips and anus. Child does not like baths. Very offensive sweat or stools. Diarrhea in the morning that is very acrid, irritating, and painful, causing a red, inflamed diaper rash. These infants are hot, usually with big bellies and thin limbs. They are irritable, sluggish, discontented, and restless.

Worse from: Too many covers or warm clothes, lying on stomach, 11 AM, and nursing mom eating too much pasta, bread, meat, or sweets. These foods are OK, but in moderation. **Better from:** Open air, motion, and after diarrhea.

The following remedies may be helpful, but are not the most commonly used for colic:

Argentum Nit: Colic from anxiety. The baby has gas and belching, with greenish stools. Infant may be susceptible to conjunctivitis. The mother may be anxious and have fears of "not doing it right." This is a good remedy if there is anxiety in the baby, mom, or family.

Worse from: Nursing mom eating too many sweets, formula with too much sugar, or high-fructose corn syrup. **Better from:** Fresh air, motion, passing gas, and burping.

Cinchona (also known as **China Officinalis**): Pains with belching and gas. Passing gas gives no relief from pain. Abdomen is bloated. This is a good remedy if there is anxiety in the baby, mom, or family.

Worse from: Eating, eating too fast, eating fruit, and nursing mom eating too much fruit or vegetables in the cabbage family. **Better from:** Gentle movement, bending double, or bringing knees to chest.

Ignatia: If the mother has experienced grief such as from loss of a loved one during the pregnancy. Stomach cramping with much gas, hiccups with burping, spit-up or vomit that smells sour, and agitation from nausea. The child will stiffen and bend backward. They may have rumbling in their bowels. They tend to be chilly, and very sensitive to pain. They are nervous, excitable, and weepy, sighing a lot, and yawning. They can have unpredictable reactions, hysterically crying one moment, very happy the next, furious the next, distant the next, anxious and restless the next. There is often a loss of appetite.

Worse from: The slightest touch, hiccups that are worse after eating, at the same hour of day and night, cold, odors, and mother's grief. **Better from:** Eating, lying on stomach, calm, and warmth, but not if it is hot outdoors.

Dosage: For an infant, you can crush 2 pellets between two spoons, add a drop of spring water, swish around, wait a few seconds, and then administer the water onto the baby's lips. Give every 15 minutes for four doses, if the symptoms are strong, then hourly. Otherwise, give 2–4 times a day, again depending on the severity of the symptoms. Stop when there is significant improvement. Repeat only if there is a return of symptoms. Repeat as often as needed. After six doses, if there has been no improvement, change to a different remedy.

Supportive Measures:

Make sure the infant is burped after eating. Some infants can burp well; others need more time, and need to be burped more often than just at the end of the feeding. If the infant has been crying a lot, they may swallow a lot of air, which exacerbates the problem further, therefore requiring more burping.

Swaddling the infant tightly may help. Pacifiers may help with the urge to suck. Nursing moms need to drink plenty of water, and eat well. If you are not nursing your baby and you suspect they are not doing well with dairy products or formula, try organic goat's milk, available in most health-food stores. Be willing to experiment. If your baby responds well to any remedy above, look to see what food makes the colic worse, and avoid that food.

Supportive Measures (cont):

Try to relax and have a calm environment around you and the baby at feeding time, and take all the time you need. Having a screaming baby will unnerve even the most easy-going parent—coupled with maternal hormonal ebbs and flows, sudden weeping or uncontrollable laughter is not unusual. It is also not unusual to feel worn out, sleep-deprived, overwhelmed, frustrated, powerless, insecure, at your wit's end, or inadequate. Babies do not come with a "how-to manual," but there are wonderful support groups and online parent chat rooms that may be helpful. Asking for breaks from your partner, other family members, friends, or even hired help is of greatest importance. Try to get out of the home every day, even if only for a brief time, with or without the baby. Also get out of the house with your partner, with or without the baby. Seek advice and emotional support from other parents who inspire you. Contact your homeopath if you feel your hormones are not rebalancing themselves.

Call your healthcare practitioner if:

- Your baby is not gaining weight.
- Your baby vomits excessively.
- Your baby has persistent diarrhea.
- There is an absence of urine.
- There is severe pain that does not respond to any remedies, and the baby constantly screams.

Call your healthcare practitioner if (cont):

- Your baby is under three months old and has any rise in temperature.
- Your child is over three months old and has a temperature over 103 degrees.
- Your child is under two years of age and has had a fever for more than twenty-four hours.
- Your child is over two years of age and has had a fever for more than three days.
- Your baby is pale, frightened or has a shocked look in the eyes, and passes a loose, gelatinous, blood-stained stool—go to an urgent-care facility or hospital emergency room.

THE SEVEN MOST COMMON REMEDIES FOR COLIC

	Calc Carb	Chamomilla	Colocynthis	Lycopodium	Mag Phos	Nux Vomica	Pulsatilla
Onset	Exposure to cold. Nursing mom eats beans, peas, eggs, smoked food, or wine.	Cold wind or anger. Nursing mom drinks coffee or alcohol.	Overexcitement. Nursing mom eats cheese, fruit that is unripe or rotten, or too much fruit.	Wet weather. Nursing mom eats oysters, milk, peas, beans, or raw cabbage.	Cold baths. Cold drinks.	Overfeeding. Nursing mom ingests spicy, rich food, stimulants, or alcohol.	Nursing mom ingests fatty, rich food, or ice cream.
Symptom	Frequent burping, vomiting of sour, curdled milk; abdomen hard and bloated, with easily upset digestion. Stool hard in beginning, then diarrhea full of undigested food.	Screams, shrieks, and may arch their back from pain. One cheek red and hot, the other pale. Has gas, but passing it does not relieve the pain. Can have greenish diarrhea that smells like rotten eggs.	Twists and doubles up. Pains come suddenly, are violent, severe, cutting, and usually move from left to right. May have watery, sour, and yellowish diarrhea with gas and pain.	Much loud gas and belching, even after the slightest amount of breast milk or formula. Very hungry, but doesn't nurse long.	Pain with lots of trapped gas. Burps and passes gas, but it does not relieve pain or lessen gas. May draw all limbs into body because of pain.	Trapped gas with constipation. Infant strains and grunts with no bowel movement, even though stool may be soft. May retch without vomiting.	Gas; possible vomiting long after eating. Hiccups soon after eating. Rumbling and gurgling noises in abdomen. Diarrhea alternates with constipation, and no two stools look alike.
Mood	Fearful, restless, cries out at night. Slow, easygoing baby, usually obstinate.	Wants to be held, but only for a while. Nothing pleases them. Angry, irritable, sensitive to odors and noise. Starts to nurse, then turns away. May bite at the nipple.	Extremely restless, oversensitive, and easily irritated. Infant sometimes moans.	Wakes irritable and angry. Has look of anxiety or worry with a wrinkled brow.	Irritable. Wants to be nurtured and lie in a fetal position.	Angry, irritable, tense, and fitful, with intermittent crying.	Cries a lot until picked up: weepy and clingy. Eats constantly, not because of hunger but from craving comfort. Moods change often.
Indications	Hands and feet are cold and clammy. Chilly, fair, plump babies with a large head.	Hot, thirsty, overtired, but cannot sleep because of the pain. Child may cry out in sleep.	Wants to lie on abdomen, and screams if moved.	Long and lean infants. Abdomen bloated.	Abdomen is very bloated.	Sleep may be disrupted. May have stuffed-up nose. Face pinched, and child may arch their back. Chilly.	Face may have visible small veins. Usually thirstless. May be a plump infant.
Worse	Anything cold, drafts, damp weather, movement, and the full moon.	Cold open air, wind, touch, anger, night, and especially around 9 PM.	Night.	4 AM or 4 PM–8 PM, warm rooms, strangers, and diapers or clothes that are too tight.	Cold drafts.	Morning, 3 AM, noise, odors, light, touch, and diapers or clothes that are too tight.	Warm, stuffy rooms, and evening time.
Better	Warmth, dry weather, drawing legs up, lying on back, and being constipated.	Being rocked or carried, and in mild weather. Warm (not hot) applications on abdomen.	Warmth, drawing knees up to belly. Firm pressure on abdomen by putting infant over the top of your shoulder.	Warm (not hot) applications will aid in the release of gas.	Knees to chest, warm baths, gentle pressure, rubbing, and warm covers.	Warmth, moist air, being covered up, after a bowel movement, or sometimes after vomiting.	In parent's arms, outdoors, fresh air, gentle motion, and a soothing voice.

CONSTIPATION

In order to eliminate waste material, the colon muscles contract in waves. This action, called peristalsis, carries waste into the rectum. If a baby or child is constipated, it can mean that the peristaltic action is not functioning. This happens if the muscles of the intestine are weak, if the digestive tract is immature, or if there is poor circulation or lymph drainage. If the intestines are cramped, this will produce an urge to eliminate, but nothing comes out.

Babies can develop constipation from canned baby foods that contain refined ingredients, preservatives, and fillers. Constipation may also be accompanied by gas, bloating, pain, bad breath, headaches, and spaciness. These symptoms can arise from a poor diet of refined or sugary foods, lack of fluids, lack of fiber, wheat and gluten allergies, antibiotics, yeast infections, ignoring the urge for a bowel movement, or "holding it" for long periods of time. Negative emotional states, e.g., anxiety, worry, stress, chronic depression, and irritability, can also interfere with the peristalsis and relaxation of the sphincter muscles. There should be elimination once a day, but twice is best. Anything less than once a day means that the bowels are not performing optimally. It is best if the bowels move in the morning to get the toxic waste out right away. Traveling can very easily upset the rhythm of the intestinal tract.

The use of laxatives ultimately leads to more frequent use, or the need for a stronger laxative. Laxatives make the body lazy and reliant on the laxatives to do its job. They can also unbalance bowel chemistry.

If constipation becomes chronic, consult your healthcare practitioner. Continual straining can stress organs, muscles, and surrounding tissues of the lower abdominal area or rectum.

What to observe:

What is the color and firmness of the stool? When was the last time the baby had a bowel movement? How many bowel movements do they have daily? Has there been a change in the usual type of stool? Has there been a change in diet recently? Any undue amount of stress or emotional upset? Are they straining a lot in order to pass a stool? Is there a particular position, time of day, or anything else that seems to make the bowel movements better or worse? Has the child been eating a lot of refined foods lately? Is there any blood in the stool? (If this is the case, consult your healthcare practitioner.)

The following are the most commonly indicated remedies for constipation:

Alumina: This is a major remedy for newborn constipation. There is usually little or no urge to have a bowel movement until there is a big buildup of stools. Stools are small, hard, dry balls. Pain is worse on the left side when the urge comes on. There is much intense straining and trembling, even if the stool is soft, with a cutting pain around anus during elimination. Bright-red blood may be present. This occurs in formula-fed infants whose digestion is delicate. Skin and mucous membranes are dry. The child is dull, sluggish, and lacks energy.

Worse from: Starchy foods, especially potatoes, aluminum cookware, dry weather, immediately after waking up, and excessive sitting. **Better from:** Evening time, open air, moderate movement, standing, and damp weather.

Bryonia: The child has little or no urge to have a bowel movement because of poor muscle tone and lack of hydration in the intestinal tract. The stools are large, dry, hard, and may have a burnt appearance. The child has much difficulty getting the stool out. Everything is dry—mouth, tongue, throat, rectum, etc. The tongue may have a white coating. The child is extremely thirsty, and craves cold drinks. Headaches are not uncommon. Weakness is brought about by the slightest exertion. This child does not want to be carried or moved but wants complete stillness. They are very grumpy and irritable.

Worse from: Any motion or exertion, touch, excessive warmth or light, early morning, and before a teenager's period. **Better from:** Pressure, being left alone, complete stillness, darkness or low lights, lying on painful side, cool, open air, rest, and quiet.

Calc Carb: Stubborn constipation, with no urge for a bowel movement. Oddly enough, even though constipated, this baby is actually better from constipation. Stools look like clay. All discharges smell sour. Abdomen is bloated, large, and hard. Or there may be a stool that is hard in the beginning, followed by diarrhea full of undigested food. Infant may have a large head, and be plump and large generally. Also fearful, restless, and crying out at night. Slow, easygoing baby, but usually obstinate.

Worse from: Cold damp, movement, teething, and full moon. **Better from:** Dry warmth, drawing legs up, and lying on back.

Lycopodium: The child has very little urge for a bowel movement, because there is a contraction of the sphincter muscles. When they have the urge, they can't get anything out, and there is an achy fullness with constriction in the anus. They feel like there is more to come, but it doesn't happen. The stools are small and hard. The abdomen is very bloated. There is rumbling with lots of gas. The older child will crave sweets. They have an anxious or worried look, with a wrinkled brow. They wake irritable and angry.

Worse from: Either 4 AM or 4 PM–8 PM, after eating, warm rooms, tight diapers or clothing, and strangers. **Better from:** Warm applications on the abdomen, which will aid in the release of gas.

Natrum Mur: Child has hard, dry, crumbly stools that cause anal contractions, with an unfinished sensation. Or little balls are passed with much straining. They only pass small amounts at a time. The stool may be coated with a glassy-looking mucus. The anus is sore and burning after passing a stool. They may experience rectal bleeding. Constipation may alternate with days of watery diarrhea. Mouth, throat, and rectum are dry. Child is thirsty, picky about food, and craving salt. These children tend to be serious, weepy, and sensitive. They don't like too much physical contact, and want to be left alone if they are upset.

Worse from: Between 9–11 AM, lying, sympathy, touch, pressure, and heat. **Better from:** Open air, sweating, lying down, and after a nap or rest.

Nux Vomica: Constant desire to pass a stool, with much painful straining but little or no result. They have an unfinished sensation. The stools are large, hard, and dark. Constipation alternates with diarrhea. Baby wakes in the early morning with gas pains, and may have headache and upset stomach with nausea. They are chilly. These children are very irritable, impatient, easily exhausted, and cry at the slightest cause, or they can be spiteful, stubborn, and morose if they don't get their own way.

Worse from: Early morning around 4 AM, getting chilled, uncovering, overuse of laxatives, loss of sleep, and drafts. **Better from:** Warmth, being wrapped up, moist air, hot drinks.

Silicea (also known as **Silica Terra**): Because the rectum does not have enough strength for contracting, the stool starts to come out, but then goes back in. This can also be due to spasms of the sphincter muscle. The baby strains and strains, only to pass a hard stool, and is exhausted afterward. And it never feels complete. The anus often becomes sore and oozes mucus. The child is sweaty and chilly, and the sweat smells sour. They generally lack energy and stamina. They are delicate and very sensitive to cold. This child needs lots of patient handling. They are generally subdued, but can become uncharacteristically uncooperative.

Worse from: Left side, cold air, drafts, uncovering, morning, damp, loud noises, teething, and the full moon. **Better from:** Warmth, being wrapped up, wearing a warm hat, and urination.

Dosage: Give 2 pellets every 2Đ4 hours, depending on the discomfort of the child. If there is no response after twenty-four hours, try a different remedy. As soon as there is improvement, repeat the remedy only if any symptoms return.

Supportive Measures:

The baby, nursing mother, and older child should be kept well hydrated. The nursing mother and older child should incorporate more fiber, including fruit and vegetables, and less glutinous grains or starches in the diet. Do not give the baby or child laxatives or bran products unless you have discussed it with your healthcare practitioner. Only use oat bran, which is soluble, or ground flaxseed. Check with your healthcare practitioner for the correct amount and frequency, and to make sure this is the correct action.

Small amounts of aluminum can cause constipation. If you are using aluminum cookware, it is advisable to get rid of it. Aluminum has been linked to other health issues including Alzheimer's disease. When Teflon® coating breaks down, aluminum is leached into the food, because the majority of those pans are aluminum under the Teflon®. If you can't make your own baby food, use organic baby foods in glass jars.

Call your healthcare practitioner if:

- The constipation becomes chronic.
- The child has not had a bowel movement in twenty-four hours and is having unusually strong pains.
- The child is having a hard time passing stools, and they come out white, grey, very dark, or black.
- There is blood in the stools.
- The white of the child's eyes are yellow, or there is a yellow tinge to the skin.
- There is a fever over 101 degrees, with constipation and pain.
- There is a sudden, drastic change in stool color or bowel habits.

DIARRHEA, NAUSEA, AND VOMITING

Acute diarrhea is usually caused by bacteria or a virus in the gut, food poisoning, or eating something inappropriate. It can be a serious threat to an infant, because they can dehydrate so quickly. Severe dehydration can mean a loss of fluid from tissues and blood, which in turn can damage circulation to the brain and vital organs. The baby can become listless, weak, and pale; the eyes and fontanel (soft spot on top of the head) look sunken, the urine has a strong smell, and/or the skin has no rebound (does not spring back when pressed on the shinbone).

It can be very difficult to get babies to drink water. If your baby is refusing to drink, you must ask for professional help, because shock and collapse with dehydration can cause severe damage to brain cells. Diarrhea in babies is common if there is an intolerance to breast milk, during teething, a change of diet, e.g., introducing solid foods, or consumption of too much fruit. It is imperative that the older child is kept hydrated as well. It is good to have Smart Water (available at most health-food stores) on hand at all times to prevent an imbalance of the electrolytes, which are essential for the body to function properly. A drop in electrolytes, potassium and sodium in particular, produces lightheadedness, confusion, faintness on trying to stand, paleness, and weakness in the older child. In an older child, this condition can be expressed as wanting to run away from an unpleasant situation.

If your baby or toddler is experiencing diarrhea and none of the pictures below fit, they may be teething. The remedies for teething diarrhea are: **Calc Carb, Calc Phos, Chamomilla, Dulcamara** (this remedy is not in the teething section, because it is for teething diarrhea only), **Kreosotum,** and **Podophyllum.** Check the "Teething" section, which lists specific diarrhea symptoms.

Vomiting occurs when the child has ingested a disagreeable food or drug, has whooping cough, or experiences motion sickness from a car, boat, air travel, or amusement-park ride. The entire contents of the stomach will be heaved out. Babies will spit up if they have overeaten in an attempt to satisfy their sucking instinct. This is usually nothing to be concerned about. If your baby is actually vomiting, look at the above information on colic. As with diarrhea, keep the baby or child well hydrated. Give liquids in frequent small sips, as tolerated.

Food poisoning occurs when the child has consumed contaminated meat, fish, impure water, or overripe fruit. It comes on quickly and usually violently, two to eight hours after ingestion of the offending food or drink. There is usually severe nausea, vomiting, and diarrhea. A low-grade fever and/or headache can be present. These incidents are usually over in six to eight hours, but leave a residual weakness.

Gastroenteritis—stomach flu, in lay terms—usually comes on fast and furious. The child is left weak, but on the mend after twenty-four hours. There is usually vomiting and diarrhea.

The following are the most commonly indicated remedies for diarrhea, nausea, and vomiting:

Argentum Nit:
Vomiting that is preceded by loud belching. The vomit is full of thick mucus and tastes sour or bitter. There is burning and constriction in the stomach, with pains radiating out in all directions into the abdominal cavity. There is severe bloating and passing gas. The gas is quite loud.

Diarrhea that is noisy, watery, and foul-smelling, with green stools that look like chopped spinach (or may look like flakes of green) and are passed with much gas. This kind of diarrhea is common in children who are being weaned from breast milk. There is much rumbling, gas, and bloating. The child feels warm, and tends to be anxious and fidgety.

Worse from: Heat, eating too much chocolate, sugar, or sweets; too much excitement, lying on the left side, anxiety, and heat. **Better from:** Fresh air, motion, passing gas, and belching.

Arsenicum: This is a major remedy for food poisoning.
Nausea and vomiting: There is retching after drinking ice-cold water or eating, and a sense of anxiety, burning, and rawness in the pit of the stomach. The vomit burns the esophagus and throat. Sometimes there is simultaneous vomiting and diarrhea. Abdomen sensitive to touch. Vomiting or diarrhea gives temporary relief. Child wants sips of cold water to wet the mouth, or might refuse water for fear of vomiting. Can't bear the thought of food. Later, the child will only want small amounts of food after the vomiting has subsided.

Diarrhea: Very watery, burning, brown, yellow, or black slimy stools that may contain undigested food; foul-smelling stools in small quantities that burn the anus, and cramping in the abdomen. Great weakness following passing of stools. In the later stages, the diarrhea may look like rice-water. The child is chilly, anxious, restless, cannot lie still, and is exhausted, with just enough energy to be demanding. The anxiety may grow into a fear that they are going to die.

Worse from: Midnight to 2 AM, cold food or drinks, getting chilled; after eating bad food (rotten meat, fish, or fruit), anxiety, and apprehension. **Better from:** Heat, warm applications to the abdomen.

Carbo Veg: A remedy for food poisoning.

Nausea: With sour belching, restricted breathing, and faintness. Cannot bear the sight or thought of food, as any food at all disagrees with the digestive tract. Extreme burning pains. Severe bloating makes abdominal skin feel stretched tight; child cannot bear anything tight around waist, and belly is very tender; bad breath, and a pale face that sometimes has a bluish tint. Feels faint on arising; low vitality or exhaustion with chill or cold sweats, bending over from pain, wanting fresh air though cold to the touch, and cold sweats.

Diarrhea: Lots of gas, burning in the rectum on passing acidic, foul-smelling stools followed by continued burning. This child is anxious, confused, indifferent, irritable, and sluggish.

Worse from: Just after drinking ice water, loss of fluids, rotten fish or meat (especially poultry), butter, fats, milk, and lying down. **Better from:** Cool, fresh air, fanning, elevating feet, passing gas, and burping.

Cinchona (also known as China Officinalis): A remedy for food poisoning.

Vomiting: Frequent sour-smelling vomiting of undigested food, very swollen abdomen with lots of gas and belching that gives no relief, sore and cold feeling in stomach, hiccups, and abdominal rumbling with thirst for cold water.

Diarrhea: Pale stools are acidic and profuse. There is usually undigested food, and the stools look frothy. The diarrhea is painless, but gas pains may make the child bend double. Diarrhea may be involuntary. This is a remedy for a child weakened by loss of fluids from diarrhea and vomiting. They are weak, with much sweating, and may feel faint or have ringing in the ears. The child is pale, weak, irritable, oversensitive, nervous, and may have problems sleeping, and dark circles under their eyes.

Worse from: Drafts, noise, after weaning from breast milk, bad fish, meat, fruit, milk, water, or tea; at nighttime, and after eating. **Better from:** Much quiet rest, firm pressure, bending double, and warmth.

Cuprum Metal:

Nausea and vomiting: Vomiting preceded by hiccupping. There is painful cramping, pressure, a strong, slimy, metallic taste in mouth, thirst for cold drinks, and nausea with abdominal spasms and cramps. The tummy feels tender, hot, sore, and bruised.

Diarrhea: Profuse, watery, green stools that gush out. Summer diarrhea in children. This remedy is indicated when the cramping is so intense that the child shrieks out in pain. They are chilly, and the skin feels icy-cold. The child is sensitive, nervous, stubborn, sullen, and may bite others when sick.

Worse from: Touch, movement, strong negative emotions, hot weather, lack of sleep, evening, and night. **Better from:** Light pressure of hand on abdominal area, and sweating. Drinking cold water makes them temporarily feel better.

Dulcamara: Only for teething diarrhea.

Diarrhea: May be present in a teething baby, and comes on from getting chilled. Cutting pain around the navel followed by watery, green, slimy, and mucusy stools that smell sour. Blood may be present in stools. The child is irritable, rejects things asked for, and is sensitive to pain.

Worse from: Night, end of summer when there are hot days and cold nights, or when weather suddenly gets cold; damp weather, and autumn. **Better from:** Warmth, motion, dry weather, and moving about.

Gelsemium: Only for diarrhea following a traumatic shock, grief, or fright, or anticipation of an upcoming ordeal such as stage fright or performance anxiety.

Note: Encourage this child to drink, because they do not feel thirsty and can become dehydrated from loss of fluids.

Diarrhea: Painless, involuntary stools that are yellow, cream, or tea-green in color. May have chills up and down the back. The child might tremble and ask to be held. The tongue trembles when protruded. They may have a dull headache and feel lightheaded. They are not thirsty. The hands and feet are cold. They may not be able to see or focus well. The eyelids are heavy and droopy. The limbs may feel heavy. They are weak, answer slowly, and feel tired. They are indifferent to surroundings, dull, droopy, emotionally delicate, and want to be left alone.

Worse from: Overexcitement, strong emotions, spring, shock, damp weather, and around 10 AM. **Better from:** Sweating, urinating, open air, and continued motion.

Ipecacuanha: A remedy for food poisoning.

Nausea and vomiting: Constant and unyielding nausea. They may want to vomit, but can't. If they do vomit, the nausea is not relieved. They vomit food, bile, sometimes green mucus, and/or bright-red blood. They usually have a headache, cannot stand the smell of food, and have increased salivation and horrible cutting and cramping pains. The face is pale and may have dark circles around the eyes. Child sometimes twitches and may have hiccups. Has odd sensation that stomach feels relaxed and is hanging down. May have violent itching.

Diarrhea: An infant may be given this remedy if the stomach has been overfilled, causing much crying, nausea, vomiting, and stools that are yellow or green, can be streaked with blood, and are very offensive-smelling. These children get angry when they don't get their way, and then complain a lot, with a lot of screaming and howling. Nothing pleases them.

Worse from: Eating bad food, unripe fruit, pork, ice cream, rich foods, pastries, sweets, or berries, or from stooping, heat, motion, and overeating. **Better from:** Open air, rest, and closing the eyes.

Nux Vomica: A remedy for food poisoning.

Nausea and vomiting: Constant nausea, feeling faint after vomiting, having a hard time vomiting, much retching, and sour-smelling vomit of food, bile, and bitter mucus. Stomach and intestines feel bruised and sore, and there is cramping, gas, sour and bitter belching, chill, and dry mouth.

Diarrhea: Sudden diarrhea that drives the child out of bed. They feel very faint just after the stool, then better for a short while, and almost immediately have to go again. Much gas and bloating. These children are angry, irritable, nervous, and spiteful, or very sensitive and easily offended, hypersensitive to light, odors, touch, and sound.

Worse from: Rich, spicy or junk food, fats, impure water, morning, after eating, and touch. **Better from:** Vomiting, temporarily after a stool; heat, lying or sitting, warm drinks and food after vomiting has subsided, and quiet, calm surroundings.

Phosphorus:

Vomiting: Vomits food by mouthfuls. Cold water helps burning pain in stomach, but is vomited back up as soon as it warms in the stomach. May vomit bile or blood. Vomit may look like coffee grounds. Sour taste and sour burps after food, with lots of belching.

Diarrhea: Exhausting diarrhea that may be bloody. It is watery and painless, with green mucus or a grey, bluish, pasty color. Great weakness afterward. Burning in rectum. The child is affectionate and cheerful. Later they may become fearful, easily upset, and irritable. At this stage, the child needs attention, consolation, and massage, which will make them feel much better.

Worse from: Evening, touch, warm food or drink, odors, light, and lying on left side. **Better from:** Sleep, sympathy, low lights or darkness, open air, eating and drinking cold things, and cool applications.

Podophyllum:

Nausea and vomiting: Sour, hot belching that smells like rotten eggs; vomiting hot, frothy mucus; constant gagging, heartburn, empty retching, and increased salivation. Infants vomit breast milk. Abdomen is sore and bloated.

Diarrhea: Lots of gurgling and gas in the intestines. Foul-smelling, painless, profuse, explosive gushing of green, watery stools with jelly-like mucus. Great weakness, with sinking and empty feeling following passing of stools. Also for summer diarrhea. May have a headache. The child is restless and fidgety. Their sleep is restless and fitful, with moaning and whining, and they may perspire on the head.

Worse from: Early morning from 2–4 AM, summer, acid fruits, milk, motion, open air, and hot air. **Better from:** Pressure, lying on the stomach, and lightly rubbing abdominal area on right side.

Pulsatilla:

Vomiting: Vomits food long after it was eaten. This is the main remedy for the ill effects of eating pork or excessive amounts of rich food, fats, and ice cream. The child feels as if there is a stone lodged in the stomach just below the ribs, and can still taste the food that caused the problem. Gas and belching.

Diarrhea: Stools are green and watery, but the child doesn't pass as much as they would like to; no two stools look alike; rumbling in gut, low appetite. The child is rarely thirsty. This child is tearful, moody, weeps easily, and wants lots of sympathy and company; boys may feel sorry for themselves.

Worse from: Heat, after a fright, twilight, and warm, stuffy rooms. **Better from:** Cool, fresh air, and being carried slowly and gently.

Rhus Tox:

Nausea: With bloating, after eating ice cream or drinking ice water when hot. Pains in stomach cause child to bend forward or want to lie on stomach.

Diarrhea: From drinking ice-cold water or eating ice cream when hot. Foul smelling, watery stools with blood or reddish mucus, possibly with frothiness or jelly-like mucus. The diarrhea is usually painless. The child is very restless and anxious.

Worse from: Cold damp weather, cold food or drinks, being uncovered, lying still, nighttime, and sweating. **Better from:** Warm drinks and food, bowel movements, gentle continual movement, warmth, and changing positions.

Sulphur: Remind the child needing this remedy to drink so that they do not become dehydrated.

Diarrhea: The stools are changeable—sometimes they are mushy, with undigested food, sometimes yellow and watery. The smell is very foul, like that of rotten eggs. They can wake with an urgent need that drives them to the toilet immediately upon awakening. Infants will be drowsy, with profuse sweating. Diarrhea can alternate with constipation. The anus burns, becoming red and sore. The diarrhea is usually but not always painful. If painful, the child tries to hold the stools for fear of pain. They may fall asleep after a bout of diarrhea. The child may have diarrhea from suppression of an acute condition after taking antibiotics. The child may be thirsty for large amount of cold water or drinks, but forget to drink. You may notice that the child is sleeping with the feet out from under the covers. The child is irritable, sluggish, quarrelsome, and restless.

Worse from: Heat, blowing the nose, bathing, standing, over-exertion, around 11 AM, and at the full moon. **Better from:** Cold, open air, gentle motion, and sweating.

Veratrum: A remedy for food poisoning.

Nausea and vomiting: Terrible abdominal pains and cramping, with symptoms of extreme exhaustion, deathly nausea, and desperate, unquenchable thirst for cold water that is soon vomited; intense chills and cold sweats with vomiting and diarrhea. There are beads of sweat on the forehead while vomiting or passing the stool. Projectile vomiting, violent, shuddering vomiting and retching. Vomit is acidic, slimy, and may be yellow, green, or black. May have simultaneous vomiting and diarrhea, or hiccups. Breath may be cold.

Diarrhea: Odorless, watery stools that look like rice-water, or can be watery yellow or watery green. Pain in abdomen before passing stools, weak and faint afterward, and frequent stools that blast out. Forehead, hands, feet, and abdomen are cold. Huge thirst for great quantities of cold water. The child is restless, moody, tearful, uncommunicative, and withdrawn. They can be either talkative or silent.

Worse from: Bad meats, fruits, potatoes, green vegetables, exertion, cold, wet weather or drinks, touch, pressure, and night. **Better from:** Warmth, covering, hot drinks, and lying down. Young children feel better if carried around but not rocked.

Dosage: Give 2 pellets every 15 minutes for four doses, then hourly until improvement. If there has been no improvement after seven doses, choose a new remedy. Repeat the remedy only if there is a return of any symptoms.

Supportive Measures:

Continue nursing a baby. Review the section on colic if the baby has colic with vomiting. For the older child, limit the intake of food and regular drinks. You can make a homemade fluid replacement with a fifty-fifty mix of apple (or any clear, pulp-free) juice and spring water. A mix of fresh, pulp-free watermelon juice and spring water is one of the most quick and natural ways to replenish electrolytes. Smart Water, available at health-food stores, has no sugar and can replenish the electrolytes as well. Even if the child is vomiting, encourage them to drink small sips frequently. *Giving a child bananas, applesauce, white toast, and white rice will give binding power to the intestines and slow the diarrhea.* These foods can also be offered after vomiting.

It is better for the child to eat small amounts frequently. Cut out all dairy products, and any fruit besides bananas or applesauce. Use organic foods when possible. If your child likes miso soup, it is very nourishing to the intestines after the diarrhea has stopped. Have the child get plenty of rest. After a heavy loss of fluids from vomiting and diarrhea, improvement is gradual. Do not overtax the system by reintroducing any rich or fatty foods too quickly. If the child has no appetite, encourage them to eat just a little. Some young children want to stop eating for fear of vomiting, especially if the symptoms have been severe.

For continued weakness after severe vomiting, gastroenteritis, or diarrhea:

Phosphoric Acid: The child just can't seem to get energy back. They look pale, with dark circles under their eyes, are very sweaty and chilly, and usually have a lack of appetite; but they do desire fruit and refreshing, light foods. The child is indifferent, quiet, easily overwhelmed, unable to concentrate, mildly irritable, un-communicative, and answers questions with minimal words.

Cinchona (also known as China Officinalis): This is for a child who has lost a lot of fluid from vomiting and diarrhea. They are chilly and pale, with dark circles under their eyes; their limbs are weak, and there is much sweating. They may feel faint and have ringing in the ears. The child is irritable, oversensitive, nervous, and may have problems sleeping.

Dosage: Give 2 pellets every 3–4 hours until improvement. If there is no improvement in twenty-four hours, call your healthcare practitioner.

Call your healthcare practitioner if:

- There has been no response in twenty-four hours.
- The skin has no rebound (if pressed on the shinbone, does not spring back).
- You think your baby is dehydrated because they will not nurse or drink.
- There is severe abdominal pain that worsens or does not respond to remedies within two hours.
- There is a fever above 103 degrees in older children, or if a baby under three months old has any elevated temperature.
- There is repeated blood in the stools or vomit.

Call your healthcare practitioner if (cont):

- Your child cannot stop vomiting.
- There is vomiting after a head injury.
- There is vomiting after a severe blow to the abdominal area.
- There is unexplained vomiting with severe pain around the navel or in the extreme lower right pelvic area, as this can indicate appendicitis in an older child.

THE FIVE MOST COMMON REMEDIES FOR DIARRHEA, NAUSEA, AND VOMITING

	Arsenicum	Cinchona	Ipecacuanha	Nux Vomica	Veratrum
Vomiting	Retching after eating or drinking, especially ice-cold water. Burning and rawness in pit of stomach. Vomit burns the esophagus and throat. Abdomen sensitive to touch. Feels better from vomiting or diarrhea. Wants sips of cold water to wet the mouth, or might refuse water for fear of vomiting. Can't bear the thought of food.	Frequent sour-smelling vomit with undigested food. Very swollen abdomen with lots of gas and belching, which gives no relief when passed. Sore and cold feeling in stomach, hiccups, and abdominal rumbling, with thirst for cold water.	Constant and unyielding nausea. May want to vomit, but can't. Nausea not relieved by vomiting. Vomits food, bile, or sometimes green mucus and/or bright-red blood. Headache. Can't stand smell of food. Increased salivation, horrible cutting and cramping pain. Face pale, and may have dark circles around eyes. Odd sensation that stomach feels relaxed and is hanging down. May have violent itching of skin.	Constant nausea. May feel faint. May have a hard time vomiting. Vomits food, bile, and bitter, sour-smelling mucus. Much retching. Stomach and intestines feel bruised and sore. Cramping, gas, with sour and bitter belching. Chilly, with dryness of the mouth.	Deathly nausea. Terrible abdominal pains and cramping, with extreme exhaustion. Beads of sweat on forehead while vomiting or passing stool. Projectile vomiting, violent vomiting and retching, and shuddering while vomiting. Acidic vomit that is slimy and may be yellow, green, or black. Unquenchable thirst for cold water that is soon vomited. Intense chills and cold sweats. Hiccups.
Diarrhea	Very watery, burning, brown, yellow, or black slimy stools that may contain undigested food. Foul-smelling stools in small quantities that burn the anus. Cramping in the abdomen. Great weakness follows the stool. In the later stages, the diarrhea may look like rice-water. Child is chilly.	Pale, acidic, profuse stools that contain undigested food and look frothy. Diarrhea is painless, but gas pains can make the child bend double. Diarrhea may be involuntary. Give this remedy if your child is weak from loss of fluids from diarrhea and vomiting. They are weak, with much sweating, and may feel faint and/or have ringing in ears. Pale, sometimes with dark circles under their eyes.	Stools are yellow or green, streaked with blood, and very offensive-smelling. If the stools of the child are bright green, this is from overeating.	Sudden diarrhea that drives them out of bed. They feel very faint just after the stool, then better for a short while, and almost immediately have to go again. Gas with much bloating.	Odorless, watery stools that look like rice-water but may also be yellow or green. Pain in abdomen before passing stools. Weak and faint afterward. Frequent stools that blast out. Forehead, hands, feet, and abdomen are cold. Huge thirst for great quantities of cold water.
Mood	The child is anxious and restless, can't lie still, and is exhausted, but has energy enough to be demanding. The anxiety may grow into a fear that they are going to die.	The child is weak, irritable, oversensitive, and nervous. May have problems sleeping.	These children get angry when they don't get their way, and then complain a lot. Nothing pleases them. A lot of screaming and howling.	These children are angry, irritable, nervous, and spiteful; or they are very sensitive and easily offended. Hypersensitive to light, odors, touch, and sound.	The child is restless, moody, tearful, uncommunicative, and withdrawn. May be either talkative or silent.
Worse	Midnight to 2 AM, cold food or drinks, getting chilled, cold, anxiety or apprehension; or after eating rotten meat, fish, or fruit.	Drafts, noise, after weaning from breast milk, tea, nighttime, after eating, and from bad fish, meat, fruit, milk, or impure water.	Stooping, heat, motion, overeating, and eating bad pork, unripe fruit, ice cream, rich foods, pastries, sweets, or berries.	Touch, morning, eating, or consuming rich, spicy, fatty, or junk food, or impure water.	Bad meats, fruits, potatoes, green vegetables, exertion, cold wet weather, cold drinks, touch, pressure, night.
Better	Heat, warm applications to the abdomen.	Much quiet, rest, firm pressure, bending double, and warmth.	Open air, rest, and closing the eyes.	Heat, lying down, sitting, hot drinks, after vomiting, temporarily after passing stools, and taking food after vomiting has subsided.	Warmth, being covered, hot drinks, and lying down. Young children feel better if carried around but not rocked.

EYE CONDITIONS

Any chronic or acute eye condition should be treated by your healthcare professional. When it comes to a child's vision, do not take any risks or allow any condition to go untreated. If none of the remedies have been effective within forty-eight hours, call your healthcare practitioner.

Most common acute problems with the eyes involve irritation of the conjunctiva, the area in back of the eyelid and covering the eyeball globe. This can be caused by infections, colds, dust, allergies, smoke, pollution, squinting, or swimming pools.

Blocked Tear Duct

A blocked tear duct can be due to an underdeveloped tear duct, birth trauma, infection, or injury to the face. Gentle massage of the tissues around the affected area can help, but have your healthcare professional show you how. Sometimes there is a general state of no energy, and occasionally a low-grade fever. In addition to remedies, you can apply a warm compress to the area unless the condition is worse from heat.

The most common remedies for this condition are: **Apis, Argentum Nit, Calc Carb, Graphites, Mercurius Viv, Natrum Mur, Pulsatilla, or Silica.**

Conjunctivitis (Acute)

Inflammation of the conjunctiva can be caused by the common cold, infection, dust, wind, pollution, injury, or an allergic reaction. The infection might be acute or chronic. The eye is irritated and the white part is usually bloodshot. This condition is called "pinkeye." There is usually burning pain, with discharge and intense itching. There is usually but very little swelling. If the condition is due to a common cold, there may be a lack of energy and sometimes a low-grade fever. Allergies are always a chronic condition, and should be treated by your healthcare professional.

The most common remedies for this condition are: **Aconitum, Apis, Argentum Nit, Arsenicum, Belladonna, Calc Carb, Euphrasia, Mercurius Viv, Pulsatilla, Rhus Tox, or Staphysagria.**

Newborn Eye Conditions (besides a blocked tear duct)

The most common remedies for this condition are: **Apis, Argentum Nit, Calc Carb, Graphites, Mercurius Viv, Natrum Mur, Nitric Acid, Pulsatilla, Silica.**

Sties

A sty is a small abscess in a gland on the eyelid. It has the appearance of a tiny boil. It is usually very painful. The sty begins with redness, tenderness, and sometimes swelling. A condition similar to a sty is a chalazion, a swollen oil gland at the edge of the eyelid. The swelling is red and irritated for a while before settling down to being a lump. Some optometrists believe that sties are caused by eyestrain, specifically astigmatism. If your child has recurrent sties, have their vision checked by an optometrist or ophthalmologist.

The most common remedies for this condition are: **Apis, Graphites, Hepar Sulph, Mercurius Viv, Pulsatilla, Rhus Tox, Sepia, Silica, Staphysagria,** or **Sulphur.**

Tired, Overworked Eyes

Give 2 pellets of **Zincum Metal.**

The following are the most commonly indicated remedies for eye conditions:

Aconitum: Conjunctivitis, with sudden onset. The eyes are red, inflamed, dry, hot, and sore. Eyelids are swollen, red, and hard. Can feel like sand is in the eye. Sensitive to light.
Worse from: Night, bright light, and cold winds. **Better from:** Fresh air and cool applications.

Apis: Sty, blocked tear duct, or conjunctivitis. There is much puffiness and swelling around the eye, redness and hot tears with rawness, stinging, and burning. The eyes are very bloodshot. The pains may be shooting or piercing. The discharge is clear, or full of pus. Much itching, especially at night. It may feel like there is grit under the lid, and it is hard to read in artificial light. This remedy can prevent recurrence of sties.

Worse from: Late afternoon, sun, right eye, and heat. **Better from:** Cool applications and cool air.

Argentum Nit: Conjunctivitis or blocked tear duct. There is swelling, inflammation, and redness on the inner corner of the eye. Eyelid is red, swollen, sore, and thick. Discharge is profuse and full of yellow pus. On waking, there is usually a thick crust on the edges of the eyelids, and they can become glued together. If a baby has conjunctivitis or a blocked tear duct, this will show up shortly after birth. In the older child, the eyes feel achy and strained, with splinter-like pains. The child may say that their vision is out of focus. Pupils may be dilated.

Worse from: Warm rooms, heat, and upon waking. **Better from:** Cool applications, light pressure, closing the eyes, and fresh air.

Arsenicum: Conjunctivitis. The eyes and eyelids have much burning pain, with hot, acidic tears. Eyes are bright-red and bloodshot, sometimes with dark rings or puffiness around them. The eyelids are red, crusty, and ulcerated. Extreme sensitivity to light. Under the eyelid may feel gritty, and the eyelid may go into spasms.

Worse from: Evening, cold damp, upon waking, light, and on the right side. **Better from:** Warm applications, and lying down.

Belladonna: Conjunctivitis. Sudden onset with red, hot, and swollen eyes that feel very dry. Throbbing pains in the eyeball, sometimes with a headache. Eyes are watery and bloodshot, with a glassy appearance, and pupils are dilated. The eyes feel enlarged, swollen, heavy, and congested. Great intolerance to light. Sensation that the eyes are half-closed. May have a fever. The older child may complain of double vision, or lines appearing crooked when they are reading.

Worse from: Heat, touch, noise, jarring, light, around 3 PM, and on the right side. **Better from:** Being semi-erect, resting, quiet, and low light.

Calc Carb: Conjunctivitis or blocked tear duct. Sore, watering eyes that may ooze a yellow or nasty-smelling discharge. Eyes are glued together after sleeping. Sensitivity to light, and dilated pupils. The child may experience fuzzy vision. Eyelids are itchy and swollen, with a sensation of grittiness. This condition can appear in babies after a cold, and you may notice that they are slightly squinting. Blocked tear ducts may occur from exposure to cold.

Worse from: Open air, early morning, cold, damp, with common cold, and any eye movement. **Better from:** Rest and warmth.

Euphrasia: Conjunctivitis. Profuse, hot, acidic, and burning tears. Eyes are very bloodshot and constantly watering, with a sensation of pressure, cutting pains, and sand in the eye. The eyelids are red, swollen, burning, and itchy. The eye may twitch, and the child blinks a lot. They are sensitive to light. Eyes may ooze thick, yellow pus. It is not uncommon to have a cold with this condition.

Worse from: Light, wind, cold air, lying down, evening time, and smoke. **Better from:** Open air (but not in sunlight or wind), very gently rubbing and wiping eyes, and low light.

Graphites: Blocked tear duct or sty. Oozing of hot tears. Eyelids appear heavy, red, and swollen. The lids are sore, dry, and may be cracked at the edges. Sensitive to light. Honey-colored deposits that are dry and painful to remove. Older child may complain of seeing double letters when reading.

Worse from: Cold and night. **Better from:** Warmth, open air, and low light.

Hepar Sulph: Conjunctivitis or sty. Profuse, yellow, thick, and very sticky discharge. Eyes and eyelids are inflamed. Child is extremely sensitive to touch, light, and air. Pain in upper orbit bone of the eye socket. Eyes are bloodshot. Margins of eyes may have tiny pimples or ulcerations. Eyelids get stuck together while sleeping. May have blurred vision. If a sty is present, there is much swelling and throbbing. This remedy can speed up bringing a sty to a head so that it can drain.

Worse from: Cold air, cold hands touching the eye area; nighttime, pressure, and light. **Better from:** Warmth and warm applications.

Mercurius Vivus (also known as **Mercurius Sol**): Conjunctivitis, blocked tear duct, or sty. Eyes ooze profuse, acidic, and burning discharge that can turn to yellow-green pus. The child has excess saliva and/or sweating, and bloodshot eyes with sensation of pressure. Sensitivity to light, heat, and cold. Eyelids are swollen, thick, sore, and red. Eyelids get glued together. Not uncommon to have a cold with this condition.

Worse from: Night, damp, heat, sunlight, bright lights, and drafts. **Better from:** Moderate temperature, rest, and low lights.

Natrum Mur: Blocked tear duct. Eyes itch, burn, and profusely water with acidic discharge. Child's eyes always appear wet with tears. Pain in eyeballs when looking down. Eyes are extremely sensitive to sunlight, and feel as if there is grit under the lid. Lids are heavy, red, and sore. Child constantly rubs eyes. They may complain of a headache. The older child will be very susceptible to eyestrain, and may see sparks or zigzags around objects.

Worse from: 9–11 AM, sunlight, and warmth. **Better from:** Open air, cool applications, sweating, and rest.

Nitric Acid: For constantly watering eyes in newborns. The eyelids are swollen. Their sweat, urine, and stools have a very offensive odor. They are chilly. These babies are miserable, irritable, and very sensitive to noise.

Worse from: Touch, noise, jarring, rattling sounds, motion, after eating, both cold air and hot weather, evening and night, and loss of sleep. **Better from:** Gliding motion, mild weather, plenty of sleep, being kept cool if it is hot, and wrapped up if it is cold.

Pulsatilla: Conjunctivitis, blocked tear duct, or sty. Also for sticky eyes in newborns. Profuse, thick, yellow or yellow-green, nonacidic discharge from the eyes, which may be smelly. The discharge is usually thick upon waking, and then watery for the rest of the day. Lots of discharge in the corners of the eyes. The eyes are achy, and water in cold air or wind. There is itching and burning of the lids, which causes the child to rub the eyes a lot. Eyelids get stuck together while sleeping. May have conjunctivitis with a cold. Sty is usually on the upper lid, and is often unable to come to a head.

Worse from: Evening time, warm, stuffy rooms, and warm wind. **Better from:** Temperate fresh air, and cool applications.

Rhus Tox: Conjunctivitis or sty. Inflammation with discharge of yellow pus, and much watering. Eyes are sensitive to light, sore, red, and burning, and painful with movement or any pressure. Swelling and itching of the eyelids, which feel heavy and stiff. Eyelids get stuck together while sleeping. Upon getting the eyelids unstuck, there is a gush of tears. Eyelids feel stiff and dry.

Worse from: Nighttime, moving the eyes when first waking, damp, and cold. **Better from:** Warm applications and warm drinks.

Sepia: Sty. Eyes red, sore, and burning, with a feeling of grit under the eyelid. Eyes may feel like they are falling out. Eyelids are droopy, swollen, and get glued together.

Worse from: Morning, evening, cold air, and damp. **Better from:** Warm applications, gentle pressure, and temperate fresh air.

Silicea (also known as **Silica Terra**): Blocked tear duct, sty, or a foreign body lodged in the tissue of the eye. Inflammation, soreness, yellow discharge, and a slowly developing swelling in the corner of the eye. Sensitivity to daylight. Eyes very tender to the touch, especially when closed. Gritty feeling in eyes. Sharp pain that can shoot through the eye. Sty on the upper lid, toward the inner corner. Sty emits pus. Older child may complain of letters running together when reading.

Worse from: Cold, damp, or fresh air, and touch. **Better from:** Heat, warm rooms, and rest.

Staphysagria: Conjunctivitis or sty. May develop blue rings around the orbit of the eye, or dark-blue circles under the eye. Eyeballs feel hot and dry even though there is a discharge of hot tears. Bursting pains in the eyeball. Edges of eyelids are itchy. The upper eyelid and inner corner are the most affected. The sty is very sensitive to the touch, and the eye can be very dry, especially in the morning.

Worse from: Getting angry, slight touch, cold drinks, and night. **Better from:** Warmth, rest, and much patience.

Sulphur: Conjunctivitis or sty. Eyes have much heat, burning, itching, and dryness. The eyes can be sore, with bursting pain in the eyeballs. Sensitive to light. The eyeballs may tremble, and eyelids may quiver. The eyes water easily in fresh air, but fresh air makes them feel better. Eyes are glued together upon awakening. Sensation of grittiness. The child may see a halo around lights, and may stick their feet out from underneath the covers in bed. The sty is usually on the upper lid.

Worse from: Heat, warm, stuffy rooms, heat in bed, around 11 AM and 11 PM (especially the itchiness), looking down, and washing the eyes. **Better from:** Cool applications, i.e., a cool washcloth on closed eyes, no socks on the feet while in bed, and open air.

Zincum Metal: Tired, overworked eyes. This is a condition that is brought on by squinting, which can be caused by the child not being able to see clearly—in which case they should be taken to an optometrist. Too much studying can also cause squinting and weakness of the eyes. The eyes are sore and watering, with burning tears. They can feel gritty, as if there is sand in them. Inflammation and redness of the conjunctiva and especially in the corners or the eye. Itching and soreness of the lids, which may twitch. Rolling of the eyes. Feeling of pressure in the eye socket.

Worse from: Exhaustion, mental effort, work, talking, heat, noise, too much time staring at a computer or TV, and from

5–7 PM. **Better from:** Eating, fresh air, rest, gentle rubbing, scratching, and light pressure from an eye pillow made with lavender.

Dosage: Give 2 pellets every hour until improvement. Then reduce to a few times a day until gone. If there has been no improvement after seven doses, choose a new remedy. Repeat the remedy only if there is a return of any symptoms.

Supportive Measures:

If your child wakes up with eyes caked shut, gently apply a warm, clean washcloth to moisten the crust. Never force the lids open. Keep eyes clean and free of crusts by applying warm or cool compresses several times a day. Check the remedy to find out whether warm or cool applications will feel best. Warm applications can also help a sty to open and drain.

Conjunctivitis is extremely contagious; wash hands after touching the child's eye. Do not touch the uninfected eye after you have touched the infected eye, because you can spread the infection to the other eye. Wash any cloths that have been used for compresses in hot, soapy water. Wash pillowcases on a daily basis, as well as anything else that has come in contact with the child's infected eye.

Try to encourage the child not to rub eyes, because rubbing can make the inflammation worse. You may want to purchase a bottle of Euphrasia Tincture from a health-food store or natural pharmacy. This is one of the best medicines for the relief of eye irritations. Use one drop in a quarter-cup of lukewarm spring water. Use this solution to bathe the eye; you may want to use an eyebath cup, which can be purchased at a drug store. For eye conditions in newborns and nursing babies, bathe the affected eyes in breast milk. This is an old and well-proven remedy.

Call your healthcare practitioner if:

- There is any eye condition in a newborn that does not respond to a remedy within forty-eight hours.
- The eyes are frequently bloodshot.
- There is a persistent sensation of pressure in the eyes.
- The eyelids are red, thick, crusty, and have ulcers, as this may be a condition called blepharitis, a bacterial infection.
- There is severe pain in the eyeball, with extreme hypersensitivity to light.
- The child has a fever over 103 degrees with eye symptoms, or a baby under three months has any elevated temperature.
- There is any abnormal vision. When it comes to a child's vision, do not take any risks!
- Your child is constantly squinting.
- There is a sudden partial loss of sight, blurring, or seeing floating shapes, as this can indicate a detaching retina. This is very unlikely, but possible. Go to an urgent-care center or the emergency room.

GROWING PAINS

Growing pains are the result of a child having a growing spurt. They are usually felt in the legs, but may be felt in any joint or other part of the body. The most common pains are felt in the shins, ankles, and knees up into the hamstrings. Please eliminate the possibility that the pain is from an injury; shin pain, for example, in a child who plays sports may be a shin splint and not a growing pain. Repeat the remedy only if there is a return of any symptoms. You may need to repeat the remedy if the child goes through another growing spurt. For this condition, dosages are given at the end of each remedy description.

The following are the most commonly indicated remedies for growing pains:

Calc Phos: For big growth spurts in which the child has grown tall too quickly, especially in the legs. The pains are shooting in all directions. The legs feel achy, weak, lame, and heavy and may have cramping in the calves. Hands and feet are usually cold. Can have loss of appetite. Give this remedy daily for one week.

Note: If your child is experiencing a lot of cramping in the legs while walking, you can alternate **Calc Phos** and **Mag Phos**. Give 2 pellets of one remedy one day and a dose of the other remedy the next day. Repeat until there is improvement. Then repeat only if there is a return of symptoms. If there is no improvement after ten days, contact your healthcare practitioner.

Worse from: Cold, damp, motion, exertion, upward motion, and puberty. **Better from:** Warm, dry, lying down, and rest.

Eupatorium: Pains in the back and legs. The flesh actually feels sore in these areas. Back and calves may feel bruised. Small of back can be weak. May feel as if they are getting a cold, or achy as if they are getting the flu. May feel nauseous from smell or sight of food. Give this remedy daily for one week.

Worse from: Autumn, winter, movement, open air, cold air, smell or sight of food, and from 7–9 AM. **Better from:** Sweating, lying still, staying in the house, and loose clothing.

Guaiacum: Stinging and burning pains shooting up the leg from the ankle. The hamstrings feel too short. Weakness in thighs. Stiffness and lameness in the legs. Joints are swollen, painful, and hot. Cannot bear any pressure. Prickles like that of needles in the buttocks. Secretions from the body have a foul odor. A strong desire for apples. Give this remedy daily for one week.

Worse from: Heat, pressure, touch, and motion. **Better from:** Cool applications and gentle stretching.

Phosphoric Acid: Pains at night that make the bones feel as if they were being scraped. Great weakness. Tearing pains in joints and bones. May feel as though ants are crawling under the skin of the legs. The child may stumble easily. The legs may tremble in walking. This is the most common remedy for children who grow rapidly and are overtaxed mentally and physically. Give this remedy daily for one week.

Worse from: Overexertion, whether physical, emotional, or mental, cold, night drafts, sitting, standing, and loss of vital fluids. **Better from:** Warmth, short naps, and hydration. Please keep this child well hydrated!

Silicea: The back is weak, and the child is sensitive to drafts on their backs. Legs may feel paralyzed and may have trembling when walking. Sometimes pains and weakness in hips, legs, and feet, and cramping in calves and soles of feet. Feet are very smelly and sweaty, with sore soles in the arch area. The child may have a stiff neck with a headache that begins at nape of the neck, spreads over the head, and settles over one or both eyes. There may be tingling in the soles of the feet. This child can become thin and gangly. They may become particularly prone to colds or swollen glands. Give this remedy daily for two weeks.

Worse from: Cold air, damp, fresh air, and touch. **Better from:** Heat, warm rooms, and rest.

HEAD LICE

A head louse is a six-legged, wingless, parasitic insect that uses its claws to hold on to hair strands. It stays close to the scalp and is found where the hair is thick. It will bite the skin and feast on blood, which keeps it alive. The eggs are called nits. The females attach the nits with a gluey substance onto the hair strands near the scalp. The warmth of the head allows the eggs to incubate and hatch in 7–10 days. When the nit has hatched, it leaves behind a white, glistening shell. In 7–14 days, the new lice will start breeding, beginning a new cycle.

Lice and their nits will only affect those children who are susceptible because of a weakened immune system. They are highly contagious, but not all children will succumb. It is not enough to use oils, nit combs, and hair conditioners. These will kill off the parasites, but will not correct the underlying constitutional problem that supports them. A treatment to strengthen the child's immune system is necessary, so their body will no longer be a host for these parasites. Once a child has been treated appropriately with the correct constitutional remedy from a homeopathic practitioner, it is unlikely that they will ever be a host for lice again. Please contact your homeopath to prescribe a remedy for this condition.

In the meantime, you can get rid of the lice and their nits by doing the following:

- Cut the hair as short as possible. This may seem extreme, but lice cannot live in a chilly environment.
- Massage one teaspoon of olive oil mixed with one drop of lavender oil into the scalp, and wrap the head in a hot towel for thirty minutes. Wash the oil out thoroughly and then apply a large amount of conditioner, let it set for a few minutes, then rinse thoroughly.
- Obtain a nit comb from a drug store. Comb through all the hair, starting at the scalp and working out your way out. Rinse the comb often. Dry the hair with a blow dryer. Repeat the lavender oil and nit-combing process each day for three days.

Do not use tea tree oil, because it can antidote homeopathic remedies.

NEWBORN DISCOMFORTS

A note about poisonous chemicals in children's clothing: It is important to buy toxin-free and sustainable fibers for the delicate skin of your child. The safest fibers for your child are organic cotton, industrial hemp, silk, bamboo, or wool. Most conventional children's clothing is coated with stain-, fire-, and wrinkle-resistant toxins. Nonorganic cotton is laden with several toxic insecticides and pesticides. Conventional dyes can be full of carcinogenic heavy metals such as chrome, copper, and zinc. If your baby is allergic to any of these chemicals, they can produce such symptoms as watery eyes, runny nose, or skin rashes. See the "Resources" section at the end of this book for places to buy toxin-free clothing.

What to observe in the newborn:

A baby cannot tell you how they feel, so you will have to be a very good observer and use your intuition. The following list is a helpful tool for prescribing the best remedies.

Discharges: Is the color clear, yellow, or yellow-green? Is the consistency thin or thick? Is the discharge profuse or scanty? Does it smell? If so, what does the odor remind you of?

Ears: Does the baby pull on their ears? If so, which one? Is there a fever? If so, how high is it?

Elimination: How frequently does the baby have a bowel movement? Does the baby strain or cry as if the bowel movement is painful? Does the baby pass gas? If so, what does it smell like? Are the stools formed or loose? What color is the stool? If the baby has diarrhea and there is a diaper rash, it probably means that the stools are acidic. See section on diarrhea.

What to observe in the newborn (cont.):

Eyes: Are they bright, dull, bloodshot, yellow, with dilated or contracted pupils, or with a scared look? Are there dark circles under the eyes? This can indicate an allergy; please consult your healthcare provider. Are the eyes oozing a discharge? If so, what color and consistency is it?

Frequency of occurrence: Observing what time your baby is most affected. Is there a particular time of day—morning, afternoon, evening, night, midnight, or upon awakening? Is there a particular time of month, such as during the full moon? Is there a particular time of year—winter, spring, summer, or autumn?

Mood: Is the baby good-natured, fussy, sensitive to noise, sensitive to stress in the household, irritable, restless, fearful, quiet, fretful, or calm? Do they want to be carried all the time?

Nose: Is there a discharge? If so, what color and consistency is it? Clear, yellow, yellow-green? Like an egg white, thick, thin, or stringy? Does the nose run or become stuffier at particular times of the day, or if they are inside, or outside? Does anything make it better or worse? Is the condition affecting both nostrils, or just one?

Skin: Is its appearance pale, or flushed? Is it cold or hot to the touch? Does it feel clammy, sweaty, or puffy? Is there a rash? Are there pimples or bumps? Is it dry, oily, flaky, or cracked? Is there an area that is sensitive to the touch?

Sleep: Does the baby sleep well and have good energy? Or restless and wake frequently? Are they too warm or too cool? Do they prefer to sleep with the window open? What position makes them feel most comfortable?

What to observe in the newborn (cont.):

Temperature: Does the baby like to have a lot of blankets? Does the baby sweat easily or shiver? If the baby feels hot, is there a temperature above 98.6 degrees? (If so, see section on "Fevers," page 182.)

Thirst: A baby that wants to suck all the time may be thirsty. You can give them one teaspoon of spring water, a bit at a time.

Throat: Does the baby cry when nursing? Is the exterior of the throat hot to the touch?

Tummy: Is it bloated? Does the baby cry if there is any pressure on the abdominal area, or if they are put down on their stomachs? Does the baby double up, or throw their body backwards? If you get a sense that there is stomach discomfort, is it better or worse after eating, or is there a position that makes it better or worse? See "Colic in Babies" section (page 12).

Birth or Circumcision Trauma

This is a condition that can be easily overlooked. The baby might be called fussy or hard to please. They may seem as if they are in constant pain. If a baby cries a lot, cannot sleep well, screams particularly in the dark, or cannot be appeased, talk with your healthcare practitioner. Was there any trauma, e.g., a car accident or a death in the family, etc. while the mother was pregnant? Was the mother given anesthesia, or was it a forceps delivery? Was the labor long or particularly difficult?

You can get a bottle of **Bach Flower Rescue Remedy** from any health store or natural pharmacy. Put one drop of the flower essence in one teaspoon of breast milk or water, and give the baby one drop, one hour apart, three times. This may always be used for any trauma that a baby, mother, or child has experienced. It may be a good thing to also take your child to a cranial-sacral osteopath. They are safe, gentle, and their treatments can be extremely beneficial to infants with any birth trauma issues.

The following are the most commonly indicated remedies for birth or circumcision trauma:

Aconitum: There is a look of terror in the baby's eyes, like the look of a deer facing headlights. They are fearful, anxious, restless, and sensitive to noise. This can be brought on especially after a fast labor or circumcision.

Borax: There is a look of fright. They are very sensitive to downward motion and thus startle when they are put down. They want to be carried all the time, day and night.

Nux Moschata: This kind of trauma produces a baby who is so sleepy that they cannot latch on to the breast. They nurse for a few minutes and then fall back asleep, because they are so exhausted. They are chilly and usually have colic with much gas.

Staphysagria: This remedy is especially helpful after circumcisions or any surgical intervention. The baby is incredibly sensitive to pain, noise, touch, or odors. They are sleepy all day, and awake all night.

Stramonium: The baby needing this remedy has a look of terror in their eyes, which are wide open with dilated pupils. There is inconsolable crying all night, because they do not want to be alone and are terrified of the dark. They scream bloody murder upon waking. This is a good remedy to give to baby boys after circumcision.

Dosage: Give 2 pellets every 15 minutes for one hour, then once an hour if needed. Repeat only if there is a return of symptoms. If there are no results after six doses, choose another remedy. Do not wake the child to give them a remedy.

Blocked Tear Ducts

These and other eye problems are discussed in depth in the "Eye Conditions" section (page 43).

Colds in Newborn Babies

I have included this short section as just a very brief overview. An infant with a cold is miserable, because they cannot eat and breathe at the same time. It takes a while for some newborns to breathe through their mouths.

The following are the most commonly indicated remedies for colds in newborns:

Aconitum: You had the baby out for a walk in the stroller and it was cold and windy. All of a sudden your baby has come down with a cold. This remedy is especially for winds from the north.

Belladonna: Your baby's face is suddenly red, the pupils are dilated, the skin is hot, the extremities are cool, and your baby is restless.

Bryonia: This is for a fussy baby that does not want to be moved. The baby is very thirsty and has a dry, stuffed-up nose. Usually the lips are dry as well. This baby will tend to be constipated, with dry, hard stools.

Hepar Sulph: This baby is sweaty but chilly, so they want to be kept warm and covered up at all times. If your hands are cold and you touch your baby, the baby will scream. The baby's breath rattles, and there may or may not be a cough.

Mercurius Viv (also known as **Mercurius Sol**): This baby usually has swollen glands under the ears and down the sides of the neck. You can gently feel them with your fingertips—they will be slightly swollen and may feel hard. The baby is sweaty, smelly, and usually has diarrhea. You will probably notice that the baby is drooling. This baby is sensitive to temperature changes.

Nux Vomica: This baby's nose drips during the day and if taken out in fresh air, but is dry at night. This baby usually has intestinal issues, and may be constipated and burp a lot.

Pulsatilla: This baby is weepy. One minute they are fine and the next they are unhappy. Your baby wants to be cuddled, carried slowly and gently, and to get attention. The discharge from the nose will be cream-colored. The baby will do better in fresh air. Their nose gets stuffy as soon as they are brought inside from being outside.

Dosage: Give 2 pellets every hour until there is improvement. If there are no results after six doses, choose another remedy. Repeat only if there is a return of symptoms. Do not wake your baby to give them a remedy. Remember, the more severe the illness, or if there has been a fast onset, the more frequently you will repeat a dose.

Supportive Measures:

Infant sections of drugstores have bulb syringes for sucking mucus from the baby's nose. Ask the pharmacist if you cannot find one. Since the baby cannot blow out the mucus, this can help until the remedy dispels it. Consistently get the mucus out of the nose so it is not draining down the back of the throat and eventually producing a cough. The nursing mother should avoid dairy products until this condition subsides. Seek other foods with high calcium values.

Colic is addressed in the "Colic in Babies" section (page 12).

Constipation is addressed in the "Constipation" section (page 25).

Cradle Cap

Cradle cap is a condition in which a baby's scalp develops scaly skin. This turns into scabby areas with matted hair. This results from elimination of toxins and should not be repressed. Rubbing organic extra-virgin olive or coconut oil onto the area loosens the scabs. You need to consult your homeopath for a constitutional consultation for your baby.

Diaper Rash

The following are the most commonly indicated remedies for diaper rash:

Graphites: The skin is dry, inflamed, raw, itchy, and cracked. The diaper rash tends to be in the folds of the skin. There is a thick, sticky, honey-colored oozing that may form yellow crusts. The baby will not want a warm bath.

Hepar Sulph: The skin oozes pus that smells like old, rotten cheese. The skin is very tender. These babies are extremely sensitive, physically and emotionally. This remedy tends to be chilly, so a warm bath will feel good. Make sure your hands are warm when touching your baby, or they will scream. They are extremely chilly and adverse to cold.

Petroleum: The skin is extremely sensitive, raw, burning, itchy, and can't heal, especially in folds and around the scrotum. The skin may crack and bleed. This diaper rash will respond best if the baby is allowed to go without a diaper. They are extremely irritable, physically and emotionally.

Sulphur: Very itchy and burning-red diaper rash. There is usually a bright-red rash around the anus. The skin is raw, and can break open and bleed. Keep this baby as cool as possible. The baby will not want a hot bath.

Dosage: Give 2 pellets every four hours. If there is no response after forty-eight hours, try a different remedy. As soon as there is improvement, repeat the remedy only if there is a return of any symptoms.

Supportive Measures:

Change diapers immediately when they are wet or contain stools. Wash the area with very mild soap, and rinse with water. You can use a hairdryer on a cool or warm setting to dry the area completely. You can also use an organic egg white on dry skin to form a waterproof barrier. Calendula cream can be applied after every diaper change while the rash is present. Calendula is known for its speedy healing properties, but it can sting, so the baby may fuss at first when it is applied. The stinging will subside. Calendula cream or diaper ointment can be purchased at any health-food store or natural pharmacy. Apricot kernel oil, coconut oil, or olive oil can also be soothing. Do not use petroleum-based ointments or castor oil. Use organic products when possible.

If your baby has a white, cottage cheese-like discharge, this may be yeast infection from candida. The baby and/or nursing mother should refrain from sweets, including cutting back on fruit until the diaper rash is completely gone.

Some babies can have reactions to disposable diapers. Cotton diapers allow the skin to breathe. Allow the baby to go without a diaper as often as possible.

Call your healthcare practitioner if:

- The rash does not respond to any remedies, and causes the child discomfort.
- The baby has had diaper rash, other rashes, warts, or ear infections since birth.
- There is rash with red, raw, shiny patches, or a white cottage cheese-like discharge, as this can indicate a yeast infection.
- There is a rash with blisters that are oozing pus. This can indicated a bacterial infection, especially if there is any rise in temperature.
- There are swollen lymph glands in the groin.

Eye Conditions (besides a blocked tear duct)

See specific symptoms for each of these remedies in the "Eye Conditions" section (page 43).

Fever in Newborns

See "Fevers" section (page 182).

Hiccups

Hiccups are usually caused by nursing too fast, inadequate burping, or taking in gulps of air instead of milk. The diaphragm goes into spasm and produces hiccups. See the "Supportive measures" section of "Colic in Babies" for tips on feeding a baby. Two pellets of **Nux Vomica** may be given on an as-needed basis, if all other potential feeding problems have been eliminated. If this problem persists, contact your healthcare professional.

Jaundice

Jaundice is not uncommon in newborns, especially at high altitudes. This condition is best left for a homeopath to treat.

Newborn Nose Snuffles

This is a condition that happens when a newborn's nose becomes inflamed, producing a thickening of the mucous-membrane lining of the nose. This makes the newborn stuffed up. Consequently, the newborn cannot breathe while nursing. This can be very frustrating, because the baby needs to have nourishment but cannot nurse. Newborn snuffles are not the same as the common cold.

The following are the most commonly indicated remedies for newborn nose snuffles:

Antimonium Tart: Profuse flow of mucus, and a rattling of mucus in the chest. The baby might sneeze. The baby is irritable, weak, and wants to be carried in upright position.

    Worse from: Warmth, early morning, night, and getting overheated. **Better from:** Gentle rocking and cool, open air.

Dulcamara: Nose is completely stopped up, especially in cold, wet weather. There is thick mucus that does not discharge. Smallest amount of cold air stops up the nose. Baby wants to be kept warm, and is irritable and restless.

    Worse from: Air conditioning, being chilled, and cold, rainy weather. **Better from:** Warmth, covering up, and gentle motion.

Lycopodium: Nose is usually dry, stuffed up, and may get crusty or plugged with elastic mucus. Baby will breathe only through the mouth. They are usually irritable, and wake up irritable and angry.

    Worse from: 4–8 PM, stuffy rooms, wind, and wet weather. **Better from:** Very gently rubbing the baby's nose, fresh air, and warmth in bed.

Mercurius Viv (also known as **Mercurius Sol**): The nose is swollen and red because the nostrils are raw with thick mucus. The baby is restless, and may sneeze. You may notice that they are drooling.

Worse from: Warm rooms, being too cold or too hot, damp weather, night, and drafts. **Better from:** Moderate temperature and rest.

Nux Vomica: Nose runs during the day and is blocked up at night. The baby is sensitive to whatever the mother eats, and oversensitive in general.

Worse from: Noise, light, odors, dry and cold weather, and early morning. **Better from:** Warmth, but not warm and stuffy rooms, staying covered up, and lying down.

Sambucus: Thick mucus in nostrils with no discharge. The breathing has a rattling sound. Baby may wake with a start because they are having trouble breathing. The baby is fretful and fussy.

Worse from: Cold dry air, sleep, midnight, and from 2–3 AM. **Better from:** Gentle rocking and covering up.

Dosage: Give 2 pellets three times a day for three days. Stop sooner if there is improvement. Repeat if there is a return of symptoms. Choose a different remedy if there has been no response.

Supportive Measures:

In the infant section of a drugstore, they have bulb syringes for sucking the mucus from the baby's nose. Since the baby cannot blow out the mucus, this can help until the remedy dispels it. Clear the mucus often. The nursing mother should avoid dairy products until this condition subsides. Seek other foods with high calcium values.

Restlessness, Agitation, or Overstimulation

These can happen in a baby who has been on a long journey, becoming overly tired and unable to wind down, or a baby who may have been overexcited by too much activity or stimulation. The senses become hypersensitive to noise, sensations, smells, tastes, light, and even fresh air. The baby may scream and tremble. If your baby cannot calm down, give them 2 pellets of **Coffea**. Repeat if the baby starts becoming agitated again. Do not give it more than 3 times per occurrence.

Thrush

Thrush is a yeast infection of the mucous membranes in the mouth of a newborn. The cause is from either the mother or baby being treated with antibiotics. There are white patches on the insides of the cheeks, the gums, or the tongue. The skin is raw and tender, making it uncomfortable for the baby to nurse. The nursing mother should incorporate yogurt with live cultures into her diet, and avoid eating too many sweets or too much fruit. The mother should also be checked to make sure she does not have a breast infection or a yeast infection.

The following are the most commonly indicated remedies for thrush:

Borax: The baby cries while nursing because their mouth is so sore. Their gums are inflamed, very tender, and hot to the touch, and the tongue is dry, cracked, or indented. There is a white fungus-like growth. The thrush can bleed easily. This baby is easily frightened, does not like downward motion, and startles at the least little noise.

Kali Mur: White ulcers in the mouth. Swollen glands in the jaw and neck. The tongue has a greyish-white coating at the base, and is either dry or slimy. The gums may be shiny, translucent red. The mouth is sore.

Mercurius Viv (also known as **Mercurius Sol**): Heavy, yellow coating on tongue. Gums are swollen, tender, sore, and may bleed. Breath is foul, as is body odor and sweat. You may notice that the baby is drooling while asleep and awake. They are thirsty despite much moistness in the mouth.

Natrum Mur: Thrush is dry and white. Mouth is sore when any food touches it. There is much pain. The lips and corners of the mouth can be dry, ulcerated, and cracked. There is a frothy coating on the tongue, with bubbles on the side. The gums are red and glistening, and the breath is hot and offensive. There may be a crack in the middle of the lower lip.

Ulcerated Navel

An ulcerated navel can be relieved by giving 2 pellets of **Petroleum** once a day for 3 days. Consult your healthcare practitioner if there is no improvement, if the infant develops a fever, or if there are red streaks going out from the navel. *If there are red streaks, go to the emergency room.*

Call your healthcare practitioner if:

- Your baby is under three months old and has any rise in temperature.
- You are in doubt about any symptom your newborn has.
- If your newborn does not seem right, do not worry about wasting someone's time with overreacting. You are being responsible and making sure that your newborn is OK.

STOMACHACHES AND INDIGESTION

Stomachaches and indigestion can be caused by a number of factors, e.g., anxiety, tension, eating too fast, consuming too much sugar or fats, certain food allergies, gas, constipation, appendicitis, the onset of a stomach virus, or a strep infection. Also see sections on "Colic" (page 12), "Constipation" (page 25), and "Diarrhea, Nausea, and Vomiting" (page 30).

There can be aches or pains, cramping gas, bloating, unusual stools, or nausea from the pain. If your baby has a stomachache, you can refer to the "Colic" section (page 12). The information below will tell you the foods that make stomachaches and indigestion worse. Please avoid these foods for a couple of days after your child has recovered.

The following are the most commonly indicated remedies for stomachaches and indigestion:

Argentum Nit: Onset from anxiety or dread before a play or performance. There is much anxiety. There is a burning and gnawing pain in the pit of the stomach that radiates out in all directions, and much loud gas and belching. There is a sensation of constriction. These children are anxious, excitable, restless, fidgety, and many times they tremble.

Worse from: Eating (especially too much chocolate, sugar or sweets), heat, too much excitement, and anxiety about upcoming events. **Better from:** Fresh air, motion, passing gas, and burping.

Carbo Veg: Burning, cramping pains with much bloating, belching, and gas. The bloating is so intense that the belly is stretched tight. Belching and passing gas temporarily relieves the pain, but soon the gas builds again. The child may be nauseous. There may be sourness to the belches, and the gas is usually quite smelly. The child is extremely uncomfortable with any tight clothes around the waist. They are weak, with cold extremities, but feel hot on the inside. The child is sluggish, indifferent, and irritable.

Worse from: Fatty and rich foods, lying down, and warmth. **Better from:** Fresh air, and being fanned.

Cuprum Metal: Painful cramping and pressure. Slimy sensation in mouth, with strong metallic taste. Thirst for cold drinks, which make all symptoms feel temporarily feel better. Child is nauseous, and may vomit. They are chilly, and the skin feels icy-cold. The stomach feels tender, hot, sore, and bruised. The child is sensitive, nervous, stubborn, sullen, and may bite others when sick.

Worse from: Dairy products, touch, movement, strong negative emotions, hot weather, lack of sleep, evening, and night.
Better from: Cold water, which yields temporary results; very light pressure of hand on abdominal area, and sweating.

Dioscorea: Pain in the pit of the stomach that is burning, sharp, and cramping. Pains radiate to back, chest, and arms. There may be a constant ache around the navel. If this is the case, refer to the "Call your healthcare practitioner if" section below. Much belching, passing large quantities of offensive gas, and hiccups. Nausea with uneasy, sinking feeling in stomach. Child is irritable, nervous, and depressed.

Worse from: Overeating, ingesting old cheese, uncooked fruit, or rich pastry, bending forward, and lying down. **Better from:** Stretching, especially backwards, moving about, and standing up.

Ignatia: Onset from getting a severe scolding, being homesick, getting extremely frightened to the point of not being able to sleep, extreme emotional upset with themselves, family or friends, or from a death in the family, or of a close friend or pet. The symptoms may be odd, such as having an empty feeling in the stomach that is not relieved by eating—or feeling nauseous but hungry. There is a sinking sensation in the stomach that is relieved by taking a deep breath, and stomach cramping that is worse from even the slightest touch. There is much sour belching. The child passes a lot of gas, especially at night. This is a sensitive child that sighs a lot, does not want consolation, is tearful, or cries convulsively alone, is moody, sentimental, and oversensitive to pain, and may be quarrelsome.

Worse from: Grief, emotional upsets, cold open air, walking, touch, morning, sweets, cucumbers, onions, rice, bread, and spices. **Better from:** Warmth, eating, being left alone to work it out, and a reminder to take deep breaths.

Lycopodium: Pressing, cramping pains in stomach, with a sensation of a band around the stomach. Sour, acidic-tasting belches that only rise to the throat. Much loud passing of gas. Bloating occurs as soon as the least amount of food is eaten. The child feels hungry but doesn't eat much because they are quickly satisfied, then wake at night from hunger. Sensation of churning and coldness in stomach. Hiccups. The child is fearful of being alone, is insecure and bossy, and wakes irritable and angry.

Worse from: Onions, beans, cabbage, tight clothing, 4–8 PM, pressure, and stuffy rooms. **Better from:** Fresh air, warm drinks, belching, and warm applications on stomach.

Nux Vomica: Onset from overindulging or eating rich foods. The child may have a stomachache with hiccups. Sour and bitter belching, with much nausea. The pains are cramping, pressing, and the stomach feels bruised and sore with a feeling of fullness and heaviness after eating, as if there is a rock in the stomach. There is bloating, and the child is extremely sensitive to pressure on the stomach. The child is irritable, easily frustrated, impatient, sensitive to noise and odors, and easily offended.

Note: Look to this remedy if a child has been hit in the stomach and has a decreased appetite.

Worse from: Eating, especially rich foods, tight clothing, early morning, and cold open air. **Better from:** Warm drinks, rest, and warmth in bed.

Pulsatilla: Onset from fats, ice cream, rich foods, and pork. Stomach feels heavy, with pressing pains. Much belching with the taste of the food just eaten, which remains long after the food is eaten. Gas with rumbling and pain in the abdominal area. Gnawing hunger. Mouth feels dry, without thirst. The child may be chilly, but want the window open for fresh air. The symptoms and emotions are very changeable. The child is clingy, weepy, and whiny. Young boys will feel sorry for themselves.

Worse from: Rich foods, pork, fatty foods, night, stuffy rooms, getting cold or wet, morning upon awakening, and twilight. **Better from:** Fresh air, movement, and crying.

Dosage: Give 2 pellets every 15 minutes, for four doses, then hourly until improvement. If there has been no improvement after six doses, choose a new remedy. As soon as there is improvement, repeat the remedy only if there is a return of any symptoms.

Supportive Measures:

Ginger or fennel tea can soothe the stomach. Keep the child well hydrated, even with only a few sips of liquid at a time. Do not let the child overeat, or eat fried, spicy, heavy, or rich foods. Do not force a child to eat if they are not hungry. Offer nutritious and light snacks. Soups or pureed vegetables are particularly good when the child is sick or recovering. Some stomachaches come from eating too fast. Encourage your child to eat slowly, and chew food thoroughly. Make sure mealtimes are as stress-free as possible. The child may be able to pass gas more easily by lying on their back and bringing their knees to their chest. Sometimes a heating pad or a hot-water bottle makes a stomachache feel better. Do not use a hot-water bottle if the stomach is sensitive to pressure.

Call your healthcare practitioner if:

- Your child has no appetite for more than three days.
- The child develops a fever over 101 degrees, or your infant under three months old develops any fever.
- Your child is getting dehydrated from vomiting or severe diarrhea.

Call your healthcare practitioner if (cont):

- Your child is losing weight.
- There is severe pain that does not respond to remedies after two hours.
- Your child has been hit in the stomach and has a decreased appetite and severe pain that does not respond to a remedy.
- There is pain around the navel that moves to the extreme bottom-right side of the pelvic area, with or without vomiting. These are signs of appendicitis. *Go to an emergency room immediately.*

TEENAGE DISCOMFORTS

Being a teenager is an exciting, adventuresome, chaotic, and stressful time. Aristotle stated, "The young are permanently in a state resembling intoxication." The teen is on a hormonal roller coaster. They can be calm and sweet one week/day/hour/moment, and down in the dumps the next, easily agitated, impulsive, and on edge.

Each teen is different, and has different needs. This is true even in the same family. The name of the game is patience, and support for who the teen really is. It is good to remember that your teenager's job is to find their own identity as they move from the safe boundaries of home to the big, wide, complicated world outside. They are really trying to figure out how to negotiate their surroundings. Above all else, they need lots of acceptance, understanding, leisure time with their friends, enough sleep, and a good diet. Boundaries are needed to gently temper the spirit, but flexibility from time to time will go far in avoiding unhealthy rebellion. The best advice I ever received for dealing with the teen years was, "Pick your battles."

A high school counselor once told me a story about an underachieving student. He asked the student, "What would you like to be when you are an adult?" The reply was, "I want to be a snowboarder, dude." At this point, most adults would roll their eyes and proceed to tell the teen that this is unrealistic, not financially viable, etc., etc. At this particular high school, however, the teens learn quite quickly that whatever comes out of their mouth will be taken seriously. The counselor informed the student that a world-class snowboarder rides the back bowls of ski areas in the wild, so he would have to make a serious study of geology.

It happened that this high school was in a town with a university that allowed high school students to take certain classes. The counselor helped the student sign up for a geology class, and informed him that physical fitness is also required to be a top athlete. The student was enrolled in a local gym that was working with the high school to help teens be fit. This allowed the student to work out before or after school. This young man went on to be a photographer for Warren Miller Films, which films extreme snowboarding and skiing. He fulfilled his dreams. By receiving guidance without judgment, this teen became a success. It is a real gift to your teen to help them come into themselves, without judgment about who you think they should be—and to help them get the education and/or training needed to become a successful, fulfilled, and happy adult.

A Quick Overview of the Teen Brain

The teen's awkwardness, both mental and physical, can be most annoying. The brain from ages twelve to twenty-five years of age is in a constant, intense state of rewiring and upgrading, so that transmissions can speed up to accommodate more conscious, sophisticated, and complicated ways of thinking. The brain is constantly redefining itself, so to speak. This is why teens can seem so spaced out and aloof at times. All it takes is some added stress, lack of sleep, or a social or emotional challenge to make the brain misfire, creating inconsistent, uncharacteristic, and sometimes foolish behavior.

Research shows that teens highly value rewards, giving little thought or attention to consequences. Cultural anthropologists have concluded that adolescents worldwide strongly desire thrills and uniqueness. And they are sometimes willing to take appalling risks to get them. Successful adaptation and flexibility is the name of the game for teens transitioning into the world they will face as adults. Some studies indicate that the teen brain reacts to peer rejection just as strongly as if there were a threat to their physical existence. This is why they can exhibit extreme reactions to social ups and downs.

Studies show that teens perform optimally when they get at least nine and a quarter hours of sleep each night. It makes sense, with all of the brain restructuring and hormones releasing, that teens need extra sleep. In one study, a high school's bell times were postponed to begin at 9 AM. As a result, the teachers stated that their students were more alert, less moody, and better prepared to learn. Test scores improved, and there were fewer visits to the nurse's office. If your teen is not getting enough sleep during the week, allow them to catch up on the weekend. This may not be enough for some teens, but it can go a long way toward reducing their stress.

Some of the teen's acute emotional and physiological woes can be addressed by choosing a well-indicated remedy. Any time the symptoms are not resolving, please seek the services of a professional homeopath. Sometimes professional counseling may be in order as well. Refer to the "Moodiness" section below (page 99), or the "Emotional Trauma and Fears" section (page 257).

Acne

If your teen has acne, it is best addressed by your homeopath. Acne is a developmental issue that will need a constitutional analysis. The body, fueled by hormonal releases, is eliminating larger amounts of substances through the skin. The fluid being excreted is called sebum, which can clog oil glands just beneath the skin. Then the sebum cannot flow, so the glands swell, become inflamed, form a pimple, and eventually rupture. The more areas rupture, the more the body is displaying the need to detoxify. The skin is our biggest organ of elimination. It is important that the eruptions are not simply suppressed by prescription skin creams, which could lead to future health issues.

Supportive Measures:

Make sure your teen is staying hydrated. Water will help keep toxins flushed out. Eliminate fatty, refined, and junk foods, and foods with chemicals and artificial dyes. Sugar and white flour should be avoided. Use natural soaps when cleansing.

Cellphones

There are still confusion and conflicting studies about the use of cellphones. The research does indicate that a child's brain from ages five to twenty receives more cellphone radiation than an adult because of their thinner skulls and smaller brains. Studies also show a decrease in sperm count for up to four hours after the use of a cellphone. Other studies following those who have used a cellphone for ten years reveal that the users are at a higher risk of developing tumors on a nerve connecting the ear to the brain.

These data alone raise enough red flags to warrant your concern as a parent. Please do some research, and share it with your teen so that they can be informed. The best possible scenario is to hold off as long as possible before your teen has a cellphone, and provide a landline for them to use when at home. It is best to have the cellphone (or any other device) as far away from the brain as possible. Young children should not talk or play games on a cellphone.

Eyestrain and Tired or Overworked Eyes

These conditions are brought on by squinting, which can be caused by the teen not being able to see clearly—in which case they should be taken to an optometrist. If your teen has been overstudying, this can cause not only squinting but a weakness of the eyes as well.

This condition will respond to **Zincum Metal**. The eyes are sore and watery, with burning tears. They can feel gritty, as if there is sand in them, inflammation and redness of the conjunctiva and especially in the corners. There is itching and soreness of the lids (which may twitch), rolling of the eyes, and a feeling of pressure in the eye socket.

Worse from: Exhaustion, mental effort, work, talking, heat, noise, too much time staring at a computer or TV, and between 5–7 PM. **Better from:** Eating, fresh air, rest, gentle rubbing, scratching, and light pressure from an eye pillow made with lavender. Dosage: Give 2 pellets on an as-needed basis.

Supportive Measures:

Supportive measures: Have your teen take a break at least once an hour, for about ten minutes of not looking at any screen.

Headaches

A typical acute headache is caused by tension from stress. These stresses may be caused by: eyestrain, overstudying, hormonal imbalances, poor diet, or emotional upset. The symptoms may include a sensation of constriction, soreness, burning, and many types of pain in the head, neck, or scalp. The pain may be localized, or affect the entire head. Sometimes the pain becomes so intense that they may become nauseated and end up vomiting. Migraine, cluster headaches, and persistent headaches are of a chronic nature and need to be addressed by your healthcare practitioner. Headaches in your female teen can suggest hormone imbalances.

Remedies for headaches caused by:

Anger: **Bryonia, Chamomilla, Ignatia, Lycopodium, Natrum Mur**, or **Staphysagria**

Anxiety: **Argentum Nit**

Artificial light (under which they sit all day in school): **Sepia**

Dehydration: **Cinchona**

Emotional upset: **Chamomilla, Gelsemium, Ignatia, Pulsatilla,** or **Staphysagria**. It may also be helpful to look at the "Emotional Trauma and Fears" section (page 257).

Excessive excitement: **Coffea**

Exhaustion from overactivity: **Arsenicum, Cinchona, Gelsemium, Nitric Acid, Sepia,** or **Zincum Metal**

Menses: **Sepia**

Missing a meal: **Lycopodium** or **Silicea**

Overeating (rich food): **Nux Vomica**

Overeating (fatty food): **Carbo Veg, Pulsatilla,** or **Sepia**

Overstudying: **Calc Phos, Ruta Grav,** or **Silicea**

Reading too much: **Natrum Mur,** or **Ruta Grav**

Sugar (overindulgence): **Argentum Nit**

The following are the most commonly indicated headache remedies:

Argentum Nit: For headache with onset from anticipation, apprehension, fear, fright, mental strain, too much sugar, stomach upsets, or worries. Feels like head is being squeezed in a vise. Head feels enlarged. Aching or boring pain in forehead, or on one side. Dullness and brain fatigue, with feeling of nervousness. Alleviated by pressure; they may squeeze head with hands. They feel dizzy and chilly, with possible trembling. Scalp may itch or have crawling sensations. Belching, sometimes vomiting. Craving for sweets. They are impulsive, obsessive, and want to do things in a hurry. They have much anticipation, apprehension, and can have fears of crowds, failure, or heights.

Worse from: Waking up, mental exertion, warm rooms, heat, anxiety, and dancing. **Better from:** Calm environments, cool compresses, light pressure, closing the eyes, and fresh air.

Arsenicum: For headache with onset from too much activity, burnout, poor diet, fright, or grief. Burning, throbbing pains with restlessness. Teen feels exhausted and weak, but restless; the head may be in constant motion. They are chilly and want to keep wrapped up, but want coolness on the head. The scalp is sensitive and may be itchy. May have pain over the left eye. They are irritable and anxious about their health, and can be hard to please.

Worse from: Evening, cold damp, on waking, right side, light, and after midnight. **Better from:** Keeping warmly wrapped up, lying down, and cool applications to the head.

Bryonia: Onset from first motion of the day, constipation, stress, anger, fright, or excess coffee intake. Bursting, tearing, and splitting headache with extremely tender scalp. Headache in forehead or on side. Can have pain in or over left eye and/or frontal sinuses. Headache can move to base of skull. May have constipation. Very thirsty for cold water, with dry mouth. May be sweaty. Extremely grumpy and irritable, and may be worried about schoolwork or job even though they are in pain. They do not want to move.

Worse from: Any motion or exertion, touch, bending over, opening or moving eyes, rooms that are too warm, early morning, light, anger, and before menses. **Better from:** Pressure, being left alone and completely still, low lights or dark, lying on the painful side, cool open air, rest, quiet, closing the eyes, and cold applications.

Calc Phos: Onset from overstudying, poor diet, disappointed or rejected love, or bad news. Pain and burning near the sutures of the skull. Pain at base of skull, which may go down the spine. Cold and soreness on top of head. Sensation of brain being pressed against the skull. May have icy sensation at nape of neck, and burning at roots of hair. Hard to hold head up; head may wobble. The teen may have diarrhea, and usually abdominal gas. They may be having difficulty with the intellectual challenges of some classes. They succumb easily to mental strain, which produces the headache.

Worse from: Overstudying, changes in weather, thinking about the symptoms, motion, lifting, ascending, and mental exertion. **Better from:** Cool bathing, lying down, rest, and warm, dry air.

Carbo Veg: Onset from eating too much fatty food, or if your teen has not fully recovered from a previous deep illness, e.g., a bad flu. Dull, compressed, and heavy pain in the back of the head. They are weak with cold extremities, but the head feels hot, with cold sweat on the forehead. They are sluggish, indifferent, and irritable, usually with much gastric discomfort and bloating.

Worse from: Fatty and rich foods, lying down, warmth, warm rooms, and any pressure on the head. **Better from:** Fresh air, being fanned, sitting quietly, and leaning back.

Chamomilla: Onset from emotional upsets, especially from bad temper. Throbbing pains on either side of the head. Desire to bend head backwards. Sweaty forehead and scalp during sleep. One cheek is usually red (or has a red patch) and hot, and the other cheek is pale. This symptom may be subtle, or quite obvious. They want to drink often. May have shivering, with sensation of hair standing on end. Very sensitive to pain, and susceptible to fury, screaming, and crying. They can be uncivil, and don't want to be looked at or have others near them. These headaches are caused by being angry for long periods, or experiencing rage.

Worse from: Cold open air, wind, touch, night (especially around 9 PM), and anger. They dread wind. **Better from:** Rocking, cold applications, mild weather, and being engaged so they are not dwelling on the pain. And patience!

Cinchona (also known as **China Officinalis**): Onset from loss of fluids, or anger. Intense throbbing and bursting pain that makes the brain feel bruised. Pain worse in temple area. Head feels heavy, and scalp is sensitive. These headaches may be caused by dehydration from low fluid intake, overexposure to heat, or after a bout of diarrhea or vomiting. These teens are very thirsty. They are pale and can have dark circles under their eyes. They are weak, irritable, oversensitive and nervous, and may have problems sleeping.

Worse from: Drafts, noise, jarring, being in the sun, nighttime, and after eating. **Better from:** Much quiet rest, firm pressure, rubbing, warmth, and moving head gently up and down. Encourage your teen to stay hydrated!

Coffea: Onset from overexcitement, or sudden intense emotions, especially joy. Also from disappointed or rejected love, fear, fright, fatigue, or excessive laughing. Throbbing pain, as if a nail is being driven into the head. Feels like the brain is shattered, crushed, or torn to pieces. Tension is felt over the entire head, with tight pain; the head feels too small. Temples throb, and eyes may burn. This teen is irritable and excited, and the senses are acute. Even though they may be exhausted, they cannot sleep. The nerves are overexcited, characterized by hyperactivity of the mind and body, and the pain is intolerable. The slightest movement may seem enormous.

Worse from: Noise, excessive emotion, mental exertion, touch, overeating, nighttime, and strong odors. **Better from:** Warmth, lying down, cold drinks, calm, and quiet.

Gelsemium: Onset from anger, bad news, depression, fear, fright, performance anxiety, traumatic shock, unpleasant surprises, or overexcitement. Pain begins in the neck and moves to the base of skull. It can extend over the head into the forehead and settle over the eyes. It can also become a band of pain around the head. Dull, heavy pain at the forehead and/or the back of the head, which can develop into a bursting sensation that shoots out and radiates. The brain feels bruised. Even though they are anxious and afraid, these teens become slow, weak, confused, exhausted, and sometimes trembly. They become dull, heavy, and sluggish, with a faint or lightheaded feeling. They have a hot face, with chills, and may get diarrhea. It is helpful to have them bend forward while sitting, or lie with their head slightly elevated. They need fresh air.

Worse from: Overexcitement, strong emotions, spring, shock, damp weather, cold, sun, and around 10 AM. **Better from:** Sweating, urinating, quiet surroundings, being left alone, fresh air, head being wrapped, and continued gentle motion, e.g., rocking.

Ignatia: Onset can be after intense anger, worry, disappointed or rejected love, emotional trauma, grief, fright, or abuse of coffee. Pains are intense, stabbing, and pressing, often in a small area, and usually on the right side. It feels as if a nail is piercing through the temple or behind the eye. The teen wants to lean the head forward, may feel chilly and faint, and usually sighs a lot. They can be moody, dramatic, and oversensitive to pain, and may become hysterical.

Worse from: Smelling tobacco, smoking, coffee, alcohol, touch, and consolation. **Better from:** Being left alone, eating, pressure, deep breathing, and warmth (but not intense heat).

Lycopodium: Onset from stress, anxiety, dehydration, anger, or pressure at school. Intense pressing pains in temples, as if temples are being screwed together, or a vise is squeezing them. Or they have pain that starts in the forehead behind the right eye and then may or may not move to the left eye; or pain at the base of the skull that is worse when hot. They may feel faint or lightheaded, and shake their head for no reason. They usually have much gas and bloating, and cold hands and feet. This teen has a lot of indecision. They awake irritable and angry, and easily lose self-esteem and self-confidence. They can act quite offensively to everyone around them when sick.

Worse from: Menses, not eating regularly, lying down, stooping, wet weather, severe colds, from 4–8 AM or around 4 PM; cabbage, beans, pastry, milk, and right side. **Better from:** Warm food and drinks, not too many covers; however, they do like cool applications, motion, and burping.

Natrum Mur: Onset from anger, disappointed or rejected love, fright, emotional trauma, grief, or overuse of eyes. Bursting, throbbing, blinding, and heavy headaches. Feels like hundreds of hammers are pounding on the brain, or like a band is around the head. Headaches are often over the eyes, in the forehead, or one-sided, and mostly on the right side. They are pale, with a faint feeling or lightheadedness. May have numbness, jerking, and/or visual disturbances. May have pain in frontal sinuses from inflammation. Dry mouth with thirst. If pain is intense, they may be nauseous and vomit. This remedy is for teens that are sad, nervous, have fears of being hurt or rejected, and are easily discouraged. They do not want sympathy, and have a hard time crying or expressing any strong emotion in front of others.

Worse from: Just before or after menses, puberty, on awakening, and all day until sunset; reading, especially fine print, studying for long periods, sun, bright lights, violent emotions, especially anger, wearing a hat, and around 10 AM. **Better from:** Sleep, pressure on eyes, lying with head propped up, being still, muted light or darkness, fresh air, taking breaks from reading (especially fine print), being left alone, and after perspiration.

Nitric Acid: Onset from lack of sleep, poor sleep, exhaustion, or shock. Crushing pains in head, with a sensation of a band around the head, or a full feeling. Pains come and go quickly, but recur at regular intervals, e.g., a headache that keeps coming back in the evening or at night. Skull feels sore, and scalp is sensitive. The bones in the face may be sensitive to the touch, and the eyes may feel sore. These teens are very sensitive to noise. They are very irritable, headstrong, pessimistic, sad, and can become despondent. They can get so angry that they tremble, and may use vulgar or profane language. They are unmoved by apologies and cannot forgive. They have a lot of self-pity.

Worse from: Pressure from hats, touch, evening and night, mental exertion, loss of sleep, jarring, noise, eating, changes in weather, and both cold air and hot weather. **Better from:** Gliding motions, mild weather, steady pressure, and getting adequate amounts of sleep (nine and a quarter hours a night for a teen).

Nux Vomica: Onset from too much mental exertion, anger, loss of sleep, digestive upset, overindulgence in rich food, drugs or alcohol, tension, or stress. Pain at base of the skull, or pressing pain and heaviness in forehead above the eyes, with a desire to press the head against something. Splitting headache. Brain feels bruised, and can feel as if a nail is being driven into the top of the head. May also feel like a band is around the head. Scalp is sensitive. The teen may be dizzy, as if from turning in a circle, with faint feeling or lightheadedness, and chilly, with nausea and possible vomiting. Many times they are constipated. The head may feel expanded. This teen may be driving too hard. They can be quite critical, angry, oversensitive to just about everything, and impatient. They may press their head into their hands, or lean their head into something.

Worse from: Cold, touch, anger, motion, noise, odors, sunlight, and morning. **Better from:** Warmth, staying wrapped up, napping, firm pressure, hot drinks, moist air, and lying or sitting. They may want their head wrapped.

Pulsatilla: Onset from abandonment, emotional trauma, grief, fright, overeating rich food, or overwork. One-sided headaches are mostly on the left; however, this is a headache where the pain moves around to different parts of the head. The pain is stabbing, piercing, and throbbing, with bursting and scalding sensations. The teen has watery eyes and tears on the side with the most pain. Looking up can make them feel dizzy. Top of the head feels heavy with pressure. Faint feeling, or lightheadedness. Usually they have no thirst, but may have a sweaty scalp. These teens are whiny and clingy, and feel sorry for themselves.

Worse from: Warm stuffy rooms, during menses, twilight and evening, sunlight, lying down, dehydration, excessive joy, and rich food. **Better from:** Intake of liquids, walking in open air or any motion, cool, fresh air, cool applications, pressure, gentle massage, and erect posture.

Ruta Grav: Onset from overexertion of eyes. Achy pains, as if a nail is being driven into the head. Needle-like, weary pains while reading, especially fine print. Eyes are red and feel hot. It feels as if there is a weight on their forehead. May be sensation of pressure, especially over one eyebrow. May have spasms in lower eyelid, with tears. This teen has intense feelings of weakness and despair when sick.

Worse from: Cold, stooping, going up and down steps, during menses, and pressure. **Better from:** Lying on the back, warmth, gentle massage of eyes, and movement without exertion.

Sepia: Onset from overeating rich food, during menses, from artificial light, or missing meals. Intense, stinging pain that shoots into the left eye. Heaviness and coldness on top of the head. There may be pain at base of the skull that alternates from side to side. Headaches come in shocks, and teen screams with pain. Teen is always tired, and may complain of backaches. Headache with nausea, empty feeling in stomach and sometimes vomiting. They are very sensitive, angry, sulky, irritable, and indifferent, especially to family members. Teen girls may worry and cry about their symptoms or illnesses.

Worse from: Before and during menses, lying on the painful side, mental exertion, jarring, shopping in artificial light, indoors, after cutting the hair, and cold air. **Better from:** Meals, rest, open air, gentle exercise, sitting with legs crossed, pressure, warm applications (but they do like cold drinks), and keeping busy, which keeps their mind from dwelling on their symptoms.

Silicea (also known as **Silica Terra**): Onset from dehydration, eyestrain, drafts of cold air, or overexcitement. Needle-like, tearing pains from nape of the neck to base of the skull over the top of the head and into the eye. It feels like blood is rushing into the head. Faint feeling or lightheadedness. Sweats easily. Lack of stamina. This teen is timid, weak, nervous, picky, and lacking in self-confidence, but very stubborn.

Worse from: Dehydration, having a head cold, motion, cold, closing the eyes, and drafts. **Better from:** Pressure, warmth, and wearing a hat when cold outside.

Staphysagria: Onset from anger, or repressed anger from being insulted, offended, humiliated, and sexually abused—for which it is recommended that professional help be sought for your teen. Compressed, tearing pains in forehead. Forehead feels as if there is a heavy round ball on it. Brain feels squeezed, numb, and dense, which makes it hard for them to think. Base of the skull feels hollow. This teen is very sensitive about what others say about them. They feel deep guilt, humiliation, and shame. Scolding or punishment affects them deeply. They can be gloomy, sad, nervous, and irritable.

Worse from: Thinking, walking, riding, loss of fluids, night, sexual excess, new moon, before full moon, and harsh reprimands. **Better from:** Leaning head against something, yawning, after breakfast, warmth, rest at night, being treated with patience, and very gentle pressure with a light firmness.

Zincum Metal: Onset from fright, grief, anger, and excessive study or overwork. Nervous headache. Pain is bursting, tearing, and pressing, in the forehead, at the base of the skull, or in the temples. The pain can be one-sided or on both sides. They may roll their head from side to side and bore it into the pillow. Pain may extend to the eyes and weaken their vision. The teen is mentally exhausted, very sensitive to noise, easily startled or excited, lethargic and forgetful, and weeps when angry. They may cry out in pain.

Worse from: Exhaustion, mental effort, work, talking, noise, touch during menstrual period, between 5–7 PM, and drinking wine. **Better from:** Eating, fresh air, rest, rubbing, scratching, hard pressure, and motion.

Dosage: Give 2 pellets every 15 minutes for four doses; then hourly until improvement. If there has been no improvement after seven doses, choose a new remedy. As soon as there is improvement, repeat the remedy only if there is a return of any symptoms.

Supportive Measures:

Encouraging your teen to let out whatever may be bothering them. A safe environment without judgment is critical for this. Again, too many demands on their plate, either physical or emotional, will give way to tension and stress,

Supportive Measures (cont):)

thus producing headaches. Teens are particularly sensitive to sensory and hormonal overload. Patience, encouraging them to get in touch with what works for them, and support for coming into who they are will go a long way toward keeping their tension and stress manageable.

Make sure your teen is getting enough sleep (nine and one quarter hours of sleep a night). Warm or cold applications can feel good and ease the pain. Slow, deep breathing helps with any type of pain. Rest in a quiet, dark area. Soothing music can be relaxing and take the mind off of the pain. A hot bath with one cup of Epsom salts can relax and detoxify the body. If it feels good to them, you can gently massage the scalp, neck, and shoulders.

Call your healthcare practitioner if:

- Your teen develops a high fever and intense headache.
- Headaches recur, or occur with visual disturbances or dizziness.
- Headaches are painful and persistent, and will not resolve.
- Headaches are in the temple area with swollen blood vessels, visual disturbances, blind spots, and jaw pain, especially when chewing.
- Headaches are accompanied by red face, shortness of breath, nosebleeds, lightheadedness, nausea with indigestion, or if easily exhausted. These are all signs of high blood pressure. This would be unusual for a teen, but can occur. This may also apply to an adult. Do not wait—seek immediate help.

Call your healthcare practitioner if (cont.):

- Dizziness with mental confusion, slurred speech, staggering gait, falling, numbness or weakness of a limb or one side of the whole body; feeling faint, vision disturbance, inability to communicate clearly, or jerky movements. Call 911 immediately. These may be signs of a stroke. This is most unlikely in a teen, but it's good to know these signs.

Menstrual Cramping

This is a painful condition known as dysmenorrhea. It produces muscular contractions of the uterus, and fluctuating hormonal levels. Sometimes there is only pain on the first day, but the pain can occur before, during, or at the end of the period. The pains can be mild or intense, shooting, radiating to other parts of the body, or just on one side. Emotional symptoms are important in analyzing what will work best for your daughter.

Most young women have minimal discomfort before and during their period. They may have discomfort in their back, or even headaches, in addition to cramping. They may also experience the blues, irritability, or an overwhelmed feeling. If your daughter is having severe cramping month after month, she will need to see a homeopath who can prescribe a constitutional remedy for her. This would be for a chronic condition as opposed to acute.

It is important to make your daughter feel comfortable about the changes happening in her body, emphasizing that they are healthy and normal. It is important to guide your daughter about taking good care of herself and keeping the belly warm, since most cramps are relieved by warmth. Extra rest and downtime can be very helpful for most young women. However, there are some situations where keeping busy to keep their mind off their discomforts is more helpful. Again, each teen is different.

When my daughter was seventeen years old, we had a rite-of-passage ceremony for her and four of her friends. My daughter asked a question of the five mothers there: "Looking back at your life, is there anything you would have done differently?" Every mother stated, in varying ways, that she wished she had taken better care of herself and made more downtime for herself. Most modern mothers have not only a full-time career but the responsibility of keeping a home together, making good nutritious food available, taking care of anyone who is sick, and overseeing that everyone in the family has their daily life on track at school, work, etc. Where is there time for mom? It is very important that your daughter learn to honor and take care of herself throughout life. If mothers and daughters put this into practice as much as possible, there will be better health and less stress.

What to observe:

Does the pain start before the period, on the first day, or at other times? Does the pain get worse or better once the flow has started? What are the qualities of the pain? Is it localized, or does it radiate to other areas of the body? Are there other symptoms, such as headache, nausea, diarrhea, constipation, an emotional upset at school, etc.? What is your daughter's mood?

The following are the most commonly indicated remedies for menstrual cramping where pains are acute but occasional:

Apis: Stinging pain in the ovarian region. Tenderness and soreness in the right abdominal area. Violent bearing-down pains with very little dark, slimy blood. Drowsiness. Many times they retain water. They may have a headache, and the brain feels very tired. May have stinging, burning pains in breasts. If in pain, they cry out with shrill, piercing screams. They are irritable, nervous, restless, oversensitive, and do not want to be disturbed; however, they do not want to be left alone. They are awkward, and usually drop things a lot. Teenage girls at puberty can become hysterical.

Worse from: Before the period, on the right side, tight clothing, heat in any form, touch, late afternoon, lying down, sleeping, and pressure. **Better from:** Cold applications, cool air, cool bathing, sitting up, cool drinks, and being uncovered.

Belladonna: Menses may come early, with a profuse flow of bright-red blood that feels hot. Bearing-down, throbbing, and cutting pain. The uterus feels full, as if it may fall out. Pains come and go suddenly. The teen may have a throbbing headache and flushed face. May crave lemonade, and may have extreme thirst for cold water, or no thirst at all. They can become delirious from the pain, furious with a desire to escape, and want to hit or bite something. All senses become acute, and moods are changeable.

Worse from: Right side in the ovarian area, lying down, getting overheated or chilled, touch, noise, jarring, light, 3 PM, 11 PM, and after midnight. **Better from:** Rest, light covering, sitting semi-erect, gentle walking, pressure, bending backwards, low lights, quiet, and morning.

Calc Phos: These teens are usually slow to mature, thin, and lack stamina. They get needle-like pains that give them a violent backache. They can also have an aching in the uterus, with cutting pains through to the sacrum (tailbone). They may moan from the pain. A heavy flow will easily weaken them. Often they have a burning vaginal discharge that looks like the white of an egg. They are irritable and hard to please. It is hard for them to maintain a sustained mental effort. It is very important that this teen be kept warm before and during her period.

Note: Since this teen can become very weakened by a heavy flow, use **Cinchona** if necessary (see below).

Worse from: Cold, damp, motion, exertion, ascending, puberty, and thinking of symptoms. **Better from:** Staying warm and dry, lying down, and resting.

Chamomilla: This teen can become quarrelsome and obstinate before the flow starts. These pains are brought on after an intense bout of anger or other strong emotions. There are intense, bearing-down pains when the flow begins. Pains in the uterus extend down into the thighs and are also felt in the back. The abdomen is tender. The flow is heavy, with dark-red clotted blood and an occasional gushing of bright-red blood. The pain is intolerable from the first onset, and they demand instant relief. They can restlessly roll around, moaning. They may have one red cheek and one pale cheek, but this can be subtle. They are chilly, but get overheated easily. Their abdomen is very tender. They are angry, irritable, oversensitive, especially to pain, and easily offended. They ask for something, get it, and then don't want it. They want mom, then send her away, then call her back. They have dramatic overreactions, with hypersensitivity.

Worse from: Cold open air and wind, touch, coffee, nighttime, especially around 9 PM, anger or strong emotions, noise, and heat. **Better from:** Gentle rocking, cold drinks, mild weather, and *being treated with patience.*

Cinchona (also known as **China Officinalis**): This remedy can be used to restore strength after a prolonged or heavy flow that has left the teen feeling weak and exhausted. Even after the flow and pain have stopped, the teen just can't seem to get her energy and vitality back. This remedy can be given morning and night for up to three days. If there has been no improvement after three days, consult your healthcare practitioner.

Cocculus: Sharp, pressing pains in the uterus, with dizziness and profound weakness. Period may start early in their cycle. Heavy flows, with dark blood. This teen can become so weak that she can hardly stand or talk very loudly. Make sure she is getting enough sleep. She usually has no appetite, and motion or the smell of food can make her feel nauseous. She feels chilly, and may vomit. May have hollow or empty feelings anywhere in the body, especially in the head, which may also feel heavy. Legs may tremble when walking. Very sensitive to noise, touch, anger, fear, grief, or other strong emotions. Easily startled.

Worse from: Lack of sleep, jarring, riding in a car, cold, open air, mental or physical exertion, and bending over or stooping. **Better from:** No motion, sitting or lying on side, warmth, and nine and a quarter hours of sleep a night.

Colocynthis: Pains are worse before the flow starts. Pain boring into and bearing-down in the ovarian area, and coming in waves. Usually a heavy flow. This teen wants to be doubled up and press a pillow or something hard into the pelvic area; she may lean over a chair. Pain may be so intense that she vomits. Can be brought on by intense anger. She is restless, easily offended, extremely irritable, irritated by the pains, and indignant. Her feelings are easily hurt. She will become angered as you ask questions to figure out which remedy she needs.

Note: This teen can tend to be sedentary, so regular exercise (especially doing squats) between periods will help lessen the flow and achieve better pelvic tone.

Worse from: Anger, any incident that has left her feeling indignant, drafts, getting chilled, evening, nighttime, eating, and drinking. **Better from:** The flow beginning, pressure, heat, lying doubled up or on the painful side, rest, gentle motion, a bowel movement, and passing gas.

Mag Phos: For sharp, shooting pains that come on before the flow starts, and shift around. Intense pain in ovarian area. Flow usually, but not always, begins early in the cycle. Flow is dark and stringy, and can be heavy at night. Labia may be swollen and very tender. Usually worse on the right side. The teen is thirsty for very cold drinks, but feels chilly. She is usually drowsy, dull, depressed, forgetful, and can't think clearly, study, or do mental work. It is important that this teen rest during her period.

Note: This remedy works best if dissolved in hot (not boiling) water. Allow a few pellets to dissolve in hot water. Sip every few minutes until the cramping is relieved.

Worse from: Lying on right side, motion, cold, touch, and night. **Better from:** Once flow begins—pressure, bending double, nurturing, rest, hot water bottles, and hot baths.

Nux Vomica: For spasms, bearing-down or twisting pains in the uterus that radiate into the sacrum (tailbone). These pains can sometimes be confused with a constant urge to have a bowel movement. When these teens do have a bowel movement, it feels like there is more to come, but it doesn't happen. They are usually constipated, and may be nauseous. Cramps may be felt in other parts of the body as well. Their periods can be irregular, with a flow that may be profuse or just a small amount of black blood. Their period can come too early and/or last too long. They may have urinary frequency, and may feel weak. They often desire spicy foods and stimulants, and feel chilly. They are irritable, hypersensitive, tense, critical, impatient, and very driven.

Worse from: Getting wet, cold, early morning, pressure of clothes at waist, noise, odors, touch, and overindulgence in rich food. **Better from:** Heat, loose clothes at the waist, and rest.

Pulsatilla: The pains are of a bearing-down nature and can extend into the back. The teen may experience these pains without the flow. The flow is usually light, starting and stopping. There is thick, clotted, dark blood. The flow can be very changeable and irregular. It may start late if she got her feet wet, or from emotional stress. Her symptoms are erratic, inconsistent, and changeable. She can become exhausted quite easily. She is tearful, weepy, needy, sensitive, and craves sympathy.

Worse from: Start of flow, cold and damp weather, autumn, cold food or drinks, being uncovered, drafts, lying still, on first movement after resting, and twilight into night. **Better from:** Warm drinks and food, constant gentle movement, stretching, warmth, changing positions, and sympathy.

Dosage: Give 2 pellets every 15 minutes, for four doses; then hourly until improvement. If there has been no improvement after eight doses, choose a new remedy. As soon as there is improvement, repeat the remedy only if there is a return of any symptoms.

Supportive Measures:

It is of utmost importance that your teen's belly is kept warm, and that intense physical exertion is kept to a minimum, especially in the first days of her period. If it feels good to her, place a hot water bottle, a warmed herbal pack, or a heating pad in the pelvic area. The following yoga poses help with cramps: child's pose, cat stretch, and a half-shoulder stand that takes pressure off of the uterus. Consult a yoga teacher to make sure your daughter is doing these poses correctly.

Patience is key during outbursts of emotions, but remember that abuse is not to be tolerated. Things to be avoided if your teen has severe cramps are alcohol, coffee, the herb ginseng (a male herb found in various teas and energy drinks that will actually increase cramping), hot spices, excess sugar, and excess dairy. Some cramping can be caused by a deficiency of good fatty acids. Both females and males need a certain amount of essential omega 3 and 6 fatty acids. Because of pressure to be skinny, your daughter may avoid fats entirely. But if she is deficient in these essential fats, her body cannot metabolize hormones efficiently, which can cause cramping.

It is also important to push fluids if there is a heavy flow. Be sure to give your daughter guidance about correct usage and recommended intervals for changing a tampon, to avoid toxic shock syndrome. Toxic shock syndrome is a bacterial infection that can be caused by leaving a tampon inserted for too long. Make sure your daughter follows the directions on the tampon box. (See below for symptoms.)

Call your healthcare practitioner if:

- Your teen has not started menstruating by age fifteen.
- Your teen's period suddenly stops for more than ninety days (and she is not pregnant).
- Your teen's periods become very irregular after she has had regular, monthly cycles.
- Your teen's period occurs more often than every twenty-one days, or less often than every thirty-five days.
- Your teen bleeds for more than seven days.
- Your teen is bleeding more heavily than usual, or using more than one pad or tampon every hour or two.
- Your teen is bleeding between periods.
- Your teen is having unusual severe pain during her period.
- You suspect that your daughter has toxic shock syndrome, particularly during menstruation and tampon use. The symptoms include: diarrhea, headache, high fever with or without chills, low blood pressure, muscle aches, nausea, vomiting, seizures, redness of eyes, mouth or throat, or a widespread red rash like a sunburn. Toxic shock syndrome is potentially fatal. *Go to the emergency room immediately.*

Mononucleosis

Homeopathy can help to reduce the discomfort, lessen complications, and shorten the duration of mononucleosis. Supportive measures sooner rather than later will help the teen to recover more quickly and completely. Even though mononucleosis is an acute condition, there is a deeper root cause that needs to be addressed. So in addition to giving the appropriate remedy, you will need to partner with your healthcare practitioner to give your teen support on a deeper level.

If your teen has contracted mononucleosis, they need help boosting their immune system. This may include diet, supplements, and lifestyle changes. As stated above, this is a time when their body is undergoing many changes. If your teen is not allowed all the time it takes to recover, they could seriously compromise their immune system and succumb to more serious conditions such as chronic fatigue syndrome, the Epstein-Barr virus, or an autoimmune condition.

Mononucleosis is caused by a virus that takes hold when there is stress, whether from peer pressure, scholastic pressure, or sports-performance pressure. It can also be brought on by indulging in a poor diet and lack of sleep. Mononucleosis is also known as "glandular fever" because it can affect the tonsils and the glands in the armpits, abdomen, and groin. The glands become swollen and painful. The teen may have a fever, sore throat, headaches, a swollen spleen, and sore, achy muscles. They suffer from severe fatigue and weakness, and any task wipes them out. They can also suffer from a cough, shortness of breath, chest pains, or nosebleeds. Also see the "Coughs" section (page 144) if they develop a cough. A blood test may or may not confirm the diagnosis.

The following are remedies for mononucleosis:

Apis: This remedy is particularly indicated when there are swollen glands. If they have a sore throat, the throat is constricted and inflamed, with the sensation of a splinter. The pains are stinging and burning. The right side is usually worse. The tongue, uvula and throat are swollen; the tongue is fiery-red and raw, and the mouth is dry. The throat is glassy-red or purple. There may be swelling on the outside of the throat, and the face can look puffy. The skin feels sore and sensitive, as if bruised. They want cold water to soothe the throat, but are usually not thirsty. They are very restless, sleepy, and irritable when disturbed. They may be weepy, but do not want to be touched.

Worse from: Warmth, touch, heavy blankets, pressure, swallowing solid hot or sour food, on the right side, from 3–5 PM, after sleeping, and a warm, stuffy room. **Better from:** Cool applications, cold liquids, cool air, motion, and light covering or being uncovered.

Baptisia: For when there is rapid onset with extreme exhaustion, fast deterioration, and weakness. The teen may curl up tightly on one side. They feel extremely ill. Their body feels sore and bruised, and the bed feels too hard. Their breath and discharges smell foul. They have a heavy, numb head that feels too large, and a heavy pain at the back of the head. Their eyes feel sore, with heavy eyelids. It looks as if they are drugged or drunk. The face, mouth, and tongue may be dark red or brown-red. They may have an intensely sore, red throat, mouth sores, diarrhea, or vomiting. They are very thirsty and sleepy all the time, falling asleep even while talking or answering questions. However, they can be restless. They may have nightmares, or delusions that their limbs are double or scattered in pieces, or feel as though their limbs are not connected to their body. They feel confused and dull.

Worse from: Around 6 PM, swallowing solids, open air, cold, heat with humidity, pressure, and on waking. **Better from:** Drinking liquids.

Gelsemium: In a nutshell, this remedy is for the teen who is droopy, drowsy, and dizzy. They are chilly and sensitive to cold. There is great muscular weakness, heaviness, drowsiness, fatigue, soreness, and achiness all over. The teeth may chatter, even without chills. They may have a dull headache in the back of the head, with stiffness and achiness in the neck and shoulders, and they may develop a sore throat. The limbs feel very heavy and may be cold. They might say they can't see or focus well. Often the tongue trembles when protruded. The face is hot and a dusky-red color. Their appetite is low, with very little thirst. They are weak and tired, and answer slowly. They are indifferent to surroundings, dull, droopy, emotionally delicate (or too tired to even be emotional), and want to be left alone.

Worse from: Overexcitement, strong emotions, spring, shock, damp weather, and around 10 AM. **Better from:** Sweating, urinating, quiet and low-stress surroundings, open air, reclining with the head propped up, and continued motion, e.g., rocking.

Mercurius Viv (also known as **Mercurius Sol**): The skin has a grayish look. The breath smells bad, and they may have a metallic taste in their mouth. There is excess saliva, and usually they will have drooled a slimy, clear saliva on their pillow. They may say that their bones ache; they are weary and might tremble. They are usually quite sweaty. The tongue may have a white or grey coating, and is swollen so that it shows imprints of the teeth on the sides. They are sensitive to heat and cold, and their temperature may be unstable. They are very thirsty for cold water, but it does not satisfy the thirst. The neck glands are swollen and tender. The teen is restless and nervous, constantly changing their mind.

Worse from: Night, drafts, damp weather, sweating, too much cold or heat, lying on the right side, warmth in bed, and warm drinks. **Better from:** Moderate, even temperatures, rest, lying on the stomach, and morning.

Phytolacca: The throat is dark red or bluish-red, and feels hot, burning, raw and too narrow. Much achiness at the root of the tongue and soft palate. Sensation of a lump or red-hot ball in the throat. Pain comes and goes on the right, and shoots into the ear on swallowing. Thick, choking, stringy mucus that is greyish-white or yellow causes much hawking and clearing of the throat. The teen cannot swallow anything hot. Tip of the tongue is fiery-red, and the tongue may have a yellow patch down the center. Swollen, painful glands in the neck and under the ears near jaw joints. Other joints may be painful as well. This teen usually refuses food. They can feel faint on rising, and greatly exhausted. They may moan a lot. They have very little interest in anything, and are sensitive and restless.

Worse from: Cold damp weather, weather changes, hot drinks, touch, and pressure. **Better from:** Warmth, cold drinks, rest, and lying on the stomach or left side.

Dosage: Give 2 pellets every 4 hours until there is improvement. If there has been no improvement after six doses, choose a new remedy. As soon as there is improvement, repeat the remedy only if there is a return of any symptoms.

Supportive Measures:

It is extremely important that ample time be given to rest and completely recuperate. The adolescent should not be sent back to school or put back into any stressful situation until they have recovered good stamina and endurance. This can take from three weeks to two months.

Besides affecting the glands, mono can also affect the liver, so it is important to keep the teen on a healthy, light, nutritious diet. Avoid non-homeopathic medications or alcohol, as these can compromise the liver. It is important that the parents do not give in to pressure from teachers or coaches for the child to return to school or school activities soon.

Once your teen is feeling better, you and your teen can take the opportunity to evaluate whether a lifestyle change may be needed: Where is there too much pressure on them? Do they have too much on their plate? Are they getting enough sleep? Are they making wise diet choices?

Call your healthcare practitioner if:

- Your teen is experiencing any fullness or discomfort on their left side. Sometimes the spleen can become painfully enlarged.
- Your teen develops a temperature over 103 degrees.
- Your teen has had a fever for more than three days.
- Your teen experiences swelling of the throat that is impeding their breathing. *Go to an urgent-care center or emergency room immediately.*

Moodiness

Your adolescent may experience intense moodiness from time to time. Encourage your teen to let out whatever may be bothering them. For this, a safe environment without judgment is critical. Adolescents need guidance on how to deal with different emotional states. It is important to be in a state of acceptance, and not denial. Rudeness, verbal abuse, or violence should always be addressed and not tolerated.

The following are remedies for occasional moodiness:

Chamomilla: For ill effects of a bad temper. The teen is angry, impatient, abrupt, irritable, restless, oversensitive (especially to pain), easily offended, and snappy. They moan and complain because they cannot have what they want. Otherwise, they may be adverse to talking, and being spoken to, touched, or looked at. They ask for something, get it, and then don't want it, or complain about it.

Ignatia: For anxiety after a bout of rage, grief, worry, fright, or humiliation. They are nervous, excitable, introspective, easily frustrated, weepy, and tearful. They sigh a lot, yawn, grieve quietly, do not want sympathy, and may become antisocial. This can come on after the trauma of grief, shock, a strong reprimand, or if they are homesick. They can have unpredictable reactions. They can be hysterically crying one moment, laughing the next, furious the next, distant the next, or anxious and restless the next.

Natrum Mur: For anger, disappointed or rejected love, fright, or grief. These teens are sad and/or nervous, have fears of being hurt or rejected, and get easily discouraged. They are oversensitive and irritable, even irritated by sympathy. They can have a hard time sleeping, if they are in a state of grief. This teen has a hard time crying or expressing any strong emotion in front of others.

Nux Vomica: For too much mental exertion, anger, loss of sleep, tension, or stress. This teen may be driving too hard. They can be quite impatient, critical, angry, and oversensitive to just about everything. They are hypersensitive to noise, odors, light, or touch. For them, time passes too slowly. They can overreact to the tiniest physical ailment. Daily twenty-minute power naps can be quite helpful to them.

Pulsatilla: For abandonment, grief, or overwork. These teens' moods are quite changeable, even from hour to hour. They are nervous, fidgety, sensitive, affectionate, timid, whiny, and clingy. A teen boy may not be whiny, but may feel quite sorry for himself. Teen girls may feel sorry for themselves as well. These teens can go to extreme ends of pain and pleasure. They can be easily persuaded and led by peers.

Dosage: Give 2 pellets 3 times a week, for three weeks. If there has been no improvement by then, choose a new remedy. As soon as there is improvement, repeat the remedy only if there is a return of any symptoms, 3 times a week for one week. The situation with teens can shift frequently, so you may have to review their condition and come up with a new remedy from time to time.

Call your healthcare practitioner if:

- The remedies are not holding.
- The moods are for prolonged periods of time and do not respond to the most common remedies—in this case, consult your homeopath.

Osgood-Schlatter Disease

This condition affects mostly boys between ten and fifteen years of age. The cartilage and bone in the knee becomes painfully swollen and inflamed. The pain occurs where the tendon at the top of the tibia attaches to the kneecap. The pains can shoot down into the shinbone. This condition usually only affects one knee. Because this condition can be caused by growth spurts, please refer to the section on "Growing Pains" (page 51).

If the child is playing sports, it is imperative that they completely stop these activities until there is full recovery. Not stopping could permanently damage the knee and lower leg. Homeopathic remedies can address the inflammation in a safer way than a cortisone injection, which a coach or doctor may recommend. Your child's health is more important than a few moments of glory from winning a game. It is best not to chance the pain your child may have to live with for years to come. This is a condition best treated by a homeopath and a cranial-sacral osteopath.

Pap Tests

If your daughter is scared about getting a Pap test, give her 2 pellets of **Aconitum** before the procedure. If she is anxious or jittery, possibly with diarrhea, give her 2 pellets of **Gelsemi-**

um before the procedure. If she experiences soreness afterward, give **Arnica** 200C right after the procedure, and then another dose 4 hours later. If she is experiencing cramping after the procedure, she can take **Mag Phos.** This remedy works best if dissolved in hot (not boiling) water: Put a few pellets in hot water and let them dissolve. Sip every few minutes until the cramping is relieved.

Some young women are very sensitive to Pap tests. It may seem as though your daughter is overreacting, angry, and feeling as if her body has been assaulted. If this is the case, give her 2 pellets of **Staphysagria** 3 times a day, for up to three days after the procedure.

Performance Anxiety

The following are remedies for anxiety before interviews, taking college entrance exam, driver's test, etc.:

Argentum Nit: The teen asks such questions as: What if I forget my lines/the answers/my speech? What if I faint? What if I make a mistake? What if I flunk? There is lots of worrying, such as about getting to the event on time. The heart starts beating hard and fast. They are in a hurry, talk fast, and desire sweets.

Gelsemium: They say such things as: I am really scared; I feel dizzy/weak/chilly/shaky. They become indifferent to their surroundings, and look dull and droopy. They are emotionally delicate, exhausted, and want to be left alone. They usually have sticky and clammy sweat. There is no thirst, so encourage them to drink.

Lycopodium: They say such things as: I know I am going to make a fool of myself and everyone will be laughing at me; or, I know I am going to fail. They get so anxious about the upcoming situation that they lose their self-esteem and may fear that they are going to break down. They can have indigestion, gas, and/ or diarrhea. They are irritable, but don't want to be left alone. Even though they get so anxious, they love applause and thrive on appreciation.

Dosage: Give 2 pellets every 15 minutes for four doses, before the performance or test.

Supportive Measures:

Slow, deep, rhythmical breaths into the belly. A cool compress to the forehead. Before the event, have the teen sit in a quiet place and visualize, over and over again, the event going just the way they would like it to be. Give them spring water with 3 drops of Bach Flower Rescue Remedy, which can be found in a health-food store with the homeopathic remedies. This can be repeated as often as necessary; have them sip it for up to two hours before the event.

Poisoning

Alcohol Poisoning

Underage and inexperienced drinkers are particularly vulnerable to alcohol poisoning. The organs affected are the liver, heart, and brain. When a teen consumes excessive amounts of alcohol in a short period, their breathing slows, and the brain and other organs are deprived of oxygen. The symptoms can include confusion, sleepiness, aggression, incoherence, irrationality, trembling, excessive laughing or crying, nausea, vomiting, a severe headache, and sometimes blacking out. The symptoms can range from mild to dangerous.

If you suspect alcohol poisoning, it is not a good idea to let them sleep it off, because the blood alcohol level can continue to rise. They usually need fresh air, and to drink lots of water to flush the toxins out of the liver and rehydrate. If they can walk, it is good for them to do so. If they have been vomiting, you will need to replenish their electrolytes: You can make a homemade fluid replacement with apple (or any clear, pulp-free) juice, and water (fifty-fifty mix). Fresh, pulp-free watermelon juice with water is one of the most natural and quickest ways to replenish electrolytes. Even if the teen is vomiting, encourage them to drink small sips frequently.

Nux Vomica is the most useful remedy in this situation. It will help dispel the toxicity in the blood and liver. The stomach and intestines feel bruised and sore; the teen may have cramping, gas, and sour or bitter belching. They are chilly. There is a dryness of the mouth.

Pulsatilla can be given if they have ingested cheap wine, to help purge all the chemicals that are in these wines. They tend to be overheated, want fresh air, are usually thirstless, and may be weepy.

Dosage: Give every 15 minutes until there is improvement, and then on an as-needed basis only if symptoms return. In addition, you can also give Bach Flower Rescue Remedy, to restore a sense of balance, calm, and harmony. It reduces the effects of shock to the system from the alcohol. The teen may feel faint, and may tremble.

This remedy can be helpful if the teen is becoming hysterical or exhibiting wild or irrational behavior from the alcohol. **Bach Flower Rescue Remedy** is a very gentle yet effective remedy for this kind of situation. Add 3 drops to a glass of spring water, and have the teen sip it frequently until you see progress; repeat as long as needed. Stop when emotional stability has returned. It would be a good idea to have the teen sip on three glasses of water with **Rescue Remedy** the day after the incident.

Call your healthcare practitioner if:

- Your teen is hard to awaken, is unconscious, or has a seizure.
- They cannot stop vomiting, or are vomiting blood.
- They are experiencing slow or irregular breathing, i.e., gaps of more than eight seconds between breaths.
- They have a low body temperature (less than 98.6 degrees).

Drugs and Glue-Sniffing

If your teen is exhibiting bizarre behavior and you suspect that they have ingested a hallucinogenic or designer drug, give a dose of **Arnica** every 15 minutes and call your healthcare practitioner; or go to the emergency room if the teen is out of control or severely incoherent. Some teenagers may be tempted to sniff glue. The symptoms are skin burns, dizziness, weakness, disorientation, burning and watering of the eyes, burning in the tracheal and lung area, possible breathing difficulties, nausea, or diarrhea. The rhythm of the heartbeat can also be affected. For this, see **Arsenicum** or **Phosphorus,** below. If you suspect that your teen has overdosed, *take them to the emergency room immediately.*

Arsenicum: For burning pains in the throat, esophagus, or abdominal area. Their mouth and throat may be dry, and they are thirsty for sips of cold water. There can be severe vomiting and retching. If a chemical has come in contact with the skin, there is itching, burning, and swelling. Blisters can form. Even though there is much burning with this remedy, they feel better with warm applications, because they are usually chilly. They are extremely exhausted but anxious, with great restlessness.

Phosphorus: If the teen has burning pains. For oversensitive reaction to chemicals. Oppressed breathing with anxiety and palpitations, and congested lungs. They feel as though there is a heavy weight pressing on their chest, with tightness. There is a sensation of rawness and burning from the throat to the bottom of the ribcage. There might be palpitations or an elevated heartbeat as well, and labored breathing from the least exertion. There is a thirst for ice-cold drinks. The skin reactions are mild itching, burning, and swelling. Blisters can form and easily bleed. The teen is weak, and may become listless. They are irritable, lightheaded, oversensitive, disorientated, a bit fearful, and sluggish.

Dosage: Give 2 pellets every 15 minutes for four doses, then hourly until improvement. If there is no improvement after eight doses, choose a new remedy. As soon as there is improvement, repeat the remedy only if there is a return of any symptoms.

Supportive Measures:

Help their bodies to detoxify by giving 2,000 mg. of vitamin C daily, and have them drink eight glasses of water a day for several days. Sometimes vitamin C in high doses can cause mild and temporary diarrhea; if it does, reduce the dosage to 1,500 mg. or 1,000 mg. if necessary. Evaluate why your child is exhibiting risk-taking behaviors. Seek professional help if these situations become chronic.

Rage

Rage is a powerfully intense emotion that is expressed with sudden and extreme anger. You may feel as though your teen has reverted to the tantrums of a two-year-old. This state can be brought on by frustration, pain, overwhelm, grief, loss, low blood sugar, poor diet, brain changes, or hormone fluctuations. It is not unusual for teenagers to go through a stage that includes occasional rage—this is a normal stage of development.

A fit of rage can be quite distressing, but you should not suppress this emotion. However, rudeness, verbal abuse, or violence should always be addressed and never tolerated. If your teen is having too many bouts of rage, refer to the section on "Emotional Trauma and Fears" (page 257).

Stress

If a teen is under severe stress, their body will begin producing symptoms of illness. If your teen is unhappy at school, they can develop headaches, stomachaches, anxiety, or sleep difficulties. It is important to not let this become a chronic situation. Encourage your teen to talk to you about it. If necessary, intervene by speaking with teachers, coaches, school counselors, or professional counselors. Teens of today have many more temptations to deal with than older generations did. In this sometimes frantic-paced world, it is easy for a teen to feel a lot of pressure to perform or conform. They can easily become overwhelmed. Again, keep the lines of communication open.

In our society, some teens have no downtime, or are forced to participate in too many sports or other activities. Your son may not want to play football or be on the debate team. Your daughter may not want to play basketball or take dance lessons. Make sure your teen is not eating junk food, playing too many video games, on the computer for long periods of time, watching too much TV, or staying up too late at night. If your teen is not responding to remedies, stress could be creating an obstacle to a cure. Any teen who has suffered a great emotional shock, e.g., divorce or death, will more than likely need professional psychological help as well as a homeopath for support.

Emotional stress can be quite intense at this time of development, and homeopathic remedies can keep your teen more level and balanced. However, it is important that they are not given a remedy for every emotional upset. If your teen has been brooding for weeks, or intensely overreacting to situations, or if there is a big distress in their lives, a homeopathic remedy is in order.

Remember to tap into your support system of other parents, trusted family members, a spiritual or school counselor, or a psychologist. In many cases, tranquilizers or antidepressants deaden the feelings and have the potential to cause detrimental side effects. It is important that teens learn how to deal with and express emotions appropriately. To choose the right remedy, refer to the "Moodiness" section above, or "Emotional Trauma and Fears" (page 257).

TEETHING

There are no known serious teething complications, but it can be very difficult for some children, and unnerving for parents. The average child begins teething between four and six months of age, starting with the two lower front teeth. Children continue to get teeth up until two and a half years of age. Because the gums are inflamed and traumatized by teething, the child usually chews on their fist or other hard things. They may drool a lot, have a dry mouth, flushed cheeks, nasal congestion, and a low-grade fever. Please refer to the section on "Fevers" (page 182) to choose a remedy and help your child be more comfortable.

There may also be mild to intense pain, emotional upset, sleeping problems, unexplained fussiness, and loss of appetite. Emotional upsets can be in the form of impatience, overwhelm, irritability and temper tantrums. The child may also experience digestive upset with diarrhea. (If this is the case, see the "Diarrhea, Nausea, and Vomiting" section, page 30.)

Note: If your baby is teething and has frequent diarrhea, check the remedy **Dulcamara** in the "Diarrhea, Nausea, and Vomiting" section (page 30). Use this remedy if the remedy picture fits.

The following are the most commonly indicated remedies for teething:

Aconitum: This remedy is indicated when the symptoms come on suddenly. The child has a hot, red face and a great need to chew on something. Many times the cheek is slightly or noticeably red on the side where the new tooth is erupting. Teething is very painful, with fever and sweating. The pains are tearing and cutting. The child is thirsty for cold water, and may have a cough. The child is fretful, restless, and whiny. Their sleep may become disturbed.

Worse from: Nighttime, around midnight, noise, pressure, touch, cold dry air, and winds from the north. **Better from:** Fresh air, cold water, and rest.

Belladonna: Symptoms come on suddenly and violently. The child wakes from sleep and looks frightened. Pain is intense, throbbing, and comes and goes suddenly. There is facial aching. The pulse is strong and pounding, the head is hot, and the extremities are cold. Eyes are usually glassy, with dilated pupils, as well as red and sensitive to light. Red face, gums, and lips, with hot, dry skin. Fever can bring delirium and confusion. Restless sleep with twitching; tired, but cannot sleep. Usually not thirsty, but the toddler-aged teether likes lemonade. The child is agitated to the point of biting, restlessness, screaming, and hitting. May be afraid of the dark.

Worse from: Drafts, being touched, sudden motion, around 3 PM, noise, lying, and right-side teeth coming in. **Better from:** Sitting partially up, quiet, bending backward, rest, firm pressure, and watered-down lemonade.

Calc Carb: For difficult teething, or delayed teething (after ten months of age). Usually chilly, fair, plump, or large children. Milk intolerance. The head usually sweats. Their sweat, stools, and spit-up all smell sour. Often their glands are swollen. Their gums are also swollen, and they may grind the gums. There is watery diarrhea, with undigested food. They may have many colds, and a persistent cough that will not go away. They may have itchy eruptions on the skin, and red, swollen, itchy, and watery eyes in the open air. Sometimes they squint their eyes. Their feet may be cold, with a clammy sweat. The child is fearful, restless, and cries out at night. They are slow, easygoing babies, but usually obstinate, and may be self-willed and mischievous.

Worse from: Anything cold, drafts, damp weather, physical or mental exertion, and the full moon. **Better from:** Dry weather, lying on the painful side, and warmth.

Calc Phos: Painful teething, delayed teething (after ten months) or walking (after twelve months). They are usually thin, and may even be emaciated. Usually has dark hair and eyes. Painful gums that may be inflamed or pale-looking. Drools excessively. Prone to have gas and greenish stools. They become weak. The toddler may have a desire for eggs, or salty or savory things. Needs to constantly change positions. The toddler loves to go places and be out and about, but is easily exhausted from mental exertion. Sleeps on knees and elbows. They are discontent, restless, and irritable.

Worse from: Cold drafts, changeable cold or damp weather, and east winds. **Better from:** Warm dry weather, summer, and riding in a car.

Chamomilla: This remedy may be used for a child who is having much difficulty teething. It can also help if the teething is delayed. It is helpful when the child cannot tolerate the intense, severe, sharp, throbbing, and tearing pains. The screams are piercing and severe. One cheek is usually red (or has a red patch) and hot, and the other cheek is pale. This symptom can be subtle or very obvious. The side on which the new tooth is erupting is usually the hot side. They rub their face and madly chew on everything. They want to drink often. If there is a discharge from the nose, it is clear. If they have diarrhea, it is greenish, can smell like rotten egg, and is usually worse at night. May have a fever. They become overtired, but cannot sleep because of the fever; they may cry out in sleep, and toss about. Nothing pleases these children; they want to be held, but are only comforted for a short time, and then want to be put down—and then want to be held again. They scream for something, and when it is handed to them they reject it or throw it down. They are extremely irritable, easily agitated, and may moan. This remedy really helps with teething pains.

Worse from: Cold open air, wind, touch, nighttime, especially around 9 PM, and anger. **Better from:** Being held, rocked or carried, cold applications, mild weather, and patient parents.

Kreosotum: Severe pains that are worse at night. Many times they have a dry cough that is worse at night. Excessive drooling. May have green discharges from the nose, and foul breath. They can have green diarrhea, or they can be constipated, with hard, dry stools. They may struggle and scream while passing the stool. The baby is weak and delicate; new teeth may emerge with signs of decay. They are restless and tossing about all night. They moan and doze with eyes half-closed, and can only sleep when carried or caressed. They are angry, irritable, shrieking, easily brought to tears; they want something and then throw it down when it is given to them.

Worse from: Around 6 PM to 6 AM, cold, cold food, eating, and lying down. **Better from:** Cuddling, being carried, caressing, warmth, and warm food.

Mag Mur: Painful teething with many digestive problems. These children tend to be scrawny and frail. They will be constipated, only passing a small quantity of a stool that is dry little balls. They have gas, especially about an hour after feeding, and are prone to hiccups. They regurgitate white, frothy mucus, and have a hard, bloated abdomen. Milk intolerance; stools may have undigested milk, or be green diarrhea. Belching can smell like rotten eggs. The child is sensitive, anxious, and weeps easily.

Worse from: About an hour after eating, touch, noise, night, lying on the right side, and mental exertion. **Better from:** Open cool air, hard pressure, and burping.

Phytolacca: Painful teething. This child will have an irresistible desire to bite down on everything they can get their mouth around. The tip of the tongue is a bright-red color. The pains come and go suddenly, and move all over. Much jaw-clenching; may hold chin down to chest. Stringy saliva. Low appetite.

Smelly breath. Teeth may take a long time to break through. The child is tearful, irritable, nervous, and sensitive to pain.

Worse from: Damp cold weather, night, motion, and hot drinks. **Better from:** Biting on hard cool objects, lying on stomach or left side, gently rubbing gums, dry weather, rest, and warmth.

Podophyllum: For difficult teething. This child will want to press the gums together. They feel better if they can bite down on anything hard and cool. They have diarrhea that is worse early in the morning, is gushing, frothy, and green or yellow, and accompanied by loud, foul gas. In sleep they sweat on the head, but the face is cold. They have hot, glowing cheeks. You may hear a rattling in their chest. The tongue can have a mustard-colored coat, and the breath is foul. There may be moaning and whining during sleep. These children are whiny, fidgety, and restless.

Worse from: Early morning, eating, acidic fruits, motion, open air, summer, hot weather, and while bathing. **Better from:** Pressure, cool applications, and cool air. However, diarrhea is improved by lying on the stomach with heat under the abdomen.

Rheum: For difficult teething. The whole child smells sour, including their sweat, breath, vomit, and stools. Diarrhea is brown, green, and slimy. They may change their routine completely. Do not give this baby strained plums or prunes, which will upset their digestion. These babies are very irritable and restless. They eat and sleep very little. They scream and cry a lot, and their crying turns into screams at night. The scalp and hair become sopping wet. They get into strange positions in order to rest. They tend to frown. They either dislike all their favorite things and foods while teething, or only want particular ones. This remedy will help to set the digestion right again and improve their appetite.

Worse from: Uncovering any part of the body, eating, nighttime, in the morning after sleeping, plums, prunes, and unripe fruit. **Better from:** Warmth, wrapping up, and bending double.

Silicea (also known as **Silica Terra**): Painful, difficult, and de-layed teething (after ten months of age). They will often come down with a cold, cough, or diarrhea while teething. Milk in-tolerance. Fine features, skin, and hair. Weak and chilly, with sweaty head, neck, feet, and hands. Foul-smelling diarrhea that is painless but with much gas. These children are irritable, very bright, alert, sensitive, anxious, and fearful, and want to do things for themselves.

Worse from: Morning, damp, cold, bathing, and lying down, especially on left side. **Better from:** Warmth, wrapping up, dressing warmly, and dry weather.

Dosage: Give 2 pellets once an hour for four doses, if the symptoms are strong. Otherwise, give two to four times a day. As soon as symptoms lessen, give the remedy less often. Stop when there is significant improvement. Repeat only if there is a return of symptoms. Repeat as often as needed. If there is no response after six doses, try a different remedy or seek professional help from your homeopath.

Supportive Measures:

Push fluids, especially if there is a fever, to prevent de-hydration. Keep teething rings in the refrigerator so the child can have something cold to put on the gums. A peeled cold carrot is useful for children who like to have hard things to bite down on when teething. *Caution:* Use a fat and long carrot so there is no chance of the child choking, and do not leave a child unattended with a carrot. When a tooth is about to emerge, if the child will let you, very gently massage the gum to facilitate the tooth break-ing through. However, do not force it.

THE SIX MOST COMMON REMEDIES FOR TEETHING

	Belladonna	Calc Carb	Calc Phos	Chamomilla	Kreosotum	Silicea
Onset	Sudden and violent onset.	Difficult and delayed teething (after ten months old).	Painful and delayed teething and walking (after twelve months old).	Cold wind, teething, and getting very angry.	From teething.	Painful, difficult, and delayed teething (after ten months old).
Symptoms	Pain that comes and goes suddenly, intense throbbing and aching in the face. Pulse is strong and pounding. Head is hot, and extremities cold. Eyes may be glassy, with dilated pupils. Eyes red and sensitive to light. Red face, gums, and lips, with hot, dry skin.	Chilly, fair, plump children. Milk intolerance. Head sweats. Sour-smelling stools and/or spit-up. Swollen gums. May grind gums. Watery diarrhea, with undigested food. Swollen glands; child may get many colds. Feet may be cold and feel damp.	Thin, even emaciated. Usually has dark hair and eyes. Prone to diarrhea, gas, and intestinal upset during teething. Painful gums that may be inflamed or pale-looking. Cold limbs. Drools.	Pains are intense, severe, sharp, throbbing, and tearing. Screams are piercing and severe. One cheek may be red and hot, and the other pale. The teething side is usually the hot side. Any discharge from the nose is clear. Greenish diarrhea that may smell like rotten eggs.	Severe pains that are worse at night. Excessive drooling, foul breath. Baby is weak and delicate. Teeth may come in with signs of decay. May have green diarrhea, or be constipated with hard, dry stools. May struggle and scream while passing the stool.	The child will often come down with a cold, cough, or diarrhea while teething. Sweating of head, neck, hands, and feet. Milk intolerance. Fine features, skin, and hair. Weak and chilly, with sweaty feet and hands. Foul-smelling diarrhea that is painless but with much gas.
Mood	Restless and agitated to the point of biting, screaming, and hitting. May be afraid of the dark.	Fearful, restless, cries out at night. Slow, easygoing baby, usually obstinate. May be self-willed, mischievous.	Loves to go places and be out and about, but easily exhausted from mental exertion. Discontent, fretful, and irritable.	Demands things, then refuses or throws them down. Oversensitive, angry, screams, bites, kicks, is easily frustrated, and can't be consoled.	Child is angry, irritable, shrieking, and easily brought to tears. They demand something, and then throw it down.	Irritable, wanting to do things for themselves; very bright, alert, sensitive, anxious, and fearful.
Indications	Fever can bring delirium, confusion. Restless sleep with twitching. Tired, but cannot sleep. Usually no thirst.	This remedy will help with the assimilation of calcium.	Child needs to constantly change positions.	Child is hot, thirsty, and may have a fever. Overtired but cannot sleep, because of the pain. May cry out in sleep.	May have a dry cough that is worse at night. May have green discharges from the nose. Restless sleep, moaning, and dozing with eyes half-closed; child can only sleep when carried or caressed.	Delicate, weak, and chilly.
Worse	Drafts, being touched, sudden motion, 3 PM, noise, lying down. Right-side teething.	Anything cold; drafts, damp weather, physical or mental exertion, the full moon.	Changeable, cold or damp weather, cold drafts, and east winds.	Cold open air, wind, touch, nighttime, especially around 9 PM, and anger.	6 PM to 6 AM, cold, cold food, eating, and lying down.	Mornings, damp, cold, baths, and lying down, especially on the left side.
Better	Sitting partially up, quiet, bending backward, rest, firm pressure, lemons.	Dry weather, lying on painful side, warmth.	Warm, dry weather, summer, riding in the car, and lying on the side.	Being held, rocked or carried, cold applications, and mild weather.	Cuddling, being carried and caressed, warmth, and warm food.	Warmth, wrapping up, dressing warmly, and dry weather.

VACCINATIONS

The debate about vaccination is a big concern for many parents. According to the National Vaccine Information Center, a child in this country receives forty-nine doses of fourteen vaccines before the age of six years old, starting on the day of their birth. It is essential to become well informed and to research the facts, not opinions, on each side.

There is now much scientific data to draw upon. No vaccine is 100% free of side effects. Through the Freedom of Information Act, the content of the studies done on vaccines is available to the public. Thousands of reactions from vaccines are reported every year to the Vaccine Adverse Event Reporting System (VAERS), a national vaccine-safety surveillance program co-sponsored by the Centers for Disease Control and Prevention (CDC) and the Food and Drug Administration (FDA). This system provides analyzed information about adverse reactions after administration of vaccines.

It has been observed, and proven by checking medical records, that most of the children who develop complications or die from common childhood diseases already have a compromised immune response and/or are failing to thrive. In other words, these children have other health problems that make it hard for them to combat any illness whatsoever.

Homeopathy may be able to help if your child is suffering from complications of a vaccination, or from the disease itself. For instance, if your child does contract whooping cough (which happens to many children who are vaccinated), homeopathy can help shorten its duration and severity. Homeopathy can also help in the same way if a child gets chicken pox.

As parents, you need to gather information from both sides while weighing the pros and cons of each individual vaccination. The reason I have included this section is to inform parents of the potential side effects of certain vaccines. More in-depth knowledge of each vaccine can be found by researching the books and websites mentioned at the end of this section. As you make your decisions on how to deal with this issue, please take into account your beliefs, feelings, common sense, and familial medical history. You will need to make a decision you can live with. Find a healthcare provider that will support your decisions and work with you.

There is a school of thought that believes common childhood illnesses such as chicken pox, mumps, and measles are needed to jumpstart a child's immune system. They believe that the immune system is like a muscle; if sickness is allowed, it actually strengthens the child's constitution. This is much like using muscles to make a body stronger.

Giving homeopathic remedies will not reduce the effectiveness of, or interfere with, the vaccines. But the remedies will help to lessen the severity of the side effects in the nervous and immune systems. The most common initial side effects are fever, rash, and lack of energy. These may be manifest within hours, days, or even within a week or two. Sometimes a child will react mildly or not at all to the first two inoculations, and then suffer considerably from the third.

If a baby suffers side effects from a vaccination, contact your healthcare provider and report any adverse symptoms. It is imperative that they be involved in treatment immediately. Do not wait for the symptoms to become chronic!

Do not vaccinate your child when they are sick with a cold, sore throat, ear infection, cough, etc.

The best support for your child, if you decide to vaccinate, is to give them 2 pellets of **Thuja** before the appointment, and another 2 pellets immediately after you leave the doctor's office. If it seems as though the **Thuja** is not resolving the reactions, give 2 pellets of **Antimonium Tart**. If the symptoms still persist, contact your healthcare practitioner.

Some choices in giving vaccinations to your child:

- There are parents who prefer to vaccinate, and then treat any side effects that may occur.
- Some parents hold off vaccinating until the child is two years old.
- There are parents who have their children vacci-

nated one shot at a time, rather than giving many vaccinations in one shot.

- There are parents who pick and choose which vaccines to give their children.
- There are parents who do not vaccinate their children.

Common side effects from some vaccines:

Your child may or may not experience the following:

DTaP (diphtheria, whooping cough [pertussis], and tetanus): The child may develop a rash, chronic runny nose with thick mucus, congested breathing, restlessness, or screaming fits. This can occur up to weeks later.

Gardasil or HPV vaccine: For nine- to twenty-six-year-old females. This vaccine has also been given to teen boys. The side effects may include: Guillain-Barré syndrome, myalgia, paresthesia, loss of consciousness, seizures, convulsions, swollen body parts, chest pain, heart irregularities, visual disturbances, joint pain, difficulty breathing, severe rashes, persistent vomiting, menstrual irregularities, vaginal lesions, and HPV infection.

Hepatitis B: A baby's liver can become compromised. They may develop a fever, swollen lymph glands, headaches, muscle pains, abdominal pains, hypersensitivity to noise, light, etc., water retention, palpitations, and rashes. According to the Vaccination Awareness Network (UK), babies can develop abnormal liver functions from receiving this vaccine. Give 2 pellets of **Thuja 30C** as soon as possible.

Hib (Haemophilus influenza type b, for meningitis): The child can develop a fever, headaches, disorientation, screaming fits, diarrhea, vomiting, and muscle pains.

Influenza: Common side effects include fever, muscle pains, headaches, dizziness, and confusion, loss of coordination, tinnitus, depression, and tiredness. Some people get the shot and get the flu anyway. In the United States at the time of this writing, flu shots still contain thimerosal (a mercury derivative), aluminium salts, and formaldehyde. Thimerosal is a neurotoxin that can adversely affect the central nervous system. According to a study conducted in Australia, formaldehyde is not safe at any level in the body. As of the writing of this book, I have been unable to find any studies, long- or short-term, on giving children flu vaccines.

MMR (measles, mumps, and rubella): Side effects may include high fever, high-pitched screaming for hours on end, febrile convulsions, tonsillitis, chronic conditions of the bowels, muscle weakness, pains in joints, cerebral palsy, autism, and behavioral and learning difficulties.

Polio: The child can experience a fever, problems with coordination and spatial perception, back spasms, headaches, paralysis and/or rigidity, especially of the lower limbs, and allergies. **Lathyrus in a 30C potency** is the most effective remedy for relieving the side effects of this vaccine. Give 2 pellets daily for three days.

Varicella (chicken pox): Side effects reported in a four- to six-week period after vaccination are pain, redness, swelling, inflammation, fatigue, fever, chest pain, malaise, headache, dizziness, migraine, gastroenteritis, nausea, arthralgia, back pain, myalgia, depression, rash, pruritus, lymphadenopathy, and anaphylactic shock. These side effects are listed in the manufacturer's data sheet for Varilrix® vaccine. There is also some evidence that children given varicella vaccine can develop shingles, an incredibly painful virus condition, when their bodies enter puberty. The shingles virus lies dormant in the body, and eruptions are brought on by stress. The stress of hormone changes, intense growth spurts, brain restructuring, and the general stress of teen years may be enough to trigger an attack. Shingles in teens were very rare before this vaccine began to be administered. No long-term studies have been done on this vaccine.

Possible contraindications
to giving certain vaccines:

Discuss with your healthcare practitioner whether or not to give a vaccine if your child:

- Was premature, had a low birth weight, or has a birth defect, especially of the heart.
- Has had a previous adverse reaction to a vaccine.

- Has an infection, fever, cold, stomach upset, vomiting, diarrhea, respiratory dysfunction, or hay fever.
- Has seizures, a history of febrile fits or seizures, or any neurological disorder.
- Is taking antibiotics, steroids, hormones, or is on immune-suppressive therapy.
- Has an immune-suppressant illness.
- Has a family history of asthma, eczema, tuberculosis, or glue ear (a form of otitis media).
- Is sensitive to any of the ingredients in the vaccines, or has an allergy to eggs or dairy products.
- Has a history of a blood-clotting problem, or thrombocytopenia.
- Has had an inoculation of another vaccine within the last three weeks.
- Is allergic to antibiotics, e.g., penicillin.
- Has had a blood transfusion.
- Has received human immunoglobulin within the last three months. (If so, discuss whether any other vaccines should be given at this time.)
- Is having dialysis.
- Is a pregnant or breastfeeding teen.

Books for further reading and research about vaccinations:

- *What Your Doctor May Not Tell You about Children's Vaccinations,* by Stephanie Cave, MD, FAAFP, with Deborah Mitchell (Grand Central Publishing, 2004).
- *How to Raise a Healthy Child ... In Spite of Your Doctor,* by Robert S. Mendelsohn, MD (Random House, 1987).
- *Vaccines: Are They Really Safe and Effective?* by Neil Z. Miller (New Atlantean Press, 2002).
- *Homeopathic Alternatives to Immunisation: A guide for travellers and parents looking for an al-*

ternative to being immunised, by Susan Curtis, RSHom (Winter Press, Kent, UK, revised 2002 edition).

Websites for further information about vaccinations:

- www.nvic.org: Information on the risks of vaccinating or not vaccinating your child.
- www.thinktwice.com: Information services, books, list of worldwide vaccination-support groups. They provide hundreds of peer-reviewed studies from scientific and medical journals.
- www.tripprep.com: Contains health conditions and recommendations for travel to each country around the globe.

PART TWO

Winter Ailments

A NOTE ABOUT ANTIBIOTICS

Approximately 90% of all upper respiratory infections are caused by viruses, yet antibiotics are prescribed for 50% to 70% of patients who seek medical care for these conditions. Prescribing antibiotics for conditions for which there is not proven benefit is not a harmless practice; it contributes to the development of antibiotic resistance.

—T. Larrabee, Journal of Pediatric Nursing (April 17, 2002)

Misdiagnosis of otitis media [middle-ear infection] is a leading cause of inappropriate antimicrobial therapy in the United States.

—S. Dowell, S. March et al., Pediatrics (1998, p. 101)

As the years go by, I observe with greater clarity that antibiotic overuse causes immune dysfunction in many patients. It seems that the more antibiotics these patients receive, the more they need. Their immune systems appear to have a blunted ability to deal with challenges, resulting in recurrent illness.

—T. Dooley, MD, ND, Homeopathy Today (December 2002)

Antibiotics have their place. They have saved many a life. However, the Centers for Disease Control and Prevention launched a campaign in 1995 to decrease inappropriate antibiotic use, due to a concern that bacterial infections were becoming resistant to treatment by antibiotics. Please use antibiotics wisely, and share any concerns about overuse with your healthcare practitioner.

COMMON COLDS AND SINUSITIS

Colds

The common cold is caused by many different kinds of viruses. And each body is different, so symptoms will vary. In the early stages, the body will produce symptoms such as fever, chills, or sweats to fight off the virus. Then the body produces such symptoms as sneezing, runny nose, sore throat, earache, headache, tearing eyes, or cough. Mucus is formed to trap viruses and expel them from the body.

It is important not to repress symptoms of a common cold with decongestants or nasal sprays. Overcoming a cold *without* repressing it exercises the immune system and helps build resistance to future viruses. Homeopathy, if needed, helps to naturally aid the body in resolving colds, and makes your child more comfortable. A cold can be the body's way of saying that it is run-down, stressed-out, or not getting enough sleep. A cold is like a spring housecleaning; when it is over, the lymphatic system has been cleared out and the child will have better energy than before it began.

There are quite a few remedies for colds. It may be helpful to cross-reference the information below with the "Fevers" section (page 182).

Sinusitis

Sinusitis can be caused by a combination of viruses, bacteria, fungus, or allergies. There are several areas of sinuses in the head:

The **frontal sinuses,** above the brow, can get infected and cause pain, sensitivity to light, and a feeling of heaviness over the eyes and across the forehead.

The **maxillary sinuses,** beneath the eyes and beside the nose, can get infected and cause nasal congestion, pain and pressure in the cheekbones, and neuralgic pains in the teeth.

The **ethmoid sinuses,** above and behind the bridge of the nose, can get infected and cause pressure and pain at the bridge of the nose, with postnasal drip. There can also be pressure and pain behind the eyes, causing a splitting headache.

The **sphenoid sinuses** are two other sinuses deeper in the head.

The mucus discharge from sinusitis can be clear, yellow, yellow-green, or green. Chronic sinusitis is characterized by not just sinus pains but a constant postnasal drip that runs down the back of the throat. This is a condition that should be treated by your healthcare provider, because it can take a toll on the immune system and set the child up for other illnesses.

Young children do not usually get sinusitis. I have included information here for the older child and the rest of the family, who may suffer from this condition. Look to the explanation of the common-cold remedy first. Specifics for sinusitis are provided at the end of the remedy descriptions.

The following remedies are for sinusitis: **Arsenicum, Calc Carb, Hepar Sulph, Kali Bich, Lycopodium, Mercurius Viv, Natrum Mur, Nux Vomica, Pulsatilla, Sabadilla, Sepia,** or **Silicea.**

A Helpful Overview of Colds

For the first stages of a cold:

Slow Onset: Ferrum Phos
Sudden Onset: Aconitum, Belladonna

Then look to the following remedies:

Chill: Arsenicum, Hepar Sulph, Silicea
Colds with eye discharges: Allium Cepa, Dulcamara, Euphrasia, Nat Mur
Frequent sneezing: Aconitum, Allium Cepa, Cal Sulph, Hepar Sulph, Kali Bich, Lycopodium, Mercurius Viv, Natrum Mur, Nux Vomica, Rhus Tox, Silicea, Sulphur
Headache with a cold: Aconitum, Belladonna, Bryonia, Nux Vomica, Phosphorus, Pulsatilla, Silicea, Sulphur
Loss of smell and/or taste: Calc Carb, Calc Sulph, Hepar

Sulph, Kali Bich, Mercurius Viv, Natrum Mur, Phosphorus, Pulsatilla, Silicea
Slow onset: Bryonia

Remedies for various types of mucus:

Clear/frothy: Silicea
Hot: Aconitum, Sulphur
Profuse flow: Allium Cepa, Arsenicum, Dulcamara, Euphrasia (daytime only), Kali Sulph, Mercurius Viv, Natrum Mur, Nux Vomica (daytime only), Phosphorus, Rhus Tox
Watery: Allium Cepa, Arsenicum, Dulcamara (only at first), Euphrasia, Mercurius Viv (only at first), Natrum Mur, Nux Vomica, Rhus Tox (only at first)
White/Grey: Kali Mur
Yellow: Calc Carb, Calc Sulph, Dulcamara (as the cold progresses), Hepar Sulph, Kali Sulph, Lycopodium, Pulsatilla, Sulphur
Yellow/Green: Kali Bich, Mercurius Viv (as cold progresses), Rhus Tox (as the cold progresses), Sepia

If cold persists (for "old, ripe" colds), look to the following remedies:

Hepar Sulph, Kali Bich, Kali Mur, Kali Sulph, Pulsatilla, Silicea, Sulphur

Colds with strange, rare, or peculiar symptoms:

Blood-streaked mucus: Phosphorus
Burning symptoms, but with desire for warmth and warm drinks: Arsenicum
Cold in female teen that comes on before, during, or just after her period: Sepia
Cold sores with colds: Natrum Mur, Rhus Tox
Constant urge to stretch: Rhus Tox
Desire to keep nose warm by covering it up: Dulcamara
Discharge of mucus, but everything feels very dry: Bryonia

Drooling on pillow: Mercurius Viv
Gas and bloating: Lycopodium
Mucus tastes salty: Natrum Mur
Profuse flow of mucus, but feels stuffed up: Allium Cepa
Sleeps with feet out from under the covers: Sulphur
Sneezing in warm room, or during sleep: Pulsatilla
Symptoms constantly changing: Pulsatilla
Yawns a lot in open air: Euphrasia

Different Kinds of Colds:

Colds in Babies: See "Newborn Discomforts" section (page 55).
Summer Colds: Dulcamara.

What to observe:

What was the weather like before the child got sick? Was it windy, rainy, cold and damp, warm and wet, or with a dry, cold wind? Did the child get wet feet, or soaked through? Did the cold come on fast, or take a few days to develop? Is the discharge clear, yellow, yellow-green, or green? Is the discharge thick or thin, bland or acidic? Is the child having difficulty sleeping, waking frequently because their nose is so stopped up? Do they look pale, or red in the face? Do they want warm or cold drinks or food, or no food or drink? Are they experiencing a low-grade fever, or a headache? Are they feeling unusually warm, or chilly? Is one nostril more stuffed up than the other? If there is pain, especially in the sinuses, what kind of pain is it, and is it more on the left or right? Does the color of the mucus vary at different times of the day? Do the ears ache? Is the throat sore? Is the chest tight? If there is achiness, what does it feel like? What is the child's temperament?

The following are the most commonly indicated remedies for colds and sinusitis (this information applies to adults as well as toddlers and older children):

Aconitum: For a cold with sudden onset after being exposed to icy north or east winds, or from shock or fright. This remedy is most useful in the first twenty-four hours, and at the very first sign of symptoms. The child goes down fast, and chills come on fast. They have shivers followed by a sudden high fever and sweating. The skin is dry and hot, and there is a thirst for cold drinks. Frequent sneezing with clear, hot mucus dripping from the nose, or the nose may be dry and stopped up. The eyes feel hot, dry, burning, and aching, and may be bloodshot. There may be roaring in the ears and a throbbing headache. The pupils may be contracted. The child is restless, fearful, anxious, and screaming, and may have nightmares with restless or no sleep.

Worse from: Nighttime, around midnight, midday, noise, cold drafts, light, and pressure. **Better from:** Fresh air, rest, sweating, and warm applications.

Note: After taking **Aconitum,** the symptoms may change to those of a regular cold. You may need to go to another remedy if the cold does not clear or if the symptom picture changes for the worse. Retake the case.

Allium Cepa: Onset from damp, windy, cold weather, or getting feet wet. Sensations like those experienced when cutting an onion. Lots of sneezing with much hot, watery, and acidic mucus. Sneezing brings no relief. The nose and top lip are sore from the acidic mucus. Left nostril gets stuffed up first and then the stuffiness moves right. Nose is profusely running, but still stuffed up. The eyes are light-sensitive, burning, and red. There is a watery discharge from the eyes, but it is not acidic. The child is hot, thirsty, and wants fresh air. The throat is sore and tickles because of the acidic postnasal drip, which may cause laryngitis. They may have an achy or dull pain in forehead, eyes, and sometimes the whole face. Sometimes there is a severe, aching pain at the nape of the neck. The child has a good temperament, but is anxious.

Worse from: Warm stuffy rooms, damp, cold, evening, and spring. **Better from:** Fresh air, cool rooms, and cool applications.

Arsenicum: Onset from getting chilled, wet weather, overheating, or overexertion. Nose drips with profuse, burning, watery mucus, especially from the right nostril. There is much sneezing; however, the nose feels stopped up with a burning, dry sensation. The nose and top lip are sore and red from the burning mucus. There is a raw, burning feeling where the back of the nose joins the throat. The child has a strong thirst for drinks, but drinks in sips. Eyes may be red, dry, and burning. Dull, throbbing headache with light sensitivity. These colds tend to move into the chest. There are a lot of burning symptoms, and the child is chilly, weak, and exhausted. The baby wants to be carried, is needy, demanding, and does not want to be left alone, but may be restless in bed. The face is pale with an anxious look, and may be covered with a cold sweat. The child is anxious, irritable, oversensitive, needy, and demanding. The older child may fear they are dying or will not get better.

Sinusitis remedy: For frontal and maxillary sinuses that are blocked, with burning in sinuses and dull and throbbing pain. **Kali Mur** may be needed if **Arsenicum** is not holding or resolving this condition. It is a remedy that follows **Arsenicum** well. See **Kali Mur,** below.

Worse from: Physical exertion, after midnight, cold air, and cold drinks. **Better from:** Warmth, warm drinks, lying down, fresh air, company, and reassurance that they are going to get better (for an older child).

Belladonna: Sudden violent onset, from getting head wet, cold and dry wind, or from getting a haircut. Glands are swollen and may be painful. Nose is dry, red, swollen, and may have blood-streaked mucus. Face is flushed bright red, and pupils are usually dilated. Skin is hot and dry. If the child has a high fever, they may be confused and delirious. If they are thirsty, they crave cold water or lemonade. Eyes may be glassy and sparkling, with a wild look. The child may smell imaginary odors. The sleep is restless. There may be headache. The child is irritable, and all senses are acute and heightened. They can become agitated to the point of biting, screaming, and hitting.

Note: This is another remedy to be used in the initial stages of a cold. You may need to go to another remedy if the cold does not clear, or if the symptoms change. Review the case.

Worse from: Noise, light, odors, drafts, touch, sudden motion, and around 3 PM. **Better from:** Sitting semi-erect or standing up, quiet, and rest in dark rooms with light covers.

Bryonia: Onset from cold winds. The cold comes on slowly. The nose is stuffed up, but only has a small amount of watery discharge, or no discharge at all. Great thirst for large quantities of liquids. Very dry nose, mouth, lips, and throat. The child complains of feeling dry everywhere in the body. Eyelids are sore, red, and swollen. Eyeballs have sore pains. Bursting headache with shooting pains. Symptoms are worse with any movement. This is a cold that often quickly descends into the chest. The baby does not want to be picked up or carried. The child needs to have the room warm, but not hot. The child is very grumpy, irritable, does not want to move, and wants to be left alone. The older child might be anxious about missing school while feeling ill; however, they want to be at home.

Worse from: Movement, around 9 PM, touch, warmth, spring, and autumn. **Better from:** Lying completely still, pressure, quiet, cool open air, cool applications, and drinks.

Calc Carb: Onset from changes in the weather. The children who respond to this remedy catch colds easily. Their mucus is smelly and yellow. The nose is stuffed up, with loss of smell. However, the child may complain that they smell an offensive odor. The nostrils become dry, sore, and ulcerated. The nose and upper lip become swollen. The child is very thirsty, and hoarseness is not unusual. They are sluggish, stubborn, sensitive, and tearful.

Sinusitis remedy: When there is pain at the root of the nose (where the roof of the mouth meets the top of the throat). Child may complain of an offensive smell like that of rotten plants. Nose is stuffed up during day, but it runs at night. May have nosebleeds.

Worse from: Cold, damp, drafts, morning, exertion, fresh air, tight clothes, and milk. **Better from:** Heat, rest, and loose clothing.

Calc Sulph: Onset from changes in weather, or getting chilled and/or wet. Thick, yellow mucus that is lumpy and may have streaks of blood. Sneezing, with only one side of nose blocked at a time. Edges of the nostrils are sore. The child is dull and sluggish, with no energy. They are tearful, whiny, moaning, and complain a lot. They become anxious in the evening.

Worse from: Cold, evening, wet, drafts, hot stuffy rooms, milk, and changes in weather. **Better from:** Open air, uncovering, bathing, and locally applied heat.

Dulcamara: Onset from cold, wet weather as in autumn, when there is a sudden change from hot to cold, exposure to damp, or summer colds after getting chilled from air conditioning. These children catch cold easily, are extremely sensitive to cold and damp, and lack vital heat. The nose becomes stopped up in cold air or cold rain. At first there is a profuse watery discharge from the nose; later, the mucus becomes thick and yellow, and bloody crusts may form. The child wants to keep the nose warm, e.g., covering it with a scarf. The cold settles in the eyes, which become red and sore from a profuse watery discharge. Glands are swollen and hard. If they were chilled, soon afterward there is a strong need to urinate or pass a stool. May have a sore throat. This cold can go into the chest, or develop into flu. The child is quarrelsome, impatient, irritable, confused, and restless.

Worse from: Cold rainy weather, autumn, night, cold air, getting chilled when heated (as from air conditioning), and rest. **Better from:** Motion, warmth, dry warm air, and keeping head and nose warm.

Euphrasia: The nose runs constantly with bland and watery mucus during the day. At night, the nose becomes stopped up.

There is a constant flow of hot, acidic tears from the eyes, which irritates the skin. The eyelids are swollen, burning, and red. The conjunctiva (the white part of the eye) is usually red. There is violent sneezing. The child may have a bursting headache and be light-sensitive. The unique symptom with this remedy is that the child yawns a lot when in open air. The throat may be tickly and burning. There is frequent waking during sleep. The child is weepy, irritable, sad, and lazy.

Worse from: Morning and evening, nighttime, and being indoors. **Better from:** Fresh air, eating, and low light.

Ferrum Phos: The onset of this type of cold is slow. This remedy may be given at the first sign of a cold that doesn't have especially distinctive symptoms. There may be symptoms, but if there is nothing distinctive about them, this is the remedy. It is also a remedy for general inflammations, and most useful for the early stages of a fever. The child is weak, chilly, and thirsty for cold drinks. The face may alternate between being pale and flushed. The child may complain of a scratchy throat, or a headache in the forehead that is worse on the right side. Some children will get a nosebleed. The eyes can be bloodshot and burning. There is often a need to follow this with another remedy if the cold does not resolve. The child is talkative, excited, irritable, and averse to company.

Worse from: Nighttime, and from 4–6 AM, on the right side, touch, motion, and jarring. **Better from:** Cold applications on the head, and lying down.

Hepar Sulph: Onset from getting too cold, or from a cold wind. These children catch cold easily and are extremely sensitive to cold. They need to be wrapped up warmly, and kept warm and indoors if possible. Glands are swollen. Discharge is thick, yellow, smelly (like old cheese), and drips down the back of the throat. Nose is red, inflamed, and swollen. Even though the discharge is thick, it does flow. This is a remedy for "old, ripe colds" that are not resolving. The child sneezes a lot when uncovered, or in a draft of cold air, and then becomes stopped up. They might lose their sense of smell. Sweating of the head and neck at night. This child is extremely irritable, demanding, sensitive, and does not want to be examined or looked at.

Sinusitis remedy: When sinuses and nasal bones are very tender, and the root of the nose (where the roof of the mouth meets the top of the throat) aches. The child may complain that there is a rotten smell in the nose, and may have nosebleeds. Cold air blocks up the nose.

Worse from: Cold dry air, winter, night, touch, uncovering, exertion, and cold drafts. **Better from:** Moist heat or warm applications, hot drinks, and wrapping the head or ears.

Kali Bich: Onset from getting chilled. This remedy is for an old, ripe cold, or for second stages when the mucus gets thick. The mucus becomes smelly, acidic, yellow or greenish, sticky, ropy, and so thick that the child cannot breathe through their nose, or blow it out. The nose feels heavy and dry. The child develops ulcerations and dry crusts on the septum of the nose, which cause bleeding when loosened. Violent sneezing, worse in the morning. Thick postnasal drip can make the voice hoarse. The child feels chilly. They usually lose their sense of smell. The child may say that it feels like there is a hair on their tongue or in their nostrils. The child is very weak. They are ill-humored, low spirited, indifferent, and lazy.

Sinusitis remedy: When there is pinching pain and pressure at the root of the nose (where the roof of the mouth meets the top of the throat). The child's voice becomes very nasal-sounding. There is pain in the frontal sinuses, with bursting headache and light-sensitivity. May have diarrhea. The mucus is so sticky and thick that it can get stuck in the throat and lungs, causing hawking and coughing.

Note: It is very important *not* to give a child with this kind of cold a decongestant, because it will greatly prolong the cold.

Worse from: Pressure on the forehead and maxillary sinus area, cold, damp, spring, autumn, undressing, and from 2–3 AM. **Better from:** Warmth, wrapping up, pressure, and motion as tolerated.

Prescribing note: Kali Bich is the best remedy if the child is **Worse from** cold, but **Better from** heat. Note that **Kali Sulph,**

below, is the best remedy for the opposite—**Worse from** heat, but **Better from** cold.

Kali Mur: This remedy is used for the later stages of a stuffy head cold. The mucus is thick, white or grey, sticky, and lumpy. The child may have nosebleeds. Many times the tubes of the ears become blocked. The voice becomes hoarse. The base of the tongue has a white, grey, or greyish-white coating. The child usually loses their appetite. Much hawking from thick mucus draining down the back of the throat. The child gets is easily angered, irritable, and discontent.

    Worse from: Open air, cold drinks or applications, lying down, drafts, night, dampness, and motion. **Better from:** Cold drinks, rubbing, and warmth.

Kali Sulph: Onset from getting chilled and then overheated. This remedy is for the second stage of a cold, when the mucus has become profuse, slimy, yellow, and sticky. The nose becomes completely obstructed and feels swollen. The child loses their sense of smell. They breathe through their mouths and may snore because the nose is so blocked. They may become hoarse. They feel heavy, weary, irritable, and anxious. The child will ask for something, and then reject it.

    Worse from: Heated stuffy rooms, evening, and noise. **Better from:** Motion and cool fresh air.

Lycopodium: Onset from wet weather. The nose is completely obstructed with a thick yellow or green mucus. The child is always sneezing and blowing their nose. The nose is dry, becomes ulcerated, and forms crusts. The sense of smell can be acute. They can become so stopped up that they have to breathe through their mouth during sleep. The throat is dry and tickles. Their breath is smelly. They are likely to have gas and be bloated. The child is irritable, spacey, sensitive, tearful, kicks and screams on awakening, and may throw a tantrum.

    Sinusitis remedy: When mucus becomes so stuck it is hard to blow anything out. The child has pressing and throbbing pains in the forehead and temples. The nose is dry at night. Nostrils alternate being stopped up.

Worse from: Cold drinks, cold food, and from 4–8 PM. **Better from:** Being well wrapped up, warm drinks, movement, and burping.

Mercurius Iodatus Flavus: Same symptoms as **Mercurius Viv,** below, but the majority of the symptoms are on the right side.

Mercurius Iodatus Ruber: Same symptoms as **Mercurius Viv,** below, but the majority of the symptoms are on the left side.

Mercurius Viv (also known as **Mercurius Sol**): Onset from getting chilled. Cold can start in the throat or chest and travel up to the nose and sinuses. There is sneezing with a profuse slimy, watery discharge that later becomes thick and yellow-green, and smells like old cheese. The nasal discharge, which may be blood-streaked, burns the upper lip and makes the nostrils raw. Loss of smell. The child will drool slimy, clear saliva onto their pillow. The breath smells bad, and there may be a metallic taste in the mouth. The child is usually quite sweaty. The tongue may have a white or grey coating, and shows imprints of the teeth on the sides. The child is sensitive to heat and cold, and their temperature may be unstable. They are very thirsty for cold water, but it does not satisfy the thirst. They may be hoarse or lose their voice. Usually the glands in the neck are swollen and tender. The child is weary, might tremble, and is restless, constantly changing their mind, and nervous.

Worse from: Night, drafts, damp weather, sweating, too much cold or heat, lying on right side, warmth in bed, and warm drinks. **Better from:** Moderate even temperatures, rest, lying on stomach, and morning.

Natrum Mur: This kind of cold starts out with much sneezing that is worse in the morning. The mucus is profuse and watery, like the white of a raw egg. This goes on for one to three days. Then the nose becomes dry, the mucus thickens, and the nose gets stopped up. The eyes water with burning and acidic tears, which makes them red. The child may state that the mucus tastes salty, and is very thirsty for cold water and salty foods. There is loss of smell and taste. If the child is susceptible to cold sores, they are likely to occur with this cold. The lips become dry and cracked. There may be ulcers in the nose. The child is easily frustrated, which makes them cry. They are very touchy, pouty, sulky, and easily offended. They are oversensitive to noise, odors, lights, and loud music.

Sinusitis remedy: When the child complains of achy pain in the cheek bones. Frontal sinus pain. Sinuses feel dry, but are stuffed up. Inside the nose becomes swollen and is sore, and it hurts if they blow the nose hard.

Worse from: Exertion, being uncovered, lying on the back, eating, and drafts. **Better from:** Warmth, being wrapped up, moist air, hot drinks, belching, quiet, and not moving the chest.

Nux Vomica: Onset from getting chilled in a cold, dry wind or air conditioning. Profuse flow of watery mucus in the daytime, but the nose is stuffed up at night or in open air. Or there is stuffiness that alternates between the nostrils. Violent sneezing, especially in the morning. The root of the nose (where the roof of the mouth meets the top of the throat) feels very full, and there may be a bloody nose. The child is chilly at the slightest movement, has a dull headache, and is achy all over. Very little thirst. The throat is raw. Their sleep is restless. They are oversensitive to strong odors. This child is angry, irritable, impatient, and easily frustrated.

Sinusitis remedy: If the gums and teeth become achy, and the head feels heavy. Pressing and tearing pains in frontal sinuses. Wants to press head against something. Prickling and tickling sensations inside nose. Head feels better if it is wrapped up. Sinuses feel better with gentle pressure. May be constipated, with an urge to go, but nothing comes out; or there is a sensation that there is more to come out, but nothing does.

Worse from: Early morning, getting chilled, cold open air, noise, being uncovered, mental exertion, warm rooms, loss of sleep, drafts, and anything that is too tight around the waist. **Better from:** Warmth, being wrapped up, moist air, hot drinks, and rest.

Phosphorus: Onset from getting drenched in rain. Nose is either profusely running or dry and stuffed up on alternating sides. The mucus is usually, but not always, blood-streaked. There is loss of smell and taste. The throat is usually sore, dry, and tickly. The child may become hoarse, and feels chilly but is thirsty for ice-cold drinks and food. If the child is not hungry, do not force them to eat, especially warm food or drink, as it will take them much longer to get better. Colds tend to go into the chest. There is an acute sense of smell, and there may be a dull headache over one eye. Even with a fever this child might be running around as if nothing is wrong—and then they go down hard. So you may want to keep them resting until you are sure of a complete recovery. The child is affectionate, fearful, easily upset, and irritable. This child needs attention, consolation, and massage, which will make them feel much better.

Worse from: Change of weather, wind, cold thunderstorms, odors, light, and lying on the left side. **Better from:** Sleep, sympathy, low lights or dark, eating and drinking cold things, cool applications, and open air.

Pulsatilla: This cold's onset is from getting feet wet and becoming chilled, or after the common cold has set in. Symptoms are constantly changing and shifting. If there is a fever, the temperature will be erratic. The mouth is dry, but they are likely thirstless. They are chilly but intolerant of heat, and may want the window open at night. There is an abundance of bland, thick, creamy-yellow or yellow-green mucus that is most profuse in the morning and early evening. Sneezing in warm, stuffy rooms and during sleep. Loss of taste and smell. The eyes may discharge and be crusty upon awakening. There may be a headache that comes and goes. The child must avoid milk, which they may crave. The child is clingy, whimpering, whiny, weepy, and fretful, but affectionate. Your older son might feel sorry for himself. This child needs attention and gentleness.

Sinusitis remedy: If frontal and maxillary sinuses feel heavy, with constant dull pain. The eyes water, and the eyelids may become red. Eyes may itch and burn a little. When the child lies down, the sinuses drain. When they get up, the nose becomes stopped up.

Note: If the child is not getting over this cold, look at **Kali Sulph.** It will finish off this kind of cold.

Worse from: Warm stuffy rooms, morning, twilight, getting over-heated, fatty or rich foods, and dairy products. **Better from:** Cool fresh air, cold applications and drinks, being uncovered, resting, being held, hugged, and rocked gently, and after a good cry.

Rhus Tox: The onset of this kind of cold is from getting wet, sitting on damp ground, or getting overheated after being chilled. Muscles and joints ache and are stiff, but get better from constant gentle movement. There is also aching in the bones of the nose. There is much sneezing, with profuse watery mucus that may turn thick and green. The glands are swollen, hard, and tender. The stools are usually loose. The child has a dry mouth and throat, and is thirsty for small sips of water. The tip of the nose is red and sore. Usually there is a red triangle on the very tip of the tongue. If a fever is present, the breath is so hot that it makes the nostrils sore. There is a constant urge to stretch. The child may develop a cold sore. They toss and turn all night because they cannot get comfortable. This child is anxious, weepy, helpless, mildly delirious, and extremely restless.

Worse from: Cold damp weather, autumn, cold food or drinks, being uncovered, drafts, lying still, nighttime, and on first movement after resting. **Better from:** Warm drinks and food, gentle movement, after moving for a while, stretching, warmth, changing positions, and massage.

Sabadilla: Onset from getting chilled in cold air. Profuse watery discharge, with much sneezing. The child is extremely oversensitive to odors, and has lots of itching and tickling in the nose. Nostrils alternate being stuffed up. Eyes are red and burning, with a lot of tearing up. If they have a fever, there are lots of chills and shivering that move upward. No thirst except after a chill. The head and face are hot, and feet cold. The child is very chilly. This child is miserable, nervous, easily startled, and obsessed that their condition is really dangerous.

Sinusitis remedy: When there is pain in the frontal sinuses, especially in the morning.

Worse from: Cold air, cold applications, smelling flowers or garlic, and any odors. **Better from:** Heat, warm food and drinks, open air, eating, calm, and wrapping up.

Sepia: Onset is from getting wet, snowfall, or being in frosty air. Mucus is thick, green or yellow, and ropy. It runs down the back of the throat, and the child keeps trying to hawk it back up. These are colds that often start in the throat and move up into the head. There is pain at the root of the nose (where the roof of the mouth meets the top of the throat), and crusts in the nose, and the child is very sensitive to odors but may lose sense of smell as cold progresses. Very sensitive to cold. These children drag themselves around and feel exhausted. They are sulky, negative, moody and tearful, may not care about their toys, and are indifferent to the family.

Note: This cold can come on in the female teen before, during, or just after her period. If she has a backache in her lower back and the above symptoms, this is the remedy for her.

Sinusitis remedy: For when the sinuses feel very dry, and the nose is obstructed, with pressing pains at the root of the nose. Nostrils hurt if cold air is drawn through them. Usually the left side is worse.

Worse from: Morning and evening, cold damp air, touch, and around the menstrual period. **Better from:** Eating, warmth, exercise as tolerated, cold drinks, pressure, keeping busy, and sleep.

Silicea (also known as **Silica Terra**): Onset is from getting chilled, getting feet wet, or change of weather to cold. These children catch colds quite easily. The nose is either running or alternating between dryness and being blocked. The mucus is clear and frothy. Dry, hard crusts form on the nose that bleed when loosened. There is sweating of the head and neck at night, and sneezing in the morning, especially in cold air. Glands are swollen. Sense of smell is lost. The mouth may be cracked at the corners. This child is very chilly, sensitive to drafts and changes in weather, tires easily, and lacks stamina. This child is subdued, shy, overly sensitive in all the senses and to pain, anxious, nervous, and can be stubborn and uncooperative. This remedy can be very useful for an unyielding cold where it feels as if thick mucus is blocking the ears. The ears will feel itchy and blocked, and the child may hear pops and crackles.

Sinusitis remedy: When there is soreness in the sinuses, with obstruction. The nasal bones are extremely tender. The mucus turns to a thick yellow discharge that may look and smell like pus. This is one of the best remedies for draining the sinuses.

Worse from: Left side, cold air and drafts, being uncovered, morning, damp, being consoled, loud noises, and the full moon.
Better from: Warmth, being wrapped up, wearing a warm hat, urination, yawning, and swallowing.

Sticta Pulmonaria: This is a sinusitis remedy. The onset in this case is from a sudden change in temperature. There is a dull heavy pressure in the forehead. The pain can be quite intense, gets worse as the day goes on, and lasts all day. The eyeballs feel sore, and may burn. The root of the nose (where the roof of the mouth meets the top of the throat) is blocked and feels very full. The mucous membranes are so dry that they hurt. There is a constant desire to blow, but nothing comes out. There is very little discharge, which dries quickly and forms crusts in the nose that are difficult to get out. Much sneezing. The child feels dull and lethargic at the onset, but is talkative.

Worse from: Nighttime, lying down, touch, and motion. **Better from:** Open air, moist air, a cool mist vaporizer, and pressure.

Sulphur: Onset from getting chilled. Profuse, acidic, burning, smelly, dirty, yellow mucus that is hot and makes the nostrils sore. The nose may form crusty scabs that bleed easily and cause blood-streaked mucus. Constant sneezing. The nose feels dry and is itchy. The child is usually hot, and feels better with fresh air. The nose runs when they are outdoors, but stops up when indoors. They are sensitive to odors. They are thirsty for great quantities of cold drinks, but may forget to drink. Remind the child to drink. The lips, nose, ears, eyelids, or skin can be red in spots. The room is likely to smell noticeably stale and sour. This cold is sometimes accompanied by frequent loose stools. You may notice that the child is sleeping with their feet out from under the covers. The child is irritable, sluggish, quarrelsome, and restless.

Note: This remedy is very useful if well-chosen remedies have not done much, or if the child keeps relapsing because their immune system cannot respond. **Sulphur** is used in the later stages of an acute illness where other remedies helped initially but are no longer working. This is true especially after **Mercurius Vivus** or **Lycopodium** were used. Make sure the symptoms fit the description above. This remedy should not be overused. If the child is not improving after giving this remedy, consult your healthcare practitioner.

Worse from: Heat, blowing the nose, bathing, standing, over-exertion, around 11 AM, and at the full moon. **Better from:** Cold, open air, gentle motion, and sweating.

Dosage: For all of the above cold remedies, if the onset is fast, give 2 pellets every 15 minutes for four doses, then hourly until there is improvement. If there has been no improvement after six doses, choose a new remedy. If there is a little improvement, continue with the same remedy.

If the onset has been slow, give the remedy every 1–2 hours for six doses. Repeat the remedy only if there is a return of the same symptoms. Repeat only as necessary. You may need to repeat the remedy two or three times per day for several days.

If you get no result, or if the remedy helped but did not hold, then reassess: You may not have been wrong with your choice, but the child may have moved on to needing a different remedy. Change the remedy if you have followed the above guidelines with no results, or if the symptoms clearly change. For example, **Aconitum** may be the remedy needed initially. But as the first twenty-four hours go by, symptoms may change and indicate, for instance, that the child has moved on to needing **Bryonia**.

Supportive Measures:

It is key to treat a cold *at the first sign of symptoms.* Neglected colds can turn into more serious conditions. It is important to teach your toddler how to blow their nose and clear their throats as soon as possible. This keeps the mucus discharging, and will facilitate a speedier recovery.

A tip: Teach this technique when the child is not sick. Hold one side of the nose shut with your finger, and ask the child to take a breath in through the mouth and then close the mouth. Then ask the child to blow out hard through the nose, while keeping the mouth closed. Keep a tissue handy to wipe. Repeat with the other nostril. The child can graduate to holding one nostril shut with a tissue in hand, and blowing out with the mouth closed. Repeat with the other nostril. Make sure your child is not blowing too hard, because this can put pressure on the Eustachian tube in the ear.

When your child is sick and their voice sounds throaty, ask the child to cough, and when they feel mucus in the throat, to spit it out and not swallow it again. Keep reminding the child to do this. It can keep the child from developing a severe cough. Have the child rest and take in lots of fluids. Avoid dairy products, because they increase mucus. Give lots of fruit—fresh, if possible, because it contains high amounts of vitamin C. Do not give sugary juice drinks; fresh-squeezed juice is best. If you live in a dry climate, a cool-mist vaporizer can help break up thick mucus. Or you can get the bathroom steamed up and have the child breathe the steam. If it is not too cold or rainy, take the child out into the fresh air for a walk. Be careful that they do not overdo it. You may be tempted to get an over-the-counter decongestant, but this will actually prolong the cold and make the child feel worse when it wears off. Look at the "Fevers" section (page 182) if your child has a fever.

Supportive Measures (cont):

Remember: It is very important not to use any products like Vicks VapoRub®, or lozenges with camphor, eucalyptus, or menthol. These substances can antidote the homeopathic remedies, as described in the Introduction of this book.

Call your healthcare practitioner if:

- Your baby is under three months old and has any rise in temperature.
- Your child has a temperature over 103 degrees.
- A fever persists for more than twenty-four hours in a child under two years of age.
- A fever persists for more than three days in a child over two years of age.
- A fever continues to rise despite giving a well-indicated remedy.
- Your child has a lack of reaction, trouble breathing, repeated vomiting, or convulsions.
- The child has frequent colds.
- There is a loss of appetite over a period of several days.
- You cannot get your child to drink, especially if there is a fever.
- There is stiffness in the neck.
- The child has a severe headache with vomiting.
- The child becomes delirious or unresponsive.
- There is high pitched, piercing screaming with no break.
- There is a rash.

COUGHS, CHEST INFECTIONS, CROUP, AND WHOOPING COUGH

Coughs

A cough is a body's way of clearing the delicate air passages of irritants—usually mucus. The mucus has been produced as a sticky substance to carry viruses, bacteria, inhaled particles (dust, pollen, and dead white blood cells) out of the body. It is best to not use cough medicines because they interfere with coughing, which is the natural protective mechanism of the lungs to rid themselves of mucus. If repressed, a cough can lead to deeper infections; or it will take longer for the child to get rid of the cough completely.

Homeopathy aids the child's body in ridding itself of the cough and making them more comfortable. Coughs can be hard to treat because of the wide variety of symptoms—there are many things to take into account. Be patient! Try not to get discouraged; you may need to re-evaluate the case two or three times. You may need to repeat a remedy a few times a day over the course of a few days.

Note: A neglected persistent cough can lead to or indicate other problems, so it is advisable to get an evaluation by your healthcare practitioner if the cough is not resolving.

The American Academy of Pediatrics states that over-the-counter cough and cold medicines should not be given to children under the age of six years old, because they do not work and can have dangerous side effects. There are warning labels on these products that state they should not be given to children under two years old.

A little anatomy lesson here so you can tell where the cough is originating:

Pharynx: The opening around the back of the tongue where it turns and goes into the throat.

Larynx: The throat down to the pit of the throat, just below the

Adam's apple. This is called the voice box.

Trachea: The windpipe, from the throat to just before it reaches the lungs.

Bronchus: The main tube into the lungs.

Bronchioles: The smaller tubes on both sides that carry the air in and out of the lungs.

Different kinds of coughs:

A **dry cough** is usually hacking and tickling, because the mucous membranes are dry or the mucus is tough and sticking to the air passages. The chest usually feels tight. The remedies for dry cough are: **Aconitum, Arsenicum, Belladonna, Bryonia, Causticum, Chamomilla, Ignatia, Iodium, Kali Bich, Lachesis, Nux Vomica, Phosphorus, Pulsatilla, Rumex, Spongea Tosta,** and Sticta Pulmonaria.

A **moist cough** is one with a lot of mucus in the air passages. There is a loose rattling and bubbling sound in the chest that can be heard in the cough or the breathing. Even though there is a lot of mucus, it may be hard for the child to cough it up. This kind of cough can take a while to clear and to stop sounding so awful. The remedies are: **Antimonium Tart, Hepar Sulph, Ipecacuanha, Kali Sulph, Lycopodium,** and **Pulsatilla.**

Spasmodic coughs come in fits of uncontrollable, violent, and prolonged coughing. The remedies are: **Carbo Veg, Coccus Cacti, Cuprum Metal, Drosera, Ignatia,** and **Ipecacuanha.**

Identifying the sound of a cough:

For **"machine-gun coughs"** that repeat frequently in rapid succession: **Drosera, Coccus Cacti**

Spells of rapid coughing: Rumex

Barking sound like a seal: Aconitum, Hepar Sulph

Sounds **like a saw** being driven through a pine board: **Spongia Tosta**

Hissing, with hoarseness: Antimonium Tart

With **rattling in the chest: Antimonium Tart, Coccus Cacti**

Chest infections

A chest infection can lead to various other serious conditions. Fever is associated with all of these at some point. You can look to the "Fevers" section (page 182) for further detail and to verify the best remedy.

A course of antibiotics is the preferred orthodox treatment for chest infection. Even if the condition is viral rather than bacterial, doctors want to prevent opportunistic bacteria from colonizing the already-compromised lungs. The viruses and bacteria take hold of the body because of prior susceptibility—being run down, highly stressed out, severely depressed, deeply grieved, out of balance, or sleep-deprived. Chest infections can quickly turn into serious conditions in those who are hereditarily susceptible, or in a weak infant, a teen who smokes, or someone on long-term medication.

It is most significant how the body signals its distress by producing a particular set of symptoms. The diagnosis of chest infection is generally applied to a cough with mucus in the lungs, and is usually the result of not taking enough care in the initial stages of a common cold.

Croup

Croup is an inflammation of the larynx, trachea, and sometimes also the bronchi. The air passages become narrowed by swollen mucous membranes. This gives the cough a croupy, metallic, or barking sound. The cough is sometimes described as the sound of a barking seal, or a high-pitched, hoarse dog barking. It is usually brought on by a cold or influenza in children six months to four years old.

Croup usually starts with hoarseness, and may or may not be accompanied by fever. It often starts suddenly around midnight: The child wakes in a panic because of trouble breathing; then they begin coughing. If the cough is severe, they may gag or choke. Croup is usually much worse at night and less severe during the day. It requires careful watching in the very young because the symptoms can change rapidly.

To ensure that the airways are kept open, prop the child up with a pillow. Make sure that fluid intake is kept high. You may warmly wrap the child, e.g., in a hat, mittens, and socks, completely covered in warmth, and take them into the cool night air for about five minutes. This reduces swelling in the airways. *Do not take them out if it is bitter cold, as this can shock the lungs.* A cool-mist vaporizer in the child's room can also be helpful.

If the child has been coughing and gagging for more than twenty-four hours despite initial homeopathic treatment, call your healthcare practitioner. A child who has croup several times, or does not get rid of the cough in between bouts, needs to be evaluated by your healthcare practitioner. Occasionally a child will not respond to indicated remedies, and the symptoms of croup become so alarming that hospitalization becomes the only course to take. (See the final notes in "Call your healthcare practitioner if" at the end of this section, and inform yourself about epiglottitis.)

As stated above, croup often starts suddenly around midnight. This indicates **Aconitum** as an initial remedy, but there are other symptoms that point to it as well—heat, anxiety, restlessness, or hoarseness; if the cough is dry and barking like a seal, or breaths are short and difficult. Two pellets will often ease the symptoms immediately. If symptoms persist, repeat in half an hour.

If there are no results, and the child's breathing sounds harsh, is becoming more labored, and the cough persists, give 2 pellets of **Spongia Tosta** and wait another half-hour. If your child is not asleep by then, and the breathing is still not easy and coughing continues, give 2 pellets of **Hepar Sulph.**

The main remedies for croup are **Aconitum, Hepar Sulph,** and **Spongia Tosta.** There are a few others in the cough section below. If there are no results from the above remedies, look to other remedies: **Arsenicum, Belladonna, Iodium, Ipecacuanha, Kali Bich, Lachesis, Phosphorus,** or **Rumex.**

Whooping Cough

This information is here because there have been many cases where a child develops whooping cough even after having been immunized with the DTaP vaccine (the "P" stands for pertussis, the medical term for whooping cough).

Note: *Do not attempt to treat whooping cough in a child under one year old. Seek professional help.*

Whooping cough, or pertussis, is caused by Bordetella pertussis bacteria. The "whoop" sound is a hoarse intake of breath at the end of a bout of coughing. The bacteria emit toxins that paralyze the cilia in the lungs. The cilia are like tiny hairs that line the respiratory openings. Because of the paralysis, inflammation sets in, which interferes with the clearing of normal mucus. Thick, sticky mucus builds up and produces a gagging cough.

The incubation period of whooping cough is seven to ten days. Infected children are contagious from onset up to twenty-one days after coughing has begun. Whooping cough was once known as the "hundred-day cough" because that was the typical period from onset to full recovery.

This cough is more likely to occur in the spring or summer. It usually starts with a low-grade fever, sneezing, a runny nose, and a loose cough that is worse at night. This may continue up to two weeks. The child may also be achy, and have low energy, a loss of appetite, watery eyes, and earaches. Then the mucus becomes thick, and the child cannot cough it up. The coughing fits often end in gagging and vomiting. There may be eight to ten coughs per breath. The child's face can become blue, due to the long coughing bouts and shortness of breath. There may be a look of terror on the child's face because the severity of the cough, being unable to catch their breath, or the pain of coughing causing fear and dread. This stage can last up to six weeks.

Whooping cough requires calm observation and patience. It is a long and tiring condition for both child and parent. Remedy pictures can change unexpectedly, and it is best to have expert help if the coughing persists. It is really advisable to have help from a homeopath for this condition and/or stay in close contact with your healthcare provider to provide your child with the utmost comfort. It is rare for complications to occur in a child over one year old. However, it is important to monitor progress very carefully, because the cough can become violent and damage the lungs. In the very young, it can also cause a hernia in the navel or a bowel prolapse. Complications can include pneumothorax, or collapsed lung (which requires emergency hospital treatment), pleurisy, or pneumonia. If the child persistently cries after coughing, or a sudden high fever develops, then you must seek professional help immediately. Again, this is rare—but one needs to be observant and use good judgment.

There are many remedies for whooping cough, and it is not unusual for the child to need more than two of them. The most usual choices are: **Antimonium Tart, Bryonia, Carbo Veg, Coccus Cacti, Cuprum Metal, Drosera, Ipecac, Lycopodium, Nux Vomica, Phosphorus,** and **Spongia Tosta.**

What to observe:

Based on the above explanations, what kind of cough does the child have? What is the sound of the cough—rattling, deep, hoarse, ringing, hacking, like a machine gun, hollow, or barking? Is the cough worse or better from: talking, movement, sitting up or lying down, day or night, cool or warm air, dry or moist air, hot or cold drinks, or being inside or outside? What is the sound of the child's breathing—wheezy, labored, or squeaky? If the child coughs up mucus, does it have a specific taste—metallic, sweet, or salty? Is the child taking short shallow breaths? What color is the mucus, if they can cough it up? Is it lumpy, frothy, or stringy? Do they have a sore throat? Is there a tickling in the throat? What is the child's mood? Does the child want warm or cold drinks or food, or no food or drink at all? Is the child experiencing a fever or a headache? Take their temperature.

The following are the most commonly indicated remedies for coughs:

Aconitum: Onset is sudden, from getting chilled by icy north or east winds, or from a shock or fright. This remedy is most useful in the first twenty-four hours and at the very first sign of symptoms. **Constant barking, dry, hacking, hoarse cough** around midnight. Air passages are irritated and burning. Breathing becomes quick and strained, especially on the in-breath. The child may grasp at the throat while coughing. Thirst for cold water. Waves of chills run through the body. The pupils are usually small, and the eyes have a glassy appearance. The child is fearful, may have an anguished, anxious, or shocked expression. They are restless and hard to console. The older child may fear that they are dying.

Croup remedy: For croup, unless there are symptoms clearly pointing to a different remedy, give this one first. It is for hoarse, dry, coughs with a loud, sharp quality. The child becomes panicked because it is hard to take a normal breath during the coughing attack. If your child has asthma and you are having trouble discerning between croup or an asthma attack, consult your healthcare practitioner or go to an urgent-care facility or emergency room.

Worse from: Midnight, noise, pressure, motion, light, warm rooms, touch, and dry cold air. **Better from:** Fresh air, rest, and hot applications.

Antimonium Tart: Onset after a cold or flu that has not responded to rest and care, or from anger. This is a **moist cough.** It is a **suffocating, loud, wheezy, rattling cough** with much mucus in the lungs, but little or no mucus that is brought up by coughing. Rattling sounds on both the in- and out-breaths. The child is left gasping for air and panting after coughing bouts. They must sit up to cough and catch their breath. It is very characteristic for the child to bend backwards to cough. Face is cold, pale, and bluish, with cold sweat.

The child may have nausea with a sinking feeling in the stomach, and vomit food and mucus. After coughing and vomiting the child is pale, sleepy, and nonreactive. The child is thirsty for cold water, drinking little and often. They become weak and weary to the point where it is hard to cough. Anger will increase their coughing bouts. The child is whiny, moaning, irritable, and wants to be left alone—not touched, looked at, or examined. However, they have a fear of being alone.

Whooping-cough remedy: For a cough excited by anger, and after eating. Rapid, short, labored breathing with much coughing and gasping for air. Loud sounds of mucus rattling in chest. There is so much mucus that you can even feel it when touching their chest. There is nausea, vomiting, and gagging, with the cough eventually bringing up mucus that has been swallowed. The child bends the head backwards when coughing.

Worse from: Evening and night, warm rooms, anger, during sleep, eating, cold, damp, lying down, sour food, and warm drinks. **Better from:** Getting the mucus out, sitting erect, motion, burping, vomiting, cool open air, and lying on the right side.

Arsenicum: Onset from getting chilled, after overheating or overexertion, or wet weather. **Short, dry, hacking, loose cough with very little mucus.** The small amount of mucus brought up is frothy, and may be blood-flecked and taste salty. The child is unable to lie down and must sit up, especially to cough. Rapid, whistling, and wheezy breathing, with shortness of breath. Tickling and sensation of sulphur vapors in the larynx. Cough is dry at night, and loose during the day. The chest feels either burning or cold.

The child likes frequent sips of water to lubricate their dry mouth and throat. They cannot bear the sight, smell, or thought of food. Their sleep is restless, and they may sleep with their hands above their head. The older child wants order and neatness around them. It actually makes them feel better if their room is tidy. The baby needing this remedy will want to be carried or rocked in an invigorating way. (However, do not shake the baby.) These children are restless and anxious to the point of fearing death.

Worse from: Midnight to 2 AM, lying down, especially on their back, drinking, laughing, odors, cold damp air, and ascending.

Better from: Sitting up and being propped up with lots of pillows, hot drinks, heat, dry hot applications, and sweating.

Belladonna: Onset is sudden, from cold dry winds, or getting chilled when head is wet. **Dry, short, hacking, violent cough,** with tickling in the trachea, that comes in fits and is exhausting and tormenting. Breathing will be short, shallow, and rapid. Nose and throat are dry, with tickling and burning in throat. Larynx is sore and feels as if there is a foreign body in it. Cough can be violent enough to cause bloodshot eyes. Pupils are dilated. The face is red, with radiant heat from the head. The mouth and breath are likely to be hot as well.

The child may cry before coughing, from anticipating the sharp, needle-like chest pains. Voice is hoarse or lost. The older child may grind the teeth, or crave lemonade. The child may have a fierce look on their face. They are irritable, and all senses are acute and heightened. They can become agitated to the point of biting, screaming, and hitting.

Whooping-cough remedy: For a barking cough, which may turn into a **spasmodic cough** that is worse from lying down. Pain in stomach just before coughing. Head feels as if it is going to burst open when coughing. Very little mucus is raised, which makes the larynx even drier. This sets up more tickling, and the cough becomes more violent, sometimes causing gagging that can end in vomiting.

Worse from: Nighttime, yawning, deep breathing, cold air, touch, noise, odors, jarring, light, fine dust in the air, and around 3 PM. **Better from:** Rest, light covering, sitting semi-erect, low lights, and quiet.

Bryonia: Onset from cold winds. **Hard, dry, wracking, painful cough** from a crawling, tickling sensation in the upper trachea. Every time the child moves, they cough. They will sit up and hold the chest when they cough. Coughing makes them feel like their chest is going to fly to pieces. Sharp, needle-like pains in the chest or under the right shoulder blade.

The child is short of breath, but deep breaths bring on coughing fits. They cannot bring up any mucus without much hawking and trying to clear the throat. Mucus may be blood-streaked. Great dryness, especially of lips and mouth. The child is thirsty for large quantities of liquids at a time. They may have dry constipation, and/or soreness in stomach while coughing. If there is a headache, coughing makes the head feel as if it might split open. Cough with sneezing. Child does not want to be carried or moved. Any movement aggravates them. They are very grumpy.

Whooping-cough remedy: For a **dry and spasmodic cough** that makes the child's whole body shake. Eating and drinking lead to gagging, retching, and vomiting. This child needs to have small quantities of food and drink at a time; encourage the child to eat and drink very slowly. Child does not want to be touched.

Worse from: Eating, drinking, any movement, around 9 PM, coming from outside into a warm room, deep breathing, touch, and warm food or drink. **Better from:** No movement, rest, pressure, quiet, cool open air, and drawing knees to chest.

Calc Fluorica: Onset from becoming chilled in cold, damp weather, and from changes in the weather.

Croup remedy: For a **spasmodic cough.** The child will cough up tiny lumps of yellow mucus. There is much tickling and irritation in the lungs. They have difficulty breathing, as if the throat is getting closed off.

Worse from: Lying down, motion, cold, wet, damp weather, and changes of weather. **Better from:** Rubbing, warm applications, continuous motion, and heat.

Carbo Veg: Onset from extremes of temperatures, frosty air, warm damp weather, wind on the head, or if they did not fully recover from a previous illness. Heavy, burning, sore, or weak feeling in the chest on waking. **Hollow, choking, spasmodic cough.** The mucus that comes up is thick, sticky, and yellow-green. Breathing is labored, fast, short, and wheezing, especially after a coughing fit. The breath is cold, but the child feels hot and thirsty, and wants to be fanned. Hoarseness that is worse in the evening. Sensation of sulphur fumes in the larynx. This child is weak and low in vitality. They are exhausted by even the slightest exertion. The child will be indifferent to everything, a bit confused, irritable, and sluggish.

Whooping-cough remedy: Cough is dry and spasmodic. Every coughing fit brings up a lump of mucus. The body can be ice-cold, especially the limbs. Cold sweat on face. Child becomes blue in the face when coughing. There is gagging and vomiting from coughing. The child is utterly exhausted. If your child is having a hard time responding to you, call your healthcare practitioner.

Worse from: Warmth and warm rooms, on waking, evening, walking, open air, eating, talking, and change of temperature. **Better from:** Being fanned vigorously, rest, and elevating the feet.

Causticum: Onset from dry cold air, drafts, air conditioning, or extremes of temperature. **Incessant, dry, deep, hard cough** with a feeling that they cannot cough deeply enough. Cough with hoarseness that is worse in the morning. Shortness of breath before coughing. Mucus is soapy and greasy; it slips back down and cannot be coughed up. Chest is tight and sore, with a scraping sensation. Rawness and burning in throat and trachea. The cough wakes the child at night. There may be involuntary urination on coughing. The least aggravation will make the child cry. They are sensitive, anxious, and irritable. They may not want to go to bed alone, and may be fearful of the dark or ghosts.

Worse from: Between 3–4 AM and 6–8 PM, stooping, exertion, and darkness. **Better from:** Sipping cold water, damp wet weather, pressure on chest, warmth of bed, and gentle motion.

Chamomilla: Onset from cold damp air and wind. **Dry, tickling, irritating cough** with bad temper. Rattling mucus in chest. Mucus brought up in the daytime is bitter-tasting. Suffocating tightness in chest. The child coughs during sleep, but cough does not wake them. Hoarseness and rawness in larynx. Anger provokes the cough. One cheek is usually red (or a red patch) and hot, and the other cheek is pale. This symptom can be subtle or very obvious. Child is fretful, sensitive to pain, and angry. Nothing pleases this child—they want to be held, but are only comforted for a short time. Put them down, and soon they want to be held again. They scream for something, and when it is handed to them they reject it or throw it down. They are extremely irritable. Babies want to be carried around.

Worse from: Between 9–12 PM, anger, and during sleep. **Better from:** Bending head back, patience, and being carried or rocked.

Coccus Cacti: Onset from cold air and cold wind. **Spasmodic, irritating, hacking, and tickling cough.** The child may feel like they are choking because there is so much mucus. Profuse postnasal discharge, but the throat can feel dry. They are constantly clearing their throat. They feel as though there is a thread hanging down the back of the throat. Face goes purple or red from coughing. There is much internal heat, with perspiration. Brushing teeth causes the child to cough. The child feels sad and lethargic.

Whooping-cough remedy: Spasmodic cough on first waking, ending in vomiting long, clear strings of mucus that hang from mouth. The child holds their breath for fear of another coughing attack. They may have a headache that feels as though the head is going to split open. Child is sad at 6 AM or from 2–3 PM.

Note: A drink of cold water can prevent a coughing fit. Keep a glass of it nearby. Keep their room cool.

Worse from: On waking, spending the night in a hot bed, heat, lying down, brushing teeth, morning, and wind. **Better from:** Cool air, cold drinks, walking, washing in cool water, light covering, yawning, leaning forward, and clearing mucus.

Cuprum Metal: Onset from cold air and cold wind. **Violent, spasmodic cough.** Long bouts of coughing attacks, often three at a time. Cough comes and goes at irregular intervals. Child coughs so hard that they are breathless and cannot talk, with trembling in the fingers and toes. The breath may be fast and panting. Voice may be hoarse, especially in cold air. Painful constrictions in chest. Metallic taste in the mouth. The child may stiffen. The hands and feet are usually cold. The child is nervous, uneasy, is restless in bed, and can have attacks of rage, biting and tearing things apart. Their laughter can be convulsive. They do not want people near them.

Whooping-cough remedy: When there are prolonged coughing fits that leave the child exhausted and breathless. Violent spasms in the larynx. The child gasps repeatedly, to the point that the face may have a dark-blue tint. The skin can have a bluish tint generally. There is mucus in the trachea. This cough can be so intense that it causes the child to stop breathing, stiffen, and go into convulsions or seizures. *If this is the case, seek medical help immediately.* Also see **Ipecacuanha** (below).

Worse from: Bending backwards, laughing, talking, touch, motion, deep breathing in cold air, around 3 AM, eating, and hiccups.
Better from: Sipping cold drinks, perspiration, and lying quietly.

Drosera: This is for a **spasmodic, tickling, hacking, rough, scraping, and barking cough.** The cough is **rapid, deep and incessant.** Bouts may last two or three hours. It sounds as if it is coming up from the belly. The child usually starts coughing as soon as their head hits the pillow at night; however, there is little or no coughing during the day. There is tickling in the throat, as from a stuck crumb or a feather. The trachea feels dry. Cough is dry at night. The older child has to hold their chest with both hands while coughing because of the pain, and a feeling that the chest needs support. Many times the cough ends with gagging. Constriction and pain in throat, larynx, chest, and sometimes stomach. Deep hoarseness that makes it hard to talk. Yellow mucus that may have streaks of blood. Chilliness with shivering and cold sweats. The child is anxious, irritable, extremely restless, and easily angered, but always wants someone around them.

Whooping-cough remedy: For coughing that causes breathlessness and comes in quick succession. Yellow mucus is coughed up in the morning. Fever with headache. May have nosebleeds with the cough. Every attempt to bring up mucus ends in severe retching and vomiting. The area below the ribs becomes very painful from the coughing. The chest feels tight and seized-up, to the point of not being able to talk or exhale.

Note: If your child's symptoms clearly match this description, be patient. This is a slow, deep-acting remedy. You may not see improvement in the cough for three to four days. However, this remedy will immediately help the severe vomiting, so that the child can keep food down and not lose weight.

Worse from: Laughing, talking, crying, cold food, becoming too warm in bed, lying down, vomiting, evening time and after midnight, and cold food or drink. **Better from:** Pressure and open air.

Hepar Sulph: Onset from getting too cold, or from a cold wind. This is a **moist, loose, choking, rattling cough** that comes in fits, which may end in gagging. There is much thick, yellow mucus that usually smells like old cheese. The child cries before coughing. They sweat easily during the cough. There is a rattling sound in the chest, difficult breathing, and a feeling of weakness. They are hoarse and usually lose their voice. The larynx is painful and very sensitive to cold air and any drafts. They want to be wrapped up, and cannot bear to have any part uncovered. Even putting an arm out of the covers will cause a coughing fit. The child is angry, irritable, and oversensitive, especially to pain. Make sure your hands are warm when touching this child.

Croup remedy: This follows **Aconitum** well, and is a good remedy for recurrent croup. The cough is **loose, choking, rattling, and wheezy in the day, but dry at night.** It is worse when breathing very cold air. Even though the cough is loose, the child has a hard time expectorating mucus out. The child's voice is low and weak.

Worse from: Evening until midnight, cold drinks or food, cold dry air, cold drafts, lying on the left side, being uncovered, pressure, and touch. **Better from:** Heat, wrapping up, bending the head back, moist heat, and damp weather.

Ignatia: Onset can be from a big emotional upset, especially grief or shock, or getting overly angry. Cough often comes on after a sore throat. **Dry, hacking, choking, spasmodic coughs in quick succession.** Coughing makes the child cough even more. (This is the only cough that has this odd symptom.) They take deep breaths for relief. Child is sleepy after a coughing fit. They cough as if they have inhaled dust or strong fumes. Tickling in throat, with constriction, aching, and shooting pains in chest. The child speaks in whispers, with much deep sighing. The child is very sensitive to pain, and is moody, quarrelsome, and tearful. They want to be alone, and do not want to be consoled.

Worse from: Evening, emotions, worry, fright, grief, touch, cold fresh air, walking, and lying down. **Better from:** Deep breathing, swallowing, eating, changing positions, warmth, and being left alone.

Iodium:

Croup remedy (only): **Dry, barking, spasmodic, hoarse, tickling cough.** Tickling, rawness, and dryness in trachea and chest. Larynx is dry, tight, painful, and constricted, making the child grasp the throat while coughing. Hoarseness and loss of voice. Breathing is difficult, and there is much wheezing. The mucus is hard to expectorate, and may be blood-streaked. After coughing, the child feels weak and may tremble. Glands in the neck are swollen and hard. They always feel cold to the touch, but hot externally. They may have a high and prolonged fever, and/or sweat easily. The child is anxious, worried, restless, weak, tearful, and in a bad mood.

Worse from: Heat, exertion, wet weather, warm rooms, too many covers, touch, pressure, lying on the back, and mornings. **Better from:** Cold fresh air, walking in open air, sitting up, eating, and bathing.

Ipecacuanha: This remedy is for feeble children who catch cold in warm, wet weather, or for colds with an onset from overeating candy, fruits, or ice cream. Cough is **incessant, wheezy, spasmodic, moist, and violent.** Constant constriction in chest and larynx, shortness of breath, and gasping for air. Sneezing with much mucus. The chest seems full of mucus, but it is not loosened by coughing. Oversensitivity to heat and cold. Child may have a nosebleed with bright-red blood. They feel hot inside, and cold externally. These children are anxious and demanding, and scream when they don't get what they want. They are easily frustrated, crying and screaming, and almost nothing pleases them.

Whooping-cough remedy: Violent, hollow cough that makes

the child short of breath. They turn pale, and the whole body goes rigid and stiff. The face is blue. Cough ends in gagging and vomiting of mucus that may be blood-streaked. There is much nausea, especially at the smell of food. They can bleed from the nose or mouth.

Worse from: The least motion, overeating, warmth, dampness, lying down, rich foods, and vomiting. **Better from:** Rest, inhaling cool air while warmly wrapped, open air, pressure, closing eyes, cold drinks, and expelling mucus.

Kali Bich:

Croup remedy (only): Onset from getting chilled. **Hard, dry, tickling, and metallic-sounding cough.** This cough has been described as sounding like a flag flapping back and forth in a high wind. Wheezy breathing. Tickling in larynx. Painful cough that radiates into back and shoulders. Raw, sore, and bruise-like pain in chest, and a feeling as if there is a bar across the chest. Air passages are very irritated. There are long strings of thick, sticky, and yellow mucus that are very hard to cough up. Mucus is easier to expectorate in the morning. Suffocating gagging. Much clearing of the throat. Voice becomes hoarse. The child is sluggish, weak, and a bit lethargic.

Worse from: On waking in morning, cold damp open air, stooping, sitting, and eating. **Better from:** Warmth, being wrapped up, motion, pressure, and getting mucus out.

Kali Sulph:

Whooping cough remedy (only): Onset from getting chilled after being overheated. This is for a **moist cough with much rattling and wheezing that ends in gagging,** though the child usually does not vomit. Thick, slimy, deep-yellow or yellow-green mucus that is difficult to cough up. The mucus comes up into the throat and is swallowed back down again. Tongue is coated with yellow, slimy mucus. Voice may be hoarse. Child dreads coughing, and weeps. They are angry, anxious, and irritable, and will ask for something and then reject it.

Worse from: Heated stuffy rooms, evening, and noise. **Better from:** Motion, walking, and cool fresh air.

Lachesis:

Croup remedy (only): Onset is usually in cloudy spring weather. **Choking, dry, and tickling cough.** The child has a sensation of strangulation and suffocation on dropping off to sleep, which makes them afraid to go to sleep. However, once they are asleep, the cough does not usually wake them. They feel a need to take a deep breath of cool air. Larynx is painful to touch, and feels pressure after sleeping. May lose voice. Cannot bear to have anything around the neck, or have the front of the neck touched. Sensation of a plug moving up and down with cough. Retching with no production of mucus. The child is anxious, nervous, excitable, very talkative, rambling on and on, and sensitive to touch and pain.

Worse from: Lying down, nighttime, on waking, on falling asleep, swallowing liquids, and hot drinks. **Better from:** Cold drinks, eating, especially fruits, and loose clothing, especially around the neck and waist.

Lycopodium: Onset from wet weather. Cough is **deep, moist, rattling, hollow, and tickling.** It feels as if there is a feather in the larynx. The child coughs day and night, and the cough and throat tickle disturb their sleep. There is irritation in the trachea, and short, rattling breaths. Profuse production of thick, yellow or greenish mucus with a salty taste that is difficult to cough up. Tight chest, with burning and constricted sensation. This child is very likely to be gassy and bloated. They are weak and chilly, but crave air. They are sensitive to noise and strong smells. These children are irritable and temperamental. They will kick, scream, and throw tantrums. They are difficult to deal with, and react strongly if contradicted.

Worse from: Between 4 and 8 (both AM and PM), on falling asleep, lying on the back, deep breathing, wet weather, warm rooms, going downhill, and after naps or on waking. **Better from:** Warm drinks and food, motion, early afternoon, and cool applications.

Nux Vomica: Onset is brought on by cold, dry, and windy weather. The mucus is thick and tastes sour. **DRY, violent, tickling**

cough, with tight chest, which exhausts the child. Tickling in larynx brings on a coughing fit. Cough is violent and may bring on a splitting headache. During coughing, it feels like something is tearing loose in the chest. The chest and the larynx feel painfully raw, and breathing is shallow and difficult. The voice is usually hoarse. The child will shiver if uncovered, or with movement. They are easily frustrated, which makes them cry. They are very touchy, irritable, and easily offended. They are oversensitive to noise, odors, lights, and loud music.

Worse from: Exertion, being uncovered, lying on the back, eating, and drafts. **Better from:** Warmth, being wrapped up, moist air, hot drinks, belching, quiet, and not moving the chest.

Phosphorus: Onset from getting drenched in rain, or from changes in weather. This remedy is often needed when the common cold moves into the chest. The cough is **hard, dry, tight, painful, racking, tickling, and exhausting.** Cough is **dry at first, and then becomes loose.** A tickling sensation in the throat triggers the cough. Cough creates rawness and burning from the throat to the bottom of the ribcage. The mucus is frothy, yellow, and sometimes blood-streaked, especially in the morning. It may taste sweet, sour, or salty. The cough is dry at night.

The child feels as though there is a heavy weight pressing on their chest, with tightness, burning, and much dry heat. The larynx is raw, sore, painful on talking, and feels as though it is splitting apart during a coughing fit. Hoarse and low voice. Child's whole body trembles with a coughing fit. Labored breathing with the least exertion. The child is wakened at night from the cough, and sits up to cough. There is a thirst for ice-cold drinks. Even with a fever, this child can be running around as if nothing is wrong, and then they go down hard. So you may want to keep them resting until you are sure of a complete recovery. This child is affectionate, fearful, easily upset, and irritable.

Croup remedy: This remedy is especially useful for relapsing croup, or if no other remedies have worked. The child has increased thirst for cold or iced drinks, fever, sore throat, and great weakness. They are worse in the evenings.

Whooping-cough remedy: Cough may end in retching, which causes pain in abdomen, and exhaustion. They must sit up to cough. Suffocated breathing.

Worse from: Change of weather, cold air, cold wind, cold thunderstorms, evening, strong fumes, light, exertion, lying on the left side, talking, laughing, and going from cold air into a warm room, or vice versa. **Better from:** Sleep, pressure on chest, warmth, attention, sympathy, light massage, open air, company, low lights or darkness, eating and drinking cold things, cool applications, sitting, and sleeping on the right side.

Pulsatilla: For a cold with onset from getting feet wet and becoming chilled, or for use at the end of a **Pulsatilla** cold that has progressed into a cough. The cough is both moist and dry, irritating, racking, and coming in fits. The cough keeps changing symptoms: The child has a **dry, hacking, tickling cough at night, but a loose and rattling cough during the day.** On waking, they have lots of mucus that is thick, yellow or green, gooey, bitter-tasting, and hard to cough up.

The child's breathing becomes loud and rattling as the night wears on, and wakes them. They sit up to cough. They have a smothering sensation, and anxiety on lying down. Hoarseness comes and goes, and the larynx becomes raw. They get short of breath in warm rooms, and feel pressure and soreness in the chest. They usually have no thirst. They may gag on coughing, and complain of nausea. These children are weepy, whiny, want to be carried or held, and feel noticeably better in fresh air. Just as their symptoms change, so will their mood.

Worse from: Lying down, especially on the left side, warm stuffy rooms, evening and nighttime, getting overheated, and fatty or rich foods. The child must avoid milk, though they may crave it. **Better from:** Cool fresh air, cold applications, sympathy, gentle motion, attention, and being propped up in a semi-erect position.

Rumex: Onset from cold air or changes in weather. **Suffocating, dry, tickling, painful, and choking cough that prevents sleep.** This cough starts with an incessant tickling in the throat. Every breath of cold air causes the tickling, as from a feather in the throat. Trachea and beneath collarbones feel burning, raw, and sore with pressure. They either cough in short fitful spurts or hack continuously. Lots of frothy, thin, stringy mucus that gets stuck in the back of the throat. If you gently press the outside of the throat under the Adam's apple and it produces a coughing fit, this is a strong indication for this remedy. If you have to take this child out in the cold, give them a scarf to hold against their nose and mouth to prevent coughing. Child becomes quite serious, low-spirited, indifferent to their surroundings, and restless in the evening.

Worse from: Around 11 PM, 2 AM, and 5 AM; touching throat pit, lying down, especially on the left side, changes in temperature, talking, deep breathing, inhaling cold air, undressing, being uncovered, pressure, talking, and motion. **Better from:** Covering mouth and nose, wrapping up, daytime, and sucking on non-mentholated lozenges, e.g., black-currant pastilles or lemon drops.

Spongia Tosta: Onset from dry, cold winds, or too much excitement. **Dry, constant, hollow, barking cough** that sounds like a saw going through dry wood. Everything is dry—mucous membranes, tongue, throat, and all air passages. There is soreness, burning, dryness, constriction, bruised pain, and the feeling of a plug in the larynx. The child wakes with violent coughing spasms, sweating, gasping for breath, and possibly with blue lips, feeling anxious and fearful that they are suffocating. There is a sensation of trying to breathe through a dry sponge. Mucus accumulates in the chest but cannot be brought up. The child is hoarse and can hardly talk because of weakness in the chest. Voice may give way while talking. Chest feels sore, very heavy, and bruised from coughing. Child has much anxiety, exhaustion, and is easily excitable.

Croup remedy: This remedy follows **Aconitum** and **Hepar Sulph** well. The cough is **barking and hollow-sounding,** and may be brought on just by taking in a breath of air. Chest sounds noisy and whistling. Cold drinks make the cough worse. The child wakes with burning in the chest and throat, and is anxious.

163

Worse from: Before midnight, becoming overheated, lying down in a warm room, dry cold wind, after sleep, touch, singing, too much excitement, during day, swallowing, talking, cold drinks, sweets, exertion, and the full moon. **Better from:** Warm drinks, eating small amounts of warm food, calm and quiet, lying with head low, bending forward, and moist heat.

Sticta Pulmonaria: Onset from sudden changes of temperature. **Dry, hacking, incessant, and tickling cough that prevents sleep.** Coughing and even inhaling bring on more coughing. Mucus loosens in the morning, and the cough is better during the day. There is a feeling of fullness at the root of the nose (where the roof of the mouth meets the top of the throat). The mucous membranes are painful and dry, and may feel numb. Tickling in throat, larynx, and bronchi. Breathing is oppressed. This cough lingers after colds, flu, and whooping cough. Pains in chest radiate into the back, or on the right side down to the abdomen. The child feels dull and fatigued, but talks a lot. They may feel as if they are floating in the air.

Worse from: Evening into nighttime, coughing, change of temperature, lying, inhaling, getting overly tired, and motion. **Better from:** Open air.

Dosage: If the onset is fast, give 2 pellets every 15 minutes for four doses, then hourly until there is improvement. If there has been no improvement after seven doses, choose a new remedy. If the onset has been slow, give the remedy every 1–2 hours for six doses. Repeat the remedy only if there is a return of the same symptoms. Repeat only as necessary.

You may need to keep repeating the remedy 2–3 times per day for several days. If you get no result within two days, then reassess the symptoms. You may not have been wrong with your choice, but the condition may have moved on to needing a different remedy. Change the remedy if you have followed the above guidelines with no results, or if the symptoms clearly change. For instance, Belladonna may be needed initially, but as hours or days go by, symptoms may indicate that Hepar Sulph is needed instead.

Supportive Measures:

Let the child get extra rest. Push fluids, even if they only take a few sips at a time. This will help to keep the mucus loose. Do not force the child to eat if they are not hungry. Giving the digestive system a rest encourages the body to eliminate toxic wastes. If the child asks for food, give a light diet, low in sugar and high in vitamin C, and avoid stimulants such as cola or tea.

Even if the chest is sore, encourage the child to cough; this will help to get the mucus out. Use a vaporizer (cool or hot) depending on the type of cough. If you don't have a vaporizer, give a steam treatment by running very hot water from the shower or tub spout in a closed bathroom, and have the child breathe in slow, comfortably deep breaths in there. Keep the temperature even.

If you take the child outdoors, make sure they are bundled up well. Do not repress a cough with any form of cough medicine; this blocks the immune system's natural way of expelling mucus and preventing a deeper infection. Cough medicines make the child feel better temporarily because most of them contain about 25% alcohol. With some coughs, it is helpful for the child to be propped up with pillows in a semi-erect position. Always look in "Worse from" or "Better from" for tips on what will make the child feel more comfortable; e.g., if a cough is worse lying on the back, encourage the child to lie on their side.

For tickling coughs in children over three years old, you can use lozenges that do not contain camphor, menthol, or eucalyptus, e.g., black-currant pastilles or lemon drops. Discontinue or keep dairy products to a minimum, as they cause excess mucus. Humidify the room if your home has forced-air heating. Do not use any rubs or oils containing eucalyptus, menthol, camphor, or tea tree oil. These herbs can nullify homeopathic remedies.

Homemade cough treatments:

- Lemon, honey, and glycerin are soothing for coughs that are tickling and teasing. Squeeze half a lemon into a half-cup of warm (not boiling) water. Add one teaspoon of honey and two teaspoons of glycerin. Please use pharmaceutical-grade glycerin from a pharmacy. Give one-teaspoon doses as needed.

- Thyme is traditionally used for coughs and lung problems. Make a tea by pouring one cup of boiling water over one teaspoonful of leaves and flower tops, if you have them. Brew for ten to fifteen minutes. One old recipe calls for a pinch of rosemary as well. Strain off the leaves, and add honey to taste.

- For a moist cough, drink ginger tea: Boil three to four slices of fresh ginger in two cups of water, and simmer for fifteen minutes. Licorice root tea is also good for moist coughs.

Call your healthcare practitioner if:

- Pains in the chest become persistent, especially if they are present when not coughing.
- Sharp pains shoot through the chest area when the child is moving around.
- Coughing produces blood-streaked mucus.
- A fever develops, especially when chills alternate with heat and intermittent sweating.
- Wheezing and rattling in the chest causes difficult breathing.
- There is hyperventilation (rapid breathing) or sleep apnea (breathing stops during sleep).

Call your healthcare practitioner if (cont):

- The face goes blue with the effort of coughing or breathing.
- Nausea and vomiting accompany gagging when coughing.
- There is a loss of appetite over a period of several days.
- Your child becomes excessively fatigued, or is not sleeping, because of the coughing.
- A cough lasts more than three days in an infant, or eight days in an older child.
- The cough is severe, the child can't sleep because of it, and no remedies have helped within forty-eight hours.
- Your child has a chronic cough, or a cough that does not originate from a cold or flu. Chronic coughs can be from allergies, asthma, liver problems, accidents that may have caused structural problems affecting the lungs, passive or active smoking, or a long-un-expressed emotional cause, usually grief. There may not always be a cough in children with pneumonia. *Go to the hospital if your child has a fever, is breathing rapidly, erratically or with difficulty, or is limp, lethargic, and very pale.*
- There is a high fever, rapid swelling in the larynx, or excessive drooling on the pillow because the child cannot swallow. This points to a condition called epiglottitis that affects 2–6 year olds; it is rare, but can be fatal if the airway becomes too swollen and closes off. The swelling initially causes a croupy-sounding cough, and can rapidly close the airway. Inhaling causes a raspy, noisy sound. *If you suspect this condition, take your child to the emergency room immediately.*

THE SEVEN MOST COMMON REMEDIES FOR DRY COUGHS

	Arsenicum	Belladonna	Bryonia	Nux Vomica	Phosphorus	Rumex	Spongia Tosta
Onset	Getting chilled, wet weather, getting overheated, or from overexertion.	Sudden onset from cold, dry winds, or getting chilled when head is wet.	Slow onset. Getting chilled from a cold wind, especially in spring, autumn.	Getting chilled in cold, dry, windy weather.	Onset slow and steady, from getting drenched in rain.	Onset from changes in weather, or from getting chilled in cold air.	Getting chilled from dry, cold winds, or from getting overexcited.
Symptoms	Short, hacking, tickling cough that is dry at night and loose during the day. The child sits up to cough. Wants frequent sips of water.	Violent, hacking, tormenting, exhausting cough that comes in fits. Tickling in the trachea.	Painful, tickling cough that makes the stomach sore, aggravated by movement; child sits up to cough.	Violent, tickling, exhausting cough with splitting headache.	Cough is dry, then later is loose. Cough is painful, racking, tickling, and exhausting. Child wakes at night and has to sit up to cough. Tickling sensation in throat triggers coughing.	Cough is painful, tickling, suffocative, and choking, in short, fitful spurts, or constant hacking that can prevent sleep.	Cough is constant, deep, violent, hollow, and barking, like a saw going through dry wood. Feeling as if breathing through a dry sponge.
Mood	Restless, anxious, irritable, fussy, oversensitive, needy, and demanding.	Agitated to the point of biting, screaming, or hitting. Older child may grind their teeth.	Grumpy, intolerant of being disturbed or moved, wanting to just lie still in bed and be left alone.	Easily frustrated and offended; touchy. Oversensitive to noise, odors, light, and loud music.	Needs attention and consolation; affectionate, fearful, easily upset, and irritable.	Serious, indifferent to surroundings, restless in evenings, and low-spirited.	Easily excitable, anxious, with a feeling of heaviness.
Indications	Wheezy breathing. Chest burns or feels cold. Child is chilly and does not have much mucus.	Breathing is short, shallow, and rapid. Pains are sharp and needle-like. Face red, and everything is hot. Dry nose and throat. Eyes dilated.	Shortness of breath. Needle-like pains in chest. Great dryness of mucous membranes.	Breathing is shallow and difficult. Torn-loose, raw, tight feeling in chest. Thick, sour mucus. Shivering. Hoarseness.	Cold has moved into the chest. Tightness in the chest, with sensation of a weight on the chest.	Sore, raw, burning in chest and throat. Tickling in throat, with thick, stuck mucus. Coughing from even the slightest pressure on the throat.	Gasping for breath, fear of suffocation, and a feeling of constriction. Much dryness. Soreness and burning in larynx. Stuck mucus. Sweating.
Worse	Physical exertion, after midnight, cold air, sight and smell of food, and cold drinks.	Night, yawning, deep breathing, cold air, touch, noise, jarring, light, fine dust and 3 PM.	9 PM, touch, movement, warmth, spring, autumn.	Exertion, uncovering, lying on back, eating, and drafts.	Change of weather, wind, cold, thunderstorms, odors, lying on left side, light, morning, and evening.	11 PM, 2 AM, 5 AM, touching pit of the throat, lying down on the left side, talking, deeply inhaling cool air, motion, and being uncovered.	Lying down in a warm room, dry and cold wind, touch, day, excitement, swallowing, after sleep, sweets, talking, and movement.
Better	Warmth, hot food and drink, lying down, fresh air, and company. Baby wants to be carried in an invigorating way.	Rest, light covering, sitting semi-erect, low lights, and quiet.	Lying completely still, pressure, quiet, and being left alone.	Warmth, being wrapped up, moist air, hot drinks, belching, quiet, and not moving the chest.	Sleep, sympathy, low lights or darkness, eating and drinking cold things, cool applications, and open air.	Covering mouth and nose, daytime, wrapping up, and sucking on non-mentholated lozenges.	Warm drinks, food in small amounts, calm, quiet, lying with the head low, moist heat, and bending forward.
Also For		Whooping Cough	Whooping Cough		Whooping Cough, Croup		Croup

THE FIVE MOST COMMON REMEDIES FOR MOIST COUGHS

	Antimonium Tart	Hepar Sulph	Ipecacuanha	Lycopodium	Pulsatilla
Onset	After a long bout with a cold or flu. Getting too angry.	Getting too cold, or getting chilled from a cold wind.	Warm, moist weather. Child is weak or frail, and catches a cold.	Getting chilled in wet weather.	Getting feet wet. Getting chilled at the end of a Pulsatilla cold.
Symptoms	Suffocative, loud, rattling, and weakening cough. Sits up or bends head backward to cough. Can't cough mucus up.	Choking, rattling cough that comes in fits and ends in gagging. Child cries before coughing. Sweats during cough.	Incessant and wheezy cough. Spasmodic cough.	Deep, rattling, and hollow cough with much tickling. Coughs day and night. Cannot cough up stuck mucus.	Irritating, racking cough that comes in fits. Dry and tickling cough at night; loose and moist, rattling cough during day. Symptoms keep changing.
Mood	Whiny, moaning, and irritable. Child wants to be left alone, not touched, looked at, or examined.	Angry, irritable, and oversensitive, especially to pain.	Anxious, demanding, easily frustrated, screaming and crying when they don't get what they want. Almost nothing pleases them.	Sensitive to noise and strong smells. Kicks, screams, and throws tantrums. Irritable, temperamental, and difficult if contradicted.	Weepy, whiny, and wanting to be carried. As their symptoms change, so will their mood.
Indications	Gasping for air and panting. Rattling in chest as they breathe, both in and out. Lots of mucus in lungs. May vomit.	Difficulty breathing. Rattling in chest. Hoarseness or loss of voice. Thick, yellow mucus that smells like old cheese. Chilly, weak, and sensitive to cold air.	Short of breath, gasping for air. Sneezing, with much mucus. Constriction in chest and larynx. Sensitive to heat and cold. Hot inside, but cold outside. May have bloody nose. Nausea.	Short and rattling breath, with irritation in trachea. Chest is tight and burns. Much thick, salty-tasting, yellow or greenish mucus. Gassy, bloated, weak, and chilly.	Loud and rattling breathing at night. Anxiety that they are going to smother if they lie down. Lots of thick, gooey, yellow or green mucus on waking.
Worse	Night, warm rooms, anger, sleep, eating, cold, damp, lying down, and warm drinks.	Evening until midnight, cold drinks or food, cold dry air, drafts, lying on left side, uncovering, pressure, and touch.	Least motion, overeating, warmth, dampness, lying down, rich foods, and vomiting.	Between 4–8 (both AM and PM) falling asleep, lying on the back, deep breathing, wet weather, warm rooms, after naps, and on waking.	Lying down, especially on the left side. Warm stuffy rooms, evening, nighttime, getting overheated, and fatty or rich foods.
Better	Getting the mucus out, sitting erect, motion, burping, vomiting, cool open air, and lying on right side.	Heat, wrapping up, bending head back, moist heat, and damp weather.	Rest, inhaling cool air while wrapped warmly, open air, pressure, closing eyes, and cold drinks.	Warm drinks and food, motion, early afternoons, and cool applications.	Cool, fresh air, cold applications, sympathy, gentle motion, attention, and being propped up in a semi-erect position.
Also For	Whooping Cough	Croup	Whooping Cough		

THE FIVE MOST COMMON REMEDIES FOR SPASMODIC COUGHS

	Carbo Veg	Coccus Cacti	Cuprum Metal	Drosera	Ignatia
Onset	Onset from frosty air, extreme temperatures, warm damp weather, wind on the head; or failure to completely recover from a previous illness.	Onset from cold air and cold wind.	Onset from cold air and cold wind.		May come on after a major emotional upset like grief or shock, or from getting overly angry. Often comes on after there is a sore throat.
Symptoms	Heavy, burning, sore, or weak feeling in chest on waking. Hollow, choking cough. The mucus is thick, sticky, and yellow/green when coughed up. Breathing is labored, fast, short, and wheezing, especially after a coughing fit.	Irritating, hacking, tickling cough. The child may feel they are choking because there is so much mucus. Profuse postnasal discharge, but the throat can feel dry. Face goes purple or red from coughing.	Violent cough. Long bouts of coughing attacks, often three at a time. Cough comes and goes at irregular intervals. Child coughs so hard that they are breathless and cannot talk, and tremble in the fingers and toes.	Cough is tickling, hacking, barking, rapid, incessant, and deep, as if coming up from belly. Turns into a dry cough as soon as their head hits the pillow. No coughing during the day. Hard to catch breath during coughing. Nosebleeds.	Dry, spasmodic, hacking, and choking cough. Coughs are in quick succession. Coughing makes them cough even more. (This is the only cough that has this odd symptom.) Coughing as if they have inhaled dust or strong fumes.
Mood	Child is indifferent to everything, a bit confused, irritable, and sluggish.	Child feels sad and lethargic. Child is sad at 6 AM or 2–3 PM.	Child is nervous, uneasy, and may have attacks of rage, biting and tearing things apart, or laughter that can be convulsive.	Child is anxious, irritable, extremely restless, and easily angered, but they always want someone around them.	Child is moody, quarrelsome, and tearful. They want to be alone, and do not want to be consoled.
Indications	Child's breath is cold, but they are hot and want to be fanned. Thirsty. Hoarseness, which is worse in the evening. Sensation of sulphur fumes in larynx. This child is low in vitality and weak, exhausted by even the slightest exertion.	Child is constantly clearing their throat. They feel as though there is a thread hanging down the back of the throat. There is much internal heat, with perspiration. Brushing teeth causes the child to cough.	The child may stiffen. Painful constrictions in chest. Voice may be hoarse, especially in cold air. Metallic taste in the mouth. The breath can be fast and the child may pant. The hands and feet are usually cold. Child is restless in bed.	Tickling in the throat; dry trachea. Holds chest with hands when coughing because of pain in throat, larynx, chest, and maybe stomach. Face may turn blue. Cough can end with gagging. Mucus is stringy, yellow, and may have streaks of blood. Chilly, with cold sweats and shivering.	Child takes deep breath for relief, and is sleepy after a coughing fit. Constriction, aching, and shooting pains in chest. Speaks in whispers. Tickling in throat. The child is very sensitive to pain. There is much deep sighing.
Worse	Warmth, warm rooms, on waking, evening, walking, open air, eating, talking, and changes in temperature.	On waking, nighttime in a hot bed, heat, lying down, brushing teeth, morning, and wind.	Bending backwards, laughing, deep breathing in cold air, at 3 AM, eating, and hiccups.	Laughing, talking, crying, cold food, becoming too warm in bed, lying down, vomiting, evenings, after midnight, and cold food or drink.	Evenings, emotions, worry, fright, grief, touch, cold fresh air, walking, and lying down.
Better	Being fanned vigorously, elevating the feet.	Cool air, cold drinks, walking, washing in cool water, light covers, yawning, leaning forward, and clearing mucus.	Sipping cold drinks, perspiring, and lying quietly.	Pressure and fresh air.	Deep breathing, swallowing, eating, changing positions, warmth, and being left alone.
Also For	Whooping Cough	Whooping Cough	Whooping Cough	Whooping Cough	

EARACHES

Otitis media, or inflammation of the middle ear

Otitis media occurs when there is a buildup of mucus in the Eustachian tube, behind the eardrum. The Eustachian tube connects the back of the nose to the middle ear, and transfers fluids between the two. During the common cold, this tube can become blocked with excess mucus. The pressure from the excess mucus pushes on the eardrum from within, causing pain and sometimes infection. Because young children's Eustachian tubes are small and more horizontal than an adult's tubes, this makes them more prone to ear infections. Temporary hearing loss may result.

Eighty percent of the time, an earache coming from the middle ear is caused by a virus in the mucus. Because antibiotics treat bacteria but not viruses, the American Academy of Pediatrics does not advise antibiotics as a first line of treatment for suspected ear infections. Antibiotics may need to be prescribed, but quite often the ear infection will return after the antibiotic has run its course. Homeopathic remedies do not suppress anything; they resolve acute earaches so that the problem does not keep recurring. If your child has chronic earaches, it may be due to an allergy to cow's milk, corn, or wheat. Consult your healthcare practitioner.

Sometimes there is such a buildup of mucus that an eardrum may rupture, which may bring relief from the pain. If your child's eardrum has ruptured, give 2 pellets of **Calendula** internally, 3 times a day for 3 days. Keep the child's ear clean, and it will usually resolve in about two weeks. Consult your healthcare practitioner if this has occurred. Multiple ruptures of the eardrum can permanently impair hearing; if this is the case, seek help from your healthcare practitioner.

Pressure from excessive wax, a foreign body in the ear canal, or water and chlorine from swimming pools can cause earaches also. It is not uncommon for an earache to be associated with fevers, teething, sore throats, or colds.

Some children have a painless condition called "glue ear," when a thick, sticky fluid collects behind the eardrum. This fluid can impair hearing, which can lead to delayed speech and other development. If you suspect that this might be the case, contact your homeopath. In this case, a low-potency remedy may be needed over a period of weeks to clear the condition.

What to observe:

Is the child pulling, rubbing, or scratching the ear, or poking their finger in it? Do they cry in pain when the ears are touched? Is there a discharge of any type from the ear? Is the face red, or the area around the ear? Is the child unusually fussy, fretful, and irritable, with excessive crying or screaming? Is the child experiencing a runny nose, a sore throat, or a fever? Is there a loss of appetite? Is the child having difficulty sleeping, or waking frequently? Is the child experiencing hearing loss? (This is almost always temporary.) Is there pain in the ear when swallowing, eating, blowing the nose, or lying down? Try to discern whether the right or left ear is hurting, because this can help you find the correct remedy.

What was the weather like before the child got sick? Was it windy, rainy, cold and damp, or with a dry, cold wind, or warm and wet? Did the child get wet feet, or get soaked all the way through in a rain? Did the trouble come on fast, or take a few days to develop? Does the child look pale or red in the face? Do they want warm or cold drinks or food, or no food or drink? Is the child experiencing a low-grade fever, or a headache? Are they feeling unusually warm or chilly? What is the child's mood?

The following are the most commonly indicated remedies for earache:

Aconitum: This remedy is for earaches with sudden onset, brought on by getting chilled by icy north or east winds, or from a shock or fright. It is most useful in the first twenty-four hours, and *at the very first sign of symptoms.* The pains of this kind of earache are sharp, piercing, and intense. The child may be frantic with pain, and very sensitive to noise. There can be a tickling in the ear. The external ear is usually red, swollen, hot to the touch, and the opening may look red as well. There is a thirst for cold drinks. The chills come on fast, followed by an intense and possibly high fever. The glands are usually swollen. It may feel as if there is a drop of liquid in the ear. The child is sensitive, restless, anxious, and screaming. An older child may fear they are going to die.

Worse from: Around midnight, noise, light, touch, and pressure. **Better from:** Fresh air, rest, and hot applications.

Belladonna: These earaches have a sudden and violent onset from getting the head wet and/or being in a cold, dry wind. The pain is intense, throbbing, tearing, sharp, piercing, and suddenly comes and goes; it sometimes shoots into the throat or into the neck. The pain is both internal and around the external ear. The discomforts are usually on the right side. The external ear and opening are red and hot to the touch. The eardrum bulges. The child usually has a fever, which may be high, with delirium, restlessness, and confusion.

With this kind of earache there is almost always a bright red, flushed, hot face. The head is hot, and the extremities may be cold. The pupils may be dilated, and the eyes can look glassy. Chewing anything makes the pains worse. Glands just below and behind the ear may be swollen and painful. There may be noises in the ear, and/or facial aching. The child's tongue may look like a strawberry. (For this symptom, please refer to the "Supportive measures" section below.) The sleep is restless, and the child may cry out. If they are thirsty, they crave cold water or lemonade. They are irritable, and all senses are acute and heightened. They can become agitated to the point of biting, screaming, and hitting.

This remedy is also for earaches that occur with teething.

Worse from: The right side, drafts, light, noise, odors, being touched, sudden motion, and around 3 PM. **Better from:** Sitting partially up, low lights, quiet, bending backward, rest, and any food that doesn't have to be chewed a lot.

Calc Carb: Onset is from changes in the weather. The pains are burning, achy, throbbing, and extend into the throat. Ears can also feel like the pain is pressing outward. The discharge is smelly and full of pus. The glands are swollen. Hearing is diminished, and the child may experience sounds of cracking in the ear. There may be profuse sweating around the head. The child feels very thirsty. The child with this kind of earache is sluggish, stubborn, sensitive, and tearful.

Worse from: Cold, damp, drafts, morning, exertion, blowing the nose, coughing, fresh air, tight clothes, teething, and milk. **Better from:** Heat, rest, loose clothing, and keeping the ears and neck warm.

Chamomilla: Onset can be from a cold wind, teething, or anger. The pains are very intense, intolerable, sharp, throbbing, and tearing. The ears are very sensitive to both cold winds and noise. The ears feel stopped up; they are hot, and may be red. The child usually holds the ear and screams. They may complain of a buzzing sound, or a sound of roaring water in the ear. If there is a discharge, it is clear.

With this kind of earache, one cheek is usually red and hot (or has a red patch), while the other cheek is pale. This symptom can be subtle or very obvious. The earache is usually on the right side. The child is hot and thirsty, and usually has a fever. They are very demanding of something, then they don't want it, or throw it away when given. The child demands to be carried, and screams if put down. The screams are severe and piercing, because they are frantic with pain. They are fretful, and cannot be consoled.

The child with this kind of earache may also be teething.

Worse from: Cold air or wind, touch, teething, music, night, and especially around 9 PM. **Better from:** Being held or carried, warmth, mild weather, and patience.

Ferrum Phos: The onset of this kind of earache is slow. This remedy may be given at the first sign of an earache with no other distinctive symptoms. Many symptoms are the same as with **Belladonna** earaches, but do not come on rapidly, and are not as intense. The face is red; the pains are throbbing; and usually the right side hurts worse. This is a remedy for general inflammations. The child is weak, chilly, and thirsty for cold drinks. The face may alternate between being pale and being flushed. The child may complain of a scratchy throat, or a headache in the forehead that is worse on the right side. Some children will get a nosebleed. The eyes can be bloodshot and burning, and there may be trouble sleeping. The child is talkative, excited, restless, irritable, and averse to company.

Worse from: Nighttime, especially from 4–6 AM, the right side, touch, motion, and jarring. **Better from:** Cold applications on the head, and lying down.

Hepar Sulph: Onset of these earaches is from getting too cold, or being exposed to a cold wind. There are throbbing noises with unbearable, sharp, darting, or splinter-like pains, which may radiate into the throat or jaw. This is usually a right-sided earache remedy; however, the earache can move from left to right. Hearing may be diminished, with a cracking sound when blowing the nose.

With this kind of earache, the child is chilly, sweaty, and sensitive to noise and drafts. The ears are very sensitive to the touch and to cold air. They may have swollen neck glands. It is not unusual for the child to have a throat infection or croupy cough as well. The bony structure behind the ear may be painful and inflamed. If there is a discharge, it is full of thick, yellow pus and smells like old cheese. The child does not want to be examined or looked at. The child is angry, very irritable and oversensitive (especially to pain), complains, and may throw a tantrum.

Note: When examining this child's ears, warm your hands first, because the ears will be so sensitive to cold.

Worse from: Cold air, winter, drafts, being uncovered, nighttime, and touch. **Better from:** Moist heat or warm applications, hot drinks, and wrapping the head or ears.

Kali Mur: Onset can be from recently receiving a vaccination, or from a cold causing thick, white mucus to block the Eustachian tubes. The pain is a deep soreness felt in the middle ear. The child may hear a crackling or snapping noise on blowing their nose or swallowing. The glands around the ears are swollen. There is white discharge from the nose, and a white, grey, or greyish-white coating at the base of the tongue. The Eustachian tubes can become so blocked that hearing can become diminished. The child has no appetite. They are discontent, irritable, and easily angered.

Worse from: Open air, cold drinks or applications, lying down, drafts, night, dampness, and motion. **Better from:** Cold drinks, rubbing, and warmth.

Mercurius Viv (also known as **Mercurius Sol**): Onset is slow and steady after being chilled or drenched in the rain. The pain is boring, pressing, tearing, sometimes burning, and extends from the teeth or throat to the ear. The ear feels blocked, and hearing may be impaired. Most of the discomforts are on the right side. There may be a ringing in the ears. The child will usually drool on their pillow. The tongue may have a white coating, and there may be a metallic taste. The child's breath and sweat smell foul. If there is a discharge, it is burning, thick, smelly, gluey and yellow, or green and sometimes blood-streaked. The glands are swollen and may feel hard, especially around the ear. Sometimes there are eruptions behind the ear. If there is a fever, there is a smelly sweat that does not relieve the fever. The temperature is very unstable. The child is very thirsty for cold water, but it does not satisfy the thirst. They are like a thermometer, sensitive to both heat and cold. The child is restless, nervous, and constantly changing their mind.

Worse from: The right side, nighttime, warmth of bed, sweating, damp cold, drafts, and warm drinks. **Better from:** Moderate temperature, and rest.

Pulsatilla: The onset can be from getting the feet wet and becoming chilled. Or it may appear during or after a cold. The pains are aching, needle-like, sometimes throbbing and sharp. The ears can be quite achy at night. There may be itching in the ears. The discomforts are mostly on the left side. The ear is hot and red, and the ear lobes may be swollen. Because there is a sensation of the ears feeling stopped up, hearing may be diminished. The child may say there is a pressure pushing out from the ear, creating a pulsing sound. There may be a thick creamy or yellow-green discharge. They are usually not thirsty. The child is clingy, tearful, whimpering, whiny, pathetic, and fretful, but affectionate.

Worse from: Nighttime, the left side, and a room that is too warm or stuffy. **Better from:** Open air, affection, being held, hugged, and rocked gently, and after a good cry.

Silicea (also known as **Silica Terra**): Slow onset from getting chilled, getting feet wet, or change of weather to cold. Pains are tearing, tingling, shooting, and pressing outward behind the ear. The complaints are mostly left-sided. There is usually an itching in the ear, and you may notice the child boring their finger into their ear. The ear feels plugged up, and hearing may be impaired, with roaring, crackling, popping, or hissing sounds. The child is sensitive to noise. The glands in the neck are swollen. If there is a discharge, it is offensive, thick, and sometimes blood-streaked pus that gives it the name "glue ear." This remedy can be used for an unyielding cold where thick mucus blocks the ears; it encourages the discharge and drainage of the mucus. The bony structure behind the ear can be painful and inflamed. This child is very chilly, sweaty, and sensitive to drafts and changes in weather. They tire easily, and lack stamina. This child is subdued, shy, overly sensitive (especially to pain), anxious, and nervous. However, they can also be stubborn and uncooperative.

Worse from: The left side, cold drafts and wind, open air, damp, loud noises, and the full moon. **Better from:** Warmth, warm wraps and applications, yawning, and swallowing.

Sulphur: Onset may be caused by overexertion or getting chilled. The pain is achy, needle-like, or tearing. There are noises in the ear that can be roaring, ringing, or a wet swishing. The discomforts are mostly left-sided. The ears are very red, and the external ear may itch. Discharges have a foul smell. The child is sensitive to noises, and feels hot, sweaty, and thirsty, but may forget to drink. The lips and area around the eyelids may be red. You may notice that the child is sleeping with their feet out from under the covers. The child is irritable, sluggish, quarrelsome, and restless.

Note: Sulphur is used in the later stages of an acute illness where other remedies helped initially but are no longer working. This is true especially after **Mercurius** or **Lycopodium.** Make sure the symptoms fit. This remedy should not be overused. If the child is not improving after giving this remedy, consult your healthcare practitioner.

Worse from: Heat, blowing the nose, overexertion, staying in bed, around 11 AM, and at the full moon. **Better from:** Cold, open air, and gentle motion.

Dosage: If the onset is fast, give 2 pellets every 15 minutes for four doses, then hourly until there is improvement. If there has been no improvement after seven doses, choose a new remedy. Repeat the remedy only as necessary, and only if there is a return of the same symptoms. On the first day, you may need to repeat the remedy every 1–2 hours. After the first day, you may need to repeat the remedy 3 times per day for 3 days. If you get no result within twenty-four hours, then reassess. You may not have been wrong in your choice of remedy; the condition might just have moved on to requiring a related remedy.

Change the remedy if you have followed the above guidelines with no results, or if the symptoms clearly change. For instance, Aconitum may be needed initially but, as hours or days go by, symptoms may change and indicate that Chamomilla is needed.

Supportive Measures:

Push fluids, especially if there is a fever, to prevent de-hydration. Use warm or cool applications, depending on what feels good to the child. Protect the ears from cold or wind with a hat. If the child has a head cold, tell them to not blow the nose too hard. Do not let water get in the ear. Do not let the child swim until the earache is long gone. It is advisable to stop feeding them any products made from cow's milk during this condition, because milk and cheese can cause the body to produce more mucus, which raises the level of acidity in the system. Goat's milk or products may be substituted for cow's milk products—use organic, if possible. Some children cannot tolerate cow dairy.

Earwax is secreted by the body as a protective measure; do not attempt to use Q-tips® to clear the wax during an earache. Normal amounts of wax do not cause pain. If you suspect an abnormal buildup, contact your healthcare practitioner. Do not poke anything down the ears; han-dle the head gently, since there might be tender, swollen glands around the neck. You may want to buy an otoscope, and ask your healthcare practitioner or nurse to explain what to look for.

Call your healthcare practitioner if:

- The bony area behind the ear is flaming red, hot, and extremely painful to the touch.
- Your baby is under three months old and has any rise in temperature.

Call your healthcare practitioner if (cont):

- Your child is over three months old and has a temperature over 103 degrees.
- Your child is under two years of age and has had a fever for more than twenty-four hours.
- Your child is over two years of age and has had a fever for more than three days.
- Your baby or child does not respond to bathing and homeopathic treatment to reduce a high fever.
- The earache is not clearing. An earache should start to resolve within twenty-four hours; if not, seek professional advice, especially if a high fever develops as well.
- There is profuse bleeding from the ear.
- There is stiffness in the neck.
- Your child's tongue looks like a strawberry. This can indicate scarlet fever.
- Complete hearing does not return.
- There are recurrent ear infections. The child may have narrow or slightly deformed ear canals. In this situation, it is often a good plan to combine homeopathic treatment with cranial-sacral therapy.

THE SEVEN MOST COMMON REMEDIES FOR EARACHE

	Aconitum	Belladonna	Chamomilla	Hepar Sulph	Mercurius Viv	Pulsatilla	Silicea
Onset	Sudden onset after being exposed to icy winds, fright, or shock. Most useful in first twenty-four hours and at very first sign of symptoms.	Sudden and violent onset from getting head wet, or being in a cold dry wind.	Onset can be from a cold wind, teething, or anger.	Slow onset from getting too cold, or being out in a cold wind.	Onset from getting chilled.	Onset can be from getting feet wet and becoming chilled.	Slow onset from getting chilled, getting feet wet, or change of weather to cold.
Symptoms	Pains are sharp, piercing, and intense. External ear is usually red-hot to the touch, and ear opening may look red as well. The ear may be swollen.	Pain is intense, throbbing, sharp, piercing, tearing, suddenly coming and going, and can shoot into throat or neck. Pain is inside and outside of ear. Right side is usually worse.	Pains are very intense, sharp, intolerable, throbbing, and tearing. Ears are hot, very sensitive to cold winds and noise. Child holds their ear and screams.	Throbbing noises with unbearable, sharp, darting, splinter-like pain that may radiate into throat or jaw. Usually on right side, but can move from left to right. Child is very chilly.	Pain is boring, pressing, tearing, and extends from teeth or throat to ear. Ear feels blocked, and hearing may be impaired. Usually right side is worse.	Pains are aching, needle-like, and sharp. The complaints are mostly left sided. The ear is not, red, and ear lobes can be swollen.	Pains are tearing, tingling, shooting, and pressing outward behind ear. Complaints are mostly left-sided. Usually itching in ear, and child bores finger into their ear.
Mood	Restless, sensitive, fearful, anxious, and screaming. Older child may have fear of death.	Child is restless and irritable; all senses are acute and heightened. They can become agitated to the point of biting, screaming, and hitting.	Child demands something, then doesn't want it, or throws it down. Wants to be carried, and screams if put down. Frantic with pain. Fretful and can't be consoled.	This child is extremely irritable, hypersensitive, easily angered, and does not want to be examined or looked at. May throw a tantrum.	Child is restless, constantly changing their mind, and nervous.	The child is clingy, tearful, whimpering, whiny, pathetic, and fretful. But they are affectionate.	This child is subdued, shy, anxious, and nervous. They are overly sensitive, especially to all senses and pain. They can be stubborn and uncooperative.
Indications	Sensitive to noise. Thirst for cold drinks. Chills come on fast, and high fever may follow. Glands are usually swollen. May feel as if a drop of liquid is in the ear.	External ear is red and hot. Usually high fever, with delirium. Face is usually bright red, hot, and flushed. Pupils may be dilated, and eyes may be glassy.	Ears feel stopped-up. If there is a discharge, it is clear. One cheek may be red, and the other pale. This symptom may be subtle. The child is hot and thirsty, and usually has a fever.	Ears sensitive to touch and cold air. The child is chilly and sweaty. Bony structure behind ear may be painful and inflamed. If discharge, it is thick, yellow, and smelly, like old cheese.	Child usually drools on their pillow. Breath and sweat smells foul. If discharge, it is burning, thick, smelly, gluey, yellow, or green. Glands are swollen. Unstable temperature.	Ears feel stopped-up. Hearing may be diminished. If discharge, it is thick, creamy, or yellow-green. They are usually not thirsty. May hear a pulsing sound in ear.	Ear feels plugged up, and hearing may be impaired. Child is sensitive to noise. Glands in the neck are swollen. If discharge, it is an offensive, thick pus giving the name "glue ear."
Worse	Nighttime around midnight, or midday, noise, pressure, and touch.	Chewing anything, worse on the right side, cold air, touch, noise, jarring, light, turning the head, 3 PM, and teething.	Usually the right side is worse. Cold air or wind, touch, teething, music, night, and especially around 9 PM.	Touch, being uncovered, exertion, cold drafts, wintertime, solid food, cold dry air, exertion, and at night.	On the right side, night, warmth in bed, sweating, damp cold, drafts, and warm drinks.	Nighttime, on the left side, and rooms that are too warm or stuffy.	Left side, cold drafts, wind, open air, damp, loud noises, and the full moon.
Better	Fresh air, rest, sweating, and hot applications.	Rest, light covers, sitting semi-erect, low light, quiet, food that doesn't require too much chewing, and cold water or lemonade.	Being held or carried, warmth, and mild weather.	Warm drinks, moist heat, being wrapped up, damp weather, warm applications, and covering the head and ears.	Moderate temperatures and rest.	Open air, affection, being held, hugged, and rocked gently, and after a good cry.	Warmth, warm wraps and applications, yawning, and swallowing.

FEVERS

A fever is the body's natural strategy for ridding itself of an infection. It can happen in reaction to a variety of stimuli. In some cases, a fever may be present if there is an allergic reaction, heatstroke, or extreme toxicity. A rise in temperature above 98.6 degrees F (37 degrees C) is considered a fever. There is an increased pulse rate so that the heart can pump blood faster to the organs; faster breathing to increase oxygen in the blood; and chills or perspiration to naturally cool the temperature. A raised body temperature also stimulates the body's defense mechanism to increase the production of infection-fighting white blood cells, called leukocytes.

Fevers tend to rise in the late afternoon or early evening, and drop or disappear by morning. The fever may rise and fall for a few days. Fevers should be allowed to run their natural course, and should not be repressed through the use of drugs. Hippocrates, the ancient Greek physician and father of Western medicine, said, "Give me a fever and I can cure the child." It is important to allow the self-healing process of a fever to run its course, unless the temperature is extremely high. See "Call your healthcare practitioner if:" at the end of this section for guidelines on fevers. Be sure to take the temperature with a thermometer, so you know accurately how high the fever is.

A fever in a child often precedes or accompanies an earache, sore throat, common cold, cough, teething, or the flu. It is not the goal of a homeopathic remedy to repress a fever, but rather to resolve the root cause by addressing the totality of symptoms. This will allow the fever to break naturally. A homeopathic remedy will strengthen the body and help it heal. Children who have had fevers and common childhood illnesses, e.g., chicken pox, tend to be stronger and healthier. In these cases, the immune system has learned how to fight off illnesses because they have not been repressed with drugs, unnecessary antibiotics, and vaccines.

Important Note: Do not give aspirin to a young child with a fever, because it can cause a condition called Reye's syndrome.

What to observe:

How high is the temperature? What was the onset—fear, shock, cold wind, getting chilled, overheated, wet, or too angry? Did the child get their feet wet, or get soaked through in a rain? Did the fever come on fast, or gradually? Do they look pale, or flushed? Are they thirsty and, if so, is it for cold or hot drinks? Is the child chilly, or hot? Are they restless, wiped out, or do they have plenty of energy? Does fever come and go, or is it constant? Is there a time of day that the fever is worse or better? What is the child's mood like? Do they have a headache? Are they nauseous? What makes them feel better or worse? Look at the tongue. This can be a confirmation that you have chosen the right remedy, though not a strong symptom for choosing a remedy.

The following are the most commonly indicated remedies for fevers:

Aconitum: Onset from getting chilled by icy north or east winds, or from shock or a fright. This remedy is most useful in the first twenty-four hours, and *at the very first sign of symptoms.* The temperature is high, usually starting to rise around midnight. The child may wake from a nightmare. There is dry, burning heat both inwardly and outwardly, especially of the skin, mouth, nose, eyelids, throat, lungs, and palms. The face is red. There is profuse sweat, especially of the parts on which they are lying, and they throw the covers off for relief. Waves of chills alternate with heat.

In the chill phase, there is a cold sweat, and icy coldness of the face. You can see waves of chills passing through the child's body. The tongue is coated with white, and often swollen. The pupils are usually small. The child has an intense thirst for cold water. In very high fevers, there is a marked degree of fearfulness. The child has an anguished, anxious, or shocked expression. There is excitement with fear. They are restless, tearful, and may be hard to console. They may stare off into space and have glassy eyes.

Worse from: Nighttime around midnight, noise, pressure, touch, and cold dry air. **Better from:** Fresh air, rest, warm applications, and sweating.

Apis: The onset can be from anger, fright, or grief. There is burning heat with a feeling of smothering. There are gushes of sweat. The chills come on from any movement. The face can look puffy. The tongue is fiery-red. The skin feels sore and sensitive, as if bruised. The child has no thirst during the fever but is thirsty during the chill. There is heat on one part of the body and coldness on another part. The child is very restless, sleepy, and irritable when disturbed. They may be weepy, but do not want to be touched.

Worse from: Heat, warm stuffy rooms, touch, heavy blankets, pressure, hot food, and from 3–5 PM. **Better from:** Cool applications, cold liquids, and being uncovered or lightly covered.

Arsenicum: Onset from getting chilled, after overheating or overexertion, or wet weather. The fever is high, with intense high heat and sweating. During this phase, they may be very thirsty for cold water, but they only drink in small sips, and there may be strong shivering and chills. The face is hot, but the rest of the body is cold, or there is coldness in spots. During this phase, warm drinks will make them feel better even though there is burning pain. There is a feeling of external chill along with internal burning, like hot needles or hot blood flowing.

With this kind of fever, the child goes down quickly, and continues to weaken to the point of total exhaustion. They are sensitive to cold. The face is pale with an anxious look, and may be covered with a cold sweat. The tongue is red and often has imprints of the teeth at the edge. The baby wants to be carried, is needy, demanding, and does not want to be left alone. The child is chilly, weak, and exhausted, but may be restless in bed. They are restless, anxious, irritable, oversensitive, needy, and demanding. The older child may fear they are dying or will not recover.

This is also a major flu remedy. See "Influenza" section on page 198 for more details.

Worse from: After midnight to 2 AM, change of temperature, damp wet weather, cold, and exertion. **Better from:** Warm drinks, heat, warmth in bed, elevated head, lying down, open air, and being warmly bundled.

Belladonna: The onset of this kind of fever is sudden and violent, and comes from getting the head wet and/or being in a cold dry wind, or becoming overheated. There is a high fever with a bright-red flushed face and/or ears. The heat can be so intense that you can feel it radiating off the child's body. The eyes may be glassy and sparkling, with a wild look, and the pupils are usually dilated. The skin is hot, alternating between moistness and dryness. The head is hot, and the hands and feet are cold. The sleep is restless. The child has hardly any chills. They may have a throbbing headache, and a hard, pounding pulse.

The child is not thirsty during the fever, but later may crave cold water or lemonade. The tongue is red but not swollen, and can be painful. The child's tongue may look like a strawberry. They are irritable, and all senses are acute and heightened, especially to noise, light, touch, or being jarred. They can become agitated to the point of biting, screaming, and hitting. If the child has a high fever, they may also be confused and delirious.

Worse from: The right side, cold air, touch, noise, odors, jarring, light, and around 3 PM. **Better from:** Rest, light covering, sitting semi-erect, low lights, and quiet.

Bryonia: Onset from cold winds. This fever usually comes on with a cold, and the onset is slow, sometimes developing over days. It is a dry, burning heat, during which the child has an extreme thirst for large quantities of cold water. They have chills and shivering. There is profuse, sour-smelling sweat with the least exertion. The head is hot, with a red face. The child has many complaints of dryness, e.g., dry mouth, skin, and lips. The baby does not want to be picked up or carried. The tongue can have parts coated with yellow or dark brown. They do not want to move, even the head or eyes. They want to be left alone. This child is very grumpy and irritable. The older child might be anxious about missing school while feeling ill; however, they want to be at home. They are usually very quiet.

This is also a major flu remedy. See "Influenza" section on page 198 for more details.

Worse from: Movement, around 9 PM, touch, warmth, warm rooms, spring or autumn. **Better from:** Lying completely still, pressure, quiet, and open air.

Chamomilla: Onset from cold damp air and wind. Alternating heat and chills. One part feels hot and another cold. One cheek may be red and the other cheek pale (this may be subtle), or one cheek hot and the other chilly. There is a lot of heat and sweating, especially of the head and face. This fever may last for a long time. The child is easily chilled. They are very thirsty. The tongue is whitish-yellow. They become overtired, but cannot sleep because of the fever, and may cry out in their sleep. The child is fretful, sensitive to pains, and angry. Nothing pleases them. They want to be held, but are only comforted for a short time. You put them down, and they want to be held again. They scream for something, and when it is handed to them they reject it or throw it down. They are extremely irritable. Babies want to be carried around.

Worse from: Heat, anger, around 9 AM and then again at night, after eating, from being uncovered, and open air. **Better from:** Being treated with patience, being carried or rocked, and warm, wet weather.

Cinchona (also known as **China Officinalis**): Onset from dehydration and loss of vital fluids. This can occur from fevers, diarrhea, or vomiting. Chills with thirst. The child is extremely weak and easily dehydrated, with intense thirst and headache. They can experience drenching sweats at night. The face is hot, and the hands are cold. There is a prickly-heat rash on the body.

The tongue appears to have a dirty coating, and the tip burns. If your child has become dehydrated because of a fever, this remedy will help bring back their vitality. However, if you cannot rehydrate the child, seek professional help. The child is irritable, and older children feel persecuted. This remedy is also for recurrent fevers.

Worse from: Touch, drafts, and eating fruit. **Better from:** Fresh air, rest, eating (except fruit), hard pressure, and fluids.

Eupatorium: Onset from experiencing icy cold. The key symptoms of this kind of fever are great soreness and intense aching in the bones. The fever begins with a strong thirst, and then chills and shivering follow. The child will feel better after the chills subside. In the heat phase, there is burning heat, but they do not sweat much. They usually have an intense throbbing headache that causes nausea, and they may vomit bile. They feel chilly. They may develop cracks in the corners of mouth, with a coating of yellow or white on the tongue. This child is extremely weak, and sleeps a lot. They are anxious, restless, and moaning.

This is a major flu remedy. See "Influenza" section on page 198 for more details.

Worse from: Autumn or winter, movement, open air, cold air, the smell or sight of food, and from 7–9 AM. **Better from:** Sweating, lying still, conversation, staying in the house, and getting on their hands and knees.

Ferrum Phos: For fevers of unknown origin. This is very useful for the early stages of a fever, when there are not many distinctive symptoms. The child may have a bit of a sore throat, a headache, or a bit of mucus in the nose. They don't feel well, but can't tell you much more than that. You will notice that a baby is just "off." The temperature is not as high as with **Belladonna** fevers; there is less redness, and symptoms are milder. The onset is usually gradual, but can progress readily. This fever is not sudden, as for **Belladonna** or **Aconitum.**

With this kind of fever, the child is chilly, but thirsty for cold drinks. If they have chills, they have a desire to stretch during the chill. During the heat phase, the hands are sweaty. The eyes can be a little bloodshot, with a burning sensation. The remedy may either abort the fever or cause it to be less debilitating. The child may need another remedy if the symptoms worsen, or if they are not feeling better. If this happens, reassess the case and perhaps shift to a different remedy. They are irritable, sensitive, and talkative.

Worse from: Chills around 1 PM, at night or 4–6 AM, on the right side, and from touch, motion, and jarring. **Better from:** Cold applications on the head, and lying down.

Gelsemium: The onset is gradual, and caused by damp or humid weather, traumatic shock, or fright. In a nutshell, this remedy is indicated for a child who is droopy, drowsy, and dizzy. There is heat alternating with chills. During the heat phase, there is much sweating that leaves the child exhausted and drowsy. There are chills up and down the back, with muscular soreness and achiness. The child might ask to be held because they are trembling. The tongue trembles when protruded, and can have a thick, yellow coating. The teeth may chatter, even when there are no chills. The hands and feet are cold. There is a dull headache, and sometimes a lightheaded feeling. The child is not thirsty. They may not be able to see or focus well. The eyelids are heavy and droopy, and the limbs may feel heavy. The child may become delirious during the fever, and scream upon falling asleep. They are weak, tired, and slow to respond. They are indifferent to their surroundings, dull, droopy, and emotionally delicate, and want to be left alone.

Note: Encourage this child to drink, because they will not feel thirsty.

This is also a major flu remedy. See "Influenza" section on page 198 for more details. Sometimes a child may have a lingering flu with a fever that hovers around ninety-nine degrees. If this is the case, this remedy will resolve this condition.

Worse from: Overexcitement, strong emotions, spring, shock, damp weather, and around 10 AM. **Better from:** Sweating, urinating, open air, and continued motion.

Mercurius Viv (also known as **Mercurius Sol**): Onset from getting chilled. This fever alternates between heat and chills. The child's temperature is very unstable; one moment they are too hot and throwing off the covers, and the next they are chilled to the bone. The hands and feet are cold. There is profuse, sour-smelling sweating during sleep, but the sweating gives no relief. There is a strong, unquenchable thirst for cold water. The child will drool clear saliva on their pillow. The breath smells bad, and there may be a metallic taste in the mouth. The tongue can have a yellow coating. The glands are usually swollen. The child is discontented, weary, possibly trembling, restless, nervous, and constantly changing their mind.

Worse from: Nighttime in bed, drafts, damp weather, sweating, cold or heat, and lying on the right side. **Better from:** Moderate, even temperatures, rest, lying on the stomach, and morning.

Natrum Mur: Onset can be from grief, guilt, disappointment, or fright. This remedy is for a fever with a hot face but chilly chest, feet, and hands. The fever comes and goes. The child has a loss of appetite because they feel nauseous, and may vomit. They may have a headache. They are constantly chilly, but feel worse in the sun. Any motion produces sweat. There is an extremely strong thirst for cold water, which increases as the fever goes on. Constipation often accompanies the fever. If the child is prone to get cold sores, this fever will likely produce an outbreak. They may desire salty food. The tongue may have a frothy coating with bubbles on the sides. The child is weak, irritable, and withdrawn, cries at the least little thing, and gets their feelings hurt easily.

Worse from: 9–11 AM, movement, heat, sympathy, noise, sun, and touch. **Better from:** Sweating, rest, open air, sitting up, and deep breathing.

Nux Vomica: Onset for this kind of fever is from getting chilled in a cold, dry wind, or in cold air conditioning. There is burning heat, and the skin is hot to the touch, especially the face. However, the child wants to be covered up. They are chilly at the slightest movement, or at having any part of their body uncovered. The chills dominate this fever, with shivering. The fingernails may have a bluish hue. The child is thirsty when chilly, but not thirsty when hot. Their limbs and back ache, and their digestion may be off. Their sweat may smell sour; they only sweat on one side of the body. They have no energy, and may feel heavy. There is a yellow or white coating on the back of the tongue, and the edges may have cracks. The child is easily frustrated, making them cry. They are very touchy and easily offended. They are oversensitive to noise, odors, lights, and loud music.

This is also a major flu remedy. See "Influenza" section on page 198 for more details.

Worse from: Exertion, being uncovered, lying on the back, eating, and drafts. **Better from:** Warmth, being wrapped up, moist air, hot drinks, belching, and quiet.

Phosphorus: Onset can be from getting drenched in the rain. There are fever, chills, and night sweats. Sweating is profuse and covers the whole body. There is dry, burning, intense heat inside, but not to the touch. The heat travels up the spine, alternating with shivering and chills. The chills are worse in the evening. The child is hungry, and thirsty for cold or iced drinks, especially during the chills. Early in the fever the child may appear to be well, with a sweet nature. Then they become irritable, a bit fearful, and sluggish. Any effort becomes too much, even talking. Then they get a burst of energy, and then go back down hard—so you may want to keep them resting until you are sure of a complete recovery. The tongue is dry, smooth, and can look red or have a thin coating of white. There is a headache over one eye. This child needs attention, touch, and consolation. The child is affectionate, fearful, irritable, and easily upset.

This is also a major flu remedy. See "Influenza" section on page 198 for more details.

Worse from: Changes in weather; wind, thunderstorms, odors, light, lying on the left side, and putting the hands in cold water. **Better from:** Sleep, sympathy, low lights or darkness, eating and drinking cold things, and cool applications.

Pulsatilla: The onset of this kind of fever is from getting feet wet and becoming chilled. The symptoms are constantly changing. The child might complain of feeling too hot, and then of feeling too chilly. This child craves fresh air. In the heat phase of the fever, the child throws the covers off because the heat is intolerable. They are not thirsty. One whole side of the body may feel cold, or one hand. Or the body may feel hot, but there is no fever. The temperature is erratic. The heat phase is usually in the early afternoon, and the chilly phase comes on around 4 PM. The tongue is grey. The child is clingy, whimpering, whiny, weepy, and fretful, but affectionate. Your older son might be described as feeling sorry for himself. This child needs attention and gentleness.

Note: Encourage the child to drink, because they do not feel thirsty. Avoid milk, which they may crave, because this causes excess mucus.

Worse from: Warm, stuffy rooms, evening and nighttime, getting overheated, and fatty or rich foods. **Better from:** Cool fresh air, cold applications, cold drinks, being uncovered, resting, being held, hugged, and rocked gently, and after a good cry.

Pyrogenium: This fever's onset is from cold or cold wet weather. There is a rapidly rising temperature, with aching and soreness in all the limbs, especially the legs. This fever can get high enough to produce delirium. There is profuse sweating; however, it does not help the temperature fall. Large drops of sweat form on the face during the hot phase. The chill starts between the shoulder blades, and is felt deeply in the bones and limbs. The child is cold and chilly all day and cannot get warm. There is much shivering and shaking. The temperature may go up and down. The child is hot and then cold. The breath and sweat smell foul. The tongue is red. There is extreme thirst. The child's cheeks have round areas of redness. The child is constantly changing positions to try to get comfortable. They may complain that the bed is too hard. The child is greatly debilitated but restless, anxious, and sometimes talkative.

This can sometimes be a flu remedy. See "Influenza" section on page 198 for more details.

Worse from: Sitting, morning, cold, damp, and moving the eyes. **Better from:** Pressure, heat, a warm bed, stretching, hot drinks, and hard rocking.

Rhus Tox: The onset is from getting wet, sitting on damp ground, or getting overheated after being chilled. Dry, burning fever alternates with chills. During the heat phase, there is profuse sweating from the slightest exertion, which makes them feel better. There is extreme chilliness. The child cannot bear to be uncovered because it causes shivers that make the stiffness and aching worse. They have a constant urge to stretch and yawn, but this brings on the chills again. They are sore, stiff, and achy. The glands are swollen, hard, and tender. The stools are usually loose. They have a dry mouth and throat, and are thirsty for small sips of water. They may develop a cold sore around the mouth. The tongue is coated, with red areas at the tip and sometimes the edges. The child cannot get comfortable; they toss and turn all night. The child is anxious, weepy, helpless, mildly delirious, and extremely restless.

This is a major flu remedy. See "Influenza" section on page 198 for more details.

Worse from: Cold damp weather, autumn, cold food or drinks, being uncovered, drafts, lying still, on first movement after resting, and at night. **Better from:** Warm drinks and food, constant gentle movement, stretching, warmth, changing positions, and massage.

Silicea (also known as **Silica Terra**): Onset of this kind of fever is from getting chilled, getting feet wet, or a change of weather to cold. These children do not usually have enough stamina to develop a very high fever. This is a burning fever with profuse, sour-smelling sweat, mostly on the upper part of the body. The child starts sweating upon falling asleep. They shiver easily, which makes them irritable and feel like crying. The chills of this fever are icy, intense, and creep over the whole body. The limbs are cold. The tongue may look brownish. This child tires easily, lacks stamina, and is weak and delicate. They are subdued, shy, anxious, nervous, and overly sensitive, especially to all senses and pain. However, they can also be stubborn and uncooperative.

Worse from: Cold air, changes in weather, the left side, drafts, evening into night, being uncovered, exertion, sweat, and toward morning. **Better from:** Warmth, being wrapped up, wearing a warm hat, urination, and rest.

Dosage: If the onset is fast, give 2 pellets every 15 minutes for four doses, then hourly until there is improvement. If there has been no improvement after seven doses, choose a new remedy. If the onset has been slow, give 2 pellets every 1–2 hours for six doses. Repeat the remedy only if there is a return of the same symptoms. Repeat only as necessary. You may need to repeat the remedy 2–3 times per day for a few days. If you get no result within twenty-four hours, then reassess. You may not have been wrong with your choice; the condition may simply have moved on to requiring a related remedy. Change the remedy if you have followed the above guidelines and have had no results, or if the symptoms clearly change. For instance, **Belladonna** may be needed initially but, as hours or days go by, symptoms may change and indicate that **Natrum Mur** is needed.

Supportive Measures:

Make sure the child gets extra rest. Push fluids to avoid dehydration, even if they only take a few sips at a time. A baby may refuse fluids, but may suck on a clean towel soaked in water. Try ice or frozen fruit bars for toddlers. Do not force the child to eat if they are not hungry. This gives the digestive system a rest and encourages the body to eliminate toxic wastes, aiding in recovery. If the child asks for food, give a light diet low in sugar, and avoid stimulants such as cola or caffeinated tea. Mild herbal teas are OK. Keep the child on a nutritious diet for 2–3 days after the fever has broken.

Supportive Measures (cont):

Sponge the face and forehead with lukewarm water. Even though a child has a fever, they may be extremely chilly and feel they cannot bear to be uncovered. Pile on the covers for chills, and keep them lightly covered when the heat occurs. Keep the room comfortably cool. Dress them in light clothing.

Call your healthcare practitioner if:

- Your baby is under three months old and has any rise in temperature.
- Your child is over three months old and has a temperature over 103 degrees.
- Your child is under two years of age and has had a fever for more than twenty-four hours.
- Your child is over two years of age and has had a fever for more than three days.
- Your child has a lack of reaction, trouble breathing, or convulsions, or is listless or limp.
- A rash appears on the body at the same time.
- Your child's tongue looks like a strawberry; this can indicate scarlet fever.
- Your child is refusing to drink, or keeps vomiting. Dehydration can lead to serious complications.
- If the temperature is very high, with high-pitched crying or screaming, you must take the child to the hospital. Give the remedy on your way there.

Call your healthcare practitioner if (cont):

- Adenitis is a condition where the child suffers from swollen lymph glands. In this condition, a breakdown of the immune system makes the lymph glands unable to eliminate toxicity through normal channels. Swelling then occurs, mostly affecting the glands in the throat and neck. However, the glands in the abdomen and groin may also be infected. The child will most often have a fever. The glands can be painful to touch. If children chronically have swollen neck glands, talk to your healthcare practitioner. If any swollen glands appear without fever, or if your child has persistent swollen glands and keeps getting the flu, viral infections, or a cough, contact your healthcare practitioner.

Emergency fever condition in meningitis

Meningitis is a condition for which you absolutely must seek hospital treatment. The reason for this is that the speed of its progression can be extremely alarming. Meningitis can be caused by either bacteria or a virus. Susceptibility to meningitis can be caused by head injury, a lowered immune system due to stress, frequent use of suppressive drugs, or as a result of unresolved childhood diseases such as measles or mumps. The signs to look for include:

- High fever (usually over 103 degrees)
- Headache with pain at the back of the head
- Stiffness of the neck
- Rolling the head from side to side, or arching the neck and back
- Delirium and stupor

- Vomiting and diarrhea
- High-pitched, piercing screaming
- A red rash that is blotchy and may be purplish in hue

If your child suffers from *three or more* of the above symptoms, take them to the emergency room. On your way to the hospital or urgent-care center, give either **Belladonna** (if head and upper body are hot and very flushed; child may be delirious) or **Apis** (if the child has a puffy face, and is restless and irritable, but sleepy).

Note: A fever with a wound, and/or red streaks extending out from a wound, can indicate a septic fever. Take the child to the emergency room at once.

THE SEVEN MOST COMMON REMEDIES FOR FEVER

	Aconitum	Arsenicum	Belladonna	Bryonia	Ferrum Phos	Phosphorus	Rhus Tox
Onset	Sudden onset with a high fever, after being exposed to icy winds, fright, or shock.	Getting chilled, wet weather, getting overheated, or over-exertion.	Onset sudden and violent. from getting head wet and/or being in a cold, dry wind, or getting overheated.	Slow onset (may develop over days), from getting chilled by a cold wind, especially in spring and autumn.	Onset is usually gradual, but can progress steadily. Fevers of unknown origin, which are not usually high.	Onset is slow and steady, from getting drenched in the rain. Ravenous hunger the night before onset.	Getting chilled or wet, sitting on wet ground, or getting overheated after being chilled. Overexertion.
Symptoms	Chills, then dry, burning heat inside and out. Cold sweat and icy coldness of the face. Visible waves of chills passing through the body.	Face hot and body cold, or intense high heat and sweating. Chilly on outside and burning inside, but they want heat. Thirst for small, frequent sips.	High fever, bright-red flushed face. Head is hot; hands and feet are cold. Not thirsty during fever, but craving cold water later. Head may have throbbing pains.	Chills and shivering. Dry, burning heat, with an extreme thirst for large quantities of cold water. Long fever. Achy pains over whole body. Eyeballs are sore.	Early stages of fever; very few or vague symptoms. The child generally doesn't feel well. During heat phase, hands are sweaty. Eyes can burn and be bloodshot.	Fever, chills, and night sweats. Joints feel stiff. Burning heat up the back, with profuse perspiration. Child gets a burst of energy and then goes back down. Headache over one eye.	Dry, burning fever alternating with chills. Muscle aches and stiffness. Feels bruised and sore. Constant desire to stretch and move. May get a cold sore.
Mood	If high fever, child becomes fearful. Can be hard to console. Restless, anxious, and tearful.	Restless, anxious, irritable, fussy, oversensitive, needy, and demanding.	All senses acute and heightened. Confused and delirious with high fever. Can become so agitated that they bite, scream, and hit.	Intolerant of being disturbed or moved. Wants to just lie still in bed and be left alone. Grumpy.	Irritable, sensitive, and talkative.	Needs attention and consolation. Affectionate, fearful, easily upset, and irritable.	Anxious, weepy, helpless, mildly delirious, and extremely restless.
Indications	Face red, pupils small, and eyes glassy. Profuse sweat. Intense thirst for cold water.	Much shivering. Strong chills and cold sweat. Child goes down quickly, continues to get weak, and then is totally exhausted.	Skin is hot, alternating between moistness and dryness. Eyes may be glassy and sparkling, with a wild look. Restless sleep.	Breathing is shallow and difficult. Torn-loose, raw, tight feeling in chest. Thick, sour mucus. Shivering. Hoarseness.	Chilly, but thirsty for cold drinks. Stretches during chills. This remedy may either abort fever or cause it to be less debilitating.	Craves ice water during chill. At first, may not show how sick they are. Later, it's hard to make any effort. Acute senses. Face pale, then flushed.	Much sweating from the slightest exertion. Shivers on any movement or being uncovered. Glands are hard, swollen, and tender. Child is extremely chilly.
Worse	Nighttime around midnight, noise, pressure, touch, and cold dry air.	After midnight, or around 2 AM, change of temperature, damp wet weather, cold, exertion, sight and smell of food, and cold drinks.	Right side, cold air, touch, noise, jarring, light, and around 3 PM.	Movement, 9 PM, touch, warmth, spring, autumn.	Chills at 1 PM or 4–6 AM; worse on the right side, and from touch, motion, and jarring.	Change of weather, wind, thunderstorms, odors, lying on the left side, light, morning, and evening.	Cold, damp weather, autumn, cold food or drinks, night, being uncovered, drafts, lying still, and initial movement after resting.
Better	Fresh air, rest, sweating, and warm applications.	Warmth, hot food and drink during hot phase, although there is much burning; lying down, fresh air, and elevating the head.	Rest, light covers, sitting semi-erect, low light, and quiet.	Lying completely still, pressure, quiet, and being left alone.	Cold applications on the head, and lying down.	Sleep, sympathy, low lights or darkness, eating and drinking cold things, cool applications, and open air.	Warm drinks and food, constant, gentle movement, stretching, sweating, changing positions, and massage.
Also For	Colds, earache, sore throat, and cough	Colds, flu, and cough	Colds, sore throat, earaches, and cough	Colds, flu, and cough	Sore throat and colds	Colds, sore throat, cough, and flu	Colds, sore throat, and flu

INFLUENZA

Influenza, also called "the flu," is caused by many different kinds of viruses. It may start out much like a cold, with nasal discharge, low/medium fever, achy ears, sore throat, swollen glands, or coughing. But influenza is a much more severe infection. It can also bring about aching in the muscles, joints, and bones; fever, chills, loss of appetite, exhaustion, nausea and vomiting, severe headaches, respiratory ailments, and a slow return of energy. A heavy cold may put the child down for a few days, but the flu can be debilitating.

The flu usually occurs in the winter. It is important to make sure that the child gets plenty of rest and a good diet while recovering. Otherwise, it is very easy for them to go down again. Because influenza is caused by a virus, it does not respond to antibiotics. Homeopathy can be a much more effective way to treat the symptoms. Usually a healthy baby will not get the flu unless it is a very strong strain. If a baby is immune-compromised, failing to thrive, or of low vitality, and you suspect that they have the flu, you must seek professional help. If this is the case, do not attempt to treat your child. A child with low vitality or a compromised immune system may develop secondary complications such as ear or throat infections, bronchitis, or pneumonia. *If in doubt, call your healthcare practitioner.* We have included these remedies for the older child and parents to use as a guide.

Please refer back to the sections on fevers, colds, and coughs for further information and confirmation that you are giving the correct remedy. The sooner treatment is started, the faster and more complete the recovery. Flu can cause exhaustion, depression, irritability, and lack of stamina for weeks if not properly addressed.

What to observe:

What was the weather like before the child got sick? Was it windy, rainy, cold and damp, warm and wet, with a dry cold wind, etc.? Did the child get their feet wet, or get soaked all the way through? Did the symptoms come on fast, or take a few days to develop? What is the child's mood? Do they look pale, or red in the face? Does the child want warm or cold drinks or food, or no food or drink? Are they experiencing a fever or headache? Take their temperature. Are they feeling unusually warm or chilly? Are they experiencing chills or shivering? If there is achiness, what does it feel like, and what area of the body is most affected? What positions make them feel better or worse? Are they thirsty?

The following are the most commonly indicated remedies for flu:

Arsenicum: Use this remedy when the onset is from getting chilled, overexertion or being overheated, or wet weather. The child may become delirious with high fever. The bones ache, and there is a lot of burning pain, oddly enough relieved by heat. (This is a unique symptom.) The pains may move into the chest. The face is hot, and the body is cold. The face is pale with an anxious look, and may be covered with a cold sweat.

This is a child who will feel better under a good amount of covers, so that the body is warm; however, the head will feel better with a cool application on the forehead. There is a thirst for drinks, but child drinks in sips. Acidic, burning, profuse discharge from the eyes and nose. The child is weak, chilly, and exhausted, but may be restless, tossing about and fidgety in bed. Wants to be carried, will not settle down, and does not want to be left alone. Anxious, irritable, fussy, oversensitive, needy, and demanding. The older child may fear they are dying or will not recover.

Worse from: Physical exertion, after midnight, cold air, the sight or smell of food, and cold drinks. **Better from:** Warmth, hot food and drinks, lying down, fresh air, and company.

Baptisia: This remedy is for a flu that has a rapid onset with extreme exhaustion, fast deterioration, and weakness. Onset can be from getting chilled in a cold wind, especially in autumn. There is a high fever with profuse sweating and intense thirst. The child may curl up tightly on one side. The bed feels too hard, and their body feels sore and bruised. They feel extremely ill. Breath and discharges smell foul. Heavy, numb head that feels too large. Heavy pain at back of head. Eyes feel sore, and eyelids heavy; it looks as if they are drugged or drunk. Face, mouth, and tongue may be dark red or brown-red. They may have an intensely sore red throat, mouth sores, diarrhea, or vomiting. Very thirsty. This child is sleepy all the time, and may even fall asleep while talking or answering questions. However, they can be restless. They may have delusions that their limbs are double, or scattered in pieces, or not connected to their body, and they may have nightmares. They feel confused and dull.

Worse from: Around 6 PM, swallowing solids, open air, cold, heat with humidity, and pressure on waking. **Better from:** Drinking liquids.

Bryonia: Onset from cold winds. Flu and fever mostly develop slowly over six to twelve hours. The nose has little or no discharge. The fever can continue for quite some time. The child's face is pale during chills, and deep red during fever. They have a great thirst for large quantities of cold drinks, but do not drink frequently. The lips are dry, parched, and cracked, and there is a great dryness of all the mucous membranes. The eyelids are sore, red, and swollen. If there is a cough, it is painful. The throat and chest are usually very sore as well.

This child may have a bursting headache in the front of the head, which hurts a lot when coughing. Moving the eyes causes the head to ache too, and the back of the eyeballs can be painful. There are aching pains all over the body, especially in the joints. The child is usually constipated. They are very tired, but restless, and cannot find a comfortable position. The child is very grumpy, and intolerant of being disturbed or moved, wanting to lie completely still in bed. They want to be alone. They are restless and fretful. The older child might be anxious and worried about missing school while feeling ill, at the same time that they do want to be at home.

Worse from: The least movement, or being moved, around 9 PM, touch, warmth, springtime, and autumn. **Better from:** Lying completely still, being left alone, pressure, pressing hand on head for headache, cool air, and quiet.

Eupatorium: Onset from icy cold. This flu starts out with an intense thirst for cold drinks, followed by chills and fever. This may look like a case for **Bryonia**, but the child doesn't get so agitated by slight motions. Everything aches, even the eyeballs, limbs, and back. The skin feels sore. It feels as if the bones are breaking. The head feels heavy, with pain in the back of the head and a feeling as if it will burst open. The child may feel nauseous. They will feel better after the sweat and chills subside. There is very little sweat. There is sneezing, with a watery discharge from the nose. The child may become hoarse. If they have a cough, the chest feels sore, hot, and raw; they will hold their chest when coughing. They are chilly, but want ice-cold water. The child is extremely weak, and feels beaten-up and bruised, especially in the back. Doing anything requires a great effort. The child is restless, but can't get up or move. They may moan a lot.

Worse from: Autumn, winter, movement, open air, cold air, the smell or sight of food, and from 7–9 AM. **Better from:** Sweating, lying still, conversation, staying in the house, getting on the hands and knees when coughing, and loose clothing.

Gelsemium: The onset of this type of flu is gradual, and caused by damp, humid weather, or weather that goes from cold to warm; also from spring, traumatic shock, or fright. In a nutshell, this remedy is for flu where the child is droopy, drowsy, and dizzy. The first symptoms are chills up and down the spine. The child is chilly and sensitive to cold. This is followed by great muscular weakness, heaviness, drowsiness, fatigue, soreness, and achiness all over. The teeth may chatter, even without chills. The child may be dizzy. There may be a dull headache in the back of the head, with stiffness and achiness in the neck and shoulders. Chills and sweats alternate.

There is much sneezing in the morning, with a watery discharge, and a feeling of blockage at the root of the nose (where the roof of the mouth meets the top of the throat). The child may develop a sore throat. The limbs feel very heavy, and may be cold. The eyeballs ache and are droopy, as if they are drunk. The older child might say they can't see or focus well. Many times the tongue trembles when protruded. The face is hot and a dusky-red color. Their appetite is low, with very little thirst. They are weak and tired, and answer slowly. The child might ask to be held because of the trembling. They are indifferent to their surroundings, and feel dull, droopy, emotionally delicate, or too tired to even be emotional, and want to be left alone.

Note: It is important to push fluids with this remedy, since the child has little or no thirst.

Worse from: Overexcitement, strong emotions, spring, shock, damp weather, and around 10 AM. **Better from:** Sweating, urinating, quiet and low-stress surroundings, open air, reclining with the head propped up, and continued motion, e.g., rocking.

Phosphorus: Onset of this flu is from getting drenched in the rain. An odd symptom indicating this remedy is that the child has ravenous hunger the night before coming down with the sickness. This child may have a high fever, but is sweet-tempered and content to play quietly at first; they do not yet show how sick they are. Later, however, they will be weak, sleepy, and stuffed-up in the head, with sneezing and blood-streaked mucus. They go down slowly and steadily, ending up quite sick. They have fever, chills, and night sweats. Any effort is difficult. The face may be flushed, and then turns pale.

The child is thirsty for cold drinks, and may want ice. They are usually hungry during the fever; however, if the child is not hungry, do not force them to eat—especially warm food or drink—because it will take them much longer to get better. Colds tend to go into the throat and chest. The cough is dry and tickling, and the chest feels very tight. The joints feel stiff. There may be a headache over one eye. Acute sensitivity to smells, touch, light, and sound. The child will get a burst of energy and then go back down hard, so you may want to keep them resting until you are sure of a complete recovery. The child is affectionate, fearful, easily upset, and irritable. This child needs attention, consolation, and massage, which will make them feel much better.

Worse from: Changes of weather, wind, thunderstorms, odors, light, lying on the left side, morning time, and evening.
Better from: Sleep, sympathy, low lights or darkness, eating and drinking cold things, cool applications, and open air.

Pyrogenium: Onset is from cold, or cold, wet weather. The fever rapidly rises, and there is profuse sweating. However, sweating does not help the temperature fall. Chill starts between the shoulder blades, and is felt deeply in the bones and limbs. The child feels chilly all day, and cannot get warm. There is much shivering and shaking. Their temperature goes up and down, sometimes rather quickly. They are hot, and then cold. They may complain of their heart pounding. The pulse is rapid and weak when the temperature is low, but when the temperature rises the pulse slows down. This is a unique symptom indicating this remedy.

There is an aching, bruised, sore, and beat-up feeling in the back, bones, and all the limbs, especially the legs. There is usually a throbbing and bursting headache, and sneezing upon being uncovered. The breath and sweat smell foul. The child's mouth is dry, and they are extremely thirsty for small amounts of cold water. They may complain that the bed is too hard, and they constantly change positions trying to get comfortable. Sleep is difficult. They feel greatly debilitated. The child is restless, mentally overactive, especially at night, anxious, and may be quite talkative.

Worse from: Sitting, during the chilly stage, nighttime, cold, damp, and moving the eyes. **Better from:** Pressure, heat, a warm bed, stretching, hot drinks, hot baths, hard rocking, the first movement after resting, and walking.

Rhus Tox: The onset with flu of this type is from getting wet, sitting on damp ground, overexertion, or getting overheated after being chilled. There is achy stiffness in the muscles and joints, which feels better with movement or stretching. During the heat phase of the fever, there is profuse sweating that makes the child feel better. This alternates with extreme chilliness. They cannot bear to be uncovered because it causes shivers that make the stiffness and aching much worse. The chills are brought on with even the slightest movement. The child feels bruised, sore, stiff, and achy. Their glands are swollen, hard, and tender.

The child may experience pain behind the eyes. The stools are usually loose. The mouth and throat are dry, and the child is thirsty for small quantities of fluid. The tip of the nose is red and sore. Usually there is a red triangle at the very tip of the tongue. The child stiffens up after resting, which gives them a constant urge to stretch or move; but then they become easily exhausted and need to rest. They cannot get comfortable, and toss and turn all night. They may develop a cold sore around the mouth. The child is anxious, weepy, helpless, mildly delirious, and extremely restless.

Worse from: Cold damp weather, autumn, cold food or drinks, being uncovered, drafts, lying still, initial movement after resting, and nighttime. **Better from:** Warm drinks and food, constant gentle movement, stretching, warmth, changing positions, and massage.

Dosage: If the onset is fast, give 2 pellets every 15 minutes for four doses, then hourly until there is improvement. If the symptoms have come on slowly and are not severe, give a dose every 3–4 hours. If there has been no improvement after seven doses, choose a new remedy. Repeat the remedy only if there is a return of the same symptoms. Repeat only as necessary. You may need to repeat the remedy 2–3 times per day for several days. If you get no result within two days, reassess the symptoms. You may not have been wrong with your choice of remedy, but the child may have moved on to needing a related remedy. Change the remedy if you have followed the above guidelines with no results, or if the symptoms clearly change.

Supportive Measures:

Make sure the child gets extra rest, and does not get over-stimulated, especially by TV. Push fluids to avoid dehydration, even if they only take a few sips at a time. Try ice or frozen fruit bars for toddlers. Give lots of fruit—fresh if possible, because it contains vitamin C. Do not give sugary juice drinks. Fresh-squeezed juice is best. Do not force the child to eat if they are not hungry; not eating gives the digestive system a rest and encourages the body to eliminate toxic wastes. If the child asks for food, give them a light diet, low in sugar, and avoid stimulants such as cola or caffeinated tea. Chamomile tea would be fine to give a child. Sponge the face and forehead with lukewarm water, unless the description of the remedy that your child needs says, "Worse from cold (or cool) applications." Do not send the child back to school until there is a complete return of health and they are sleeping well again.

Call your healthcare practitioner if:

- Your baby is under three months old and has any rise in temperature.
- Your child is over three months old and has a temperature over 103 degrees.

Call your healthcare practitioner if (cont):

- Your child is under two years of age and has had a fever for more than twenty-four hours.
- Your child is over two years of age and has had a fever for more than three days.
- Your child has a lack of reaction, trouble breathing, repeated vomiting, or convulsions, or is listless or limp.
- A rash appears on the body at the same time as a fever.
- Your child has a persistent fever or cough, or a cough that worsens. This can indicate a secondary infection with pneumonia.
- Swollen glands that persist.
- Recurrent flu.
- Your child is refusing to drink, or keeps vomiting. De-hydration can lead to serious complications.

For difficulty recovering from the flu:

Gelsemium: The child just cannot seem to turn the corner and regain their energy. The child will be completely exhausted, with a wiped-out expression on their face. Their appetite is low and they have very little thirst. They have great muscular weakness, answer slowly, and want to be left alone. Many times they feel lightheaded, and may have a headache. There may be a sticky perspiration on the skin.

Worse from: Overexcitement, strong emotions, spring, shock, damp weather, and around 10 AM. **Better from:** Sweating, urinating, quiet surroundings, open air, reclining with the head propped up, and continued motion, e.g., rocking.

Phosphoric Acid: This remedy is given for weakness and exhaustion. Again, the child just cannot seem to get their energy back. They have no energy. They look pale, with dark circles under their eyes. They are very sweaty and chilly. There is a lack of appetite, but a desire for fruit and other light, refreshing foods. The child is indifferent, quiet, easily overwhelmed, mildly irritable and uncommunicative, cannot concentrate, and answers with a minimal amount of words.

Worse from: Severe, acute illnesses, after eating, after arising from long periods of sleep, any exertion, and walking. **Better from:** Naps (but not long periods of sleep), fruit and other light, refreshing foods.

Dosage for **Gelsemium** and **Phosphoric Acid** only: Give 2 pellets every 3–4 hours until there is improvement. If there has been no improvement after thirty-six hours, call your healthcare practitioner.

THE SEVEN MOST COMMON REMEDIES FOR INFLUENZA

	Arsenicum	Baptisia	Bryonia	Eupatorium	Gelsemium	Phosphorus	Rhus Tox
Vomiting	Getting chilled, wet weather, getting overheated, or overexertion.	Rapid onset, with fast deterioration and high fever. From getting chilled in cold wind, and autumn winds.	Slow onset, from getting chilled by a cold wind, especially in spring and autumn.	From exposure to icy coldness. Starts with intense thirst for cold drinks, followed by chills and fever.	Gradual onset, from damp, humid weather, shock, or fright. Common in spring.	Onset slow and steady. Ravenous hunger the night before onset. Getting drenched in rain.	Getting chilled and wet. Sitting on damp ground, or overexertion.
Diarrhea	Burning pains that are relieved by heat. Very chilly, body cold, face hot; child may have high fever, and feel achy. They have a strong thirst, but take constant small sips.	Sore, heavy, and bruised feeling. Smelly sweat, mouth and stool. Profuse sweating. Face and tongue are a dusky-red color. Intense thirst.	Long fever. Infrequent but great thirst for cold drinks. Little discharge from nose. Achy all over body. Sore eyeballs. Cannot get comfortable.	Bones hurt so badly they feel broken. Muscles, limbs, and back are very achy. Skin feels sore. Head feels heavy, and eyes ache. Extremely weak.	Chills up and down spine, Then child is weak, heavy, and drowsy. May also be dizzy. Muscular soreness all over. Dull pain in head and eyes. Trembling.	Fever, chills, and night sweats. Joints feel stiff. Child gets burst of energy, and then goes back down. May have headache over one eye.	Extreme muscle aches and stiffness. The child feels bruised and sore, with a constant desire to stretch and move. Extremely chilly.
Mood	Restless, anxious, irritable, fussy, over-sensitive, needy, and demanding.	Dull, confused, drowsy, and scattered, but may be restless. May have nightmares.	Grumpy, fretful, and intolerant of being disturbed or moved. Child wants to just lie still in bed and be left alone, but is restless.	Restless with a lot of moaning. Any effort is just too much.	Indifferent to surroundings, dull, droopy, and emotionally delicate. Wants to be alone.	Needs attention and consolation. Affectionate, fearful, easily upset, and irritable.	Anxious, weepy, helpless, mildly delirious, and extremely restless.
Indications	Even though pains are burning, they want heat. They are chilly, and the sweat is cold. They are weak and tired, but restless.	The child is very ill, and looks drugged or drunk. Eyelids are heavy. Falls asleep while talking. Bed feels too hard. Tongue has yellow-brown coating.	Does not want to move, even the eyes. Mucous membranes and lips are dry, parched, and cracked. Eyelids sore, red, and swollen. Frontal headache.	Chilly, but wants cold drinks. Bursting pain in back of head that can cause nausea.	Much sweat. Eyes ache and are droopy, making them look drunk. Cannot focus. Very little thirst, and low appetite. Teeth chatter without chills.	At first the child may not show how sick they are. Then they go down; it is hard to make any effort. Senses are acute. Face is pale, then flushed.	Profuse sweating that relieves. Symptoms. Chills with any movement, or being uncovered. Hard, swollen, and tender glands. Thirst for small amounts of liquids.
Worse	Physical exertion, after midnight, cold drinks, cold air, and the sight and smell of food.	Around 6 PM, waking, swallowing solids, open air, cold, heat with humidity, and pressure.	Any movement or motion, 9 PM, touch, warmth, spring, and autumn.	From 7–9 AM, autumn, winter, open air, movement, cold air, the smell or sight of food.	Around 10 AM, over-excitement, strong emotions, spring, shock, and damp weather.	Changes of weather, wind, thunderstorms, odors, lying on the left side, light, morning, and evening.	Cold and damp weather. Drafts, autumn, cold food or drinks, being uncovered, lying still, night, and initial movement after resting.
Better	Warmth, hot food and drink, lying down, fresh air, and company.	Drinking liquids.	Lying completely still, pressure, quiet, being left alone, pressure on the head for headache, and cool air.	Sweating, lying still, loose clothing, conversation, staying in the house, being on hands and knees while coughing.	Sweating, urinating, quiet, open air, reclining with head propped up, and continued motion, especially rocking.	Sleep, sympathy, low lights or dark, eating and drinking cold things, cool applications, open air.	Warm drinks and food, warmth, constant gentle movement, stretching, changing positions, and massage.

SORE THROATS, TONSILLITIS, AND LARYNGITIS

Common sore throats and tonsillitis

A sore throat is an inflammation with pain, difficulty swallowing, and sometimes swollen glands. The tonsils are the two lymphatic sacs behind the base of the tongue, on either side of the top of the throat. They are an integral part of the lymphatic drainage system. If tonsils swell, this is a normal eliminative process for getting rid of an invading bacteria or virus. Acute tonsillitis produces swelling, inflammation of the tonsils, a sore throat, and fever that may be low-grade, medium, or high. The child may have headaches or stomachaches.

The adenoids, which are made of the same lymphatic tissue, are located above the soft palate (roof of the mouth). These may also become swollen, impeding speech and nose-breathing. Chronically swollen tonsils or adenoids should be treated by a professional. In some children the uvula can become swollen as well. The uvula is a small, v-shaped piece of flesh extending from the soft palate that hangs down at the entrance to the throat.

Children of any age may develop a sore throat. If a baby develops this condition, there may be refusal to eat, crying while nursing, and a tendency to rub the ears, which might lead you to you to think they have an earache or are teething. Vomiting may occur if a lot of mucus is being swallowed. The child may have excess mucus or saliva, bad breath, and odd tastes in their mouth. Recurring sore throats may indicate chronic postnasal drip and/or allergies. If this is the case, consult your healthcare practitioner.

Laryngitis and voice loss

Acute laryngitis is an inflammation and swelling of the vocal cords in the area of the larynx (the portion of the throat from the mouth to just below the Adam's apple, sometimes called the voice box). Laryngitis produces a change in the voice that results in hoarseness, huskiness, loud whispering, a high pitch, or complete loss of the voice. The swelling and inflammation are due to dry mucous membranes, or an accumulation of thick mucus from postnasal drip down the back of the throat. The larynx area is rich in lymph glands that can become swollen while fighting off infection. Mucus from a cold can then get stuck around the swollen vocal cords.

The cause of laryngitis with a cold can be either viral or bacterial. It is usually triggered by getting chilled or wet. Laryngitis may also be caused by overstraining the voice, by allergies, secondhand smoke, pollutants, or prolonged coughing. In some cases, it can be caused by chronic repression of emotions, or resisting the need to cry.

What to observe:

Get a flashlight and a teaspoon. Gently hold the tongue down with the spoon—not too far back on the tongue or the child will gag—and look at the throat. (Most children do not like this, so try to look quickly.) What was the weather like before the child got sick? Was it windy, rainy, cold and damp, warm and wet, with a dry cold wind, etc.? Did the child get their feet wet, or get soaked through? What is the child's mood? Did the condition come on fast, or take a few days to develop? Do they look pale, or red in the face? Does the child want warm or cold drinks or food, or no food or drink? Is the child experiencing a fever or headache? Take their temperature. Are they feeling unusually warm, or chilly? Are they experiencing chills or shivering? If there is achiness, what does it feel like, and what area of the body is most affected? What positions make them feel better or worse? Are they thirsty?

The following are the most commonly indicated remedies for common sore throat, tonsillitis, and laryngitis:

Aconitum: This remedy is for symptoms with sudden onset, brought on by getting chilled from exposure to icy north or east winds, or from a shock or fright. This remedy is most useful within the first twenty-four hours, at the very first sign of symptoms. The throat feels constricted; it is red, dry, and hot. Swallowing is difficult. Burning and needle-like pains may shoot into the ears. The child may have pain in the back of the head, or behind the outside of the ear at the jaw. They may also experience burning from the mouth to the stomach. The tonsils are swollen and dry, with a feeling of something being stuck in the throat. The tongue is coated white, and often swollen. There is a strong thirst for cold drinks. The child is restless, fearful, anxious, and screaming. They may have nightmares, with restless or no sleep. The older child may fear they are going to die.

Laryngitis: This remedy is indicated if there is sudden loss of the voice after being exposed to a cold, dry wind.

Worse from: Night around midnight, noise, pressure, touch, and cold dry air. **Better from:** Fresh air, rest, warm applications, and sweating.

Apis: The onset of this type of sore throat can be from anger, fright, or grief. There is a swollen, constricted, inflamed, dry throat with the sensation of having a splinter. The pains are stinging and burning. The tongue, uvula, and throat are swollen, and there may be swelling on the outside of the throat. The right side is usually worse. The face can look puffy. The tongue is fiery-red and raw, and the mouth is dry. The throat is glassy-red or purple. The skin feels sore and sensitive, as if bruised. The child wants cold water to soothe the throat, but is usually not thirsty. The child is very restless, sleepy, and irritable when disturbed. They may be weepy, but do not want to be touched.

Tonsillitis: The tonsils are swollen, rosy or fiery-red, and ulcerated, with whitish secretions and stinging pains.

Worse from: Warmth, on the right side, touch, heavy blankets, pressure, swallowing solid hot or sour food, from 3–5 PM, after sleep, and in a warm, stuffy room. **Better from:** Cool applications, cold liquids, cool air, motion, and being uncovered or lightly covered.

Argentum Nit: Onset from fear, fright, overindulgence in sugar, mental strain, or worry. Great amounts of thick mucus make the child constantly clear their throat. There is so much mucus that it may feel as if they are being strangled. The throat is raw and irritated. The pains are burning and splinter-like. The sensation of a splinter in the throat feels worse from swallowing, breathing, or moving the neck. Or they may feel as if there is a hair tickling the throat. The throat and uvula look dark red. The child may choke on food because there is so much mucus. The throat can feel paralyzed. The tip of the tongue is red and may be sore. There is usually a strong desire for sweets. These children are anxious, restless, fearful, fidgety, and excitable. They sometimes tremble. They do not like being alone, and dread ordeals.

Laryngitis: This kind is caused by overuse of the voice, common in singers, and includes chronic hoarseness. Singing high notes will cause coughing. There is thick, yellow-to-green mucus, and tickling in the throat.

Worse from: Mornings, heat, warm, stuffy rooms, secondhand smoke, on the left side, and from eating sugar and sweets. **Better from:** Company, coolness, and fresh air.

Baptisia: Onset can be from getting chilled in a cold wind, especially in autumn. There is extreme exhaustion and weakness, with fast deterioration. The throat and tonsils are dark red. The throat has little or no pain. However, it is so constricted that the child can only swallow liquids, and gags on solid food. They are constantly swallowing. The breath is very foul-smelling. The tonsils and soft palate are swollen. Externally, the larynx is sore to the touch, but there may be sensations of numbness on the inside. There will almost inevitably be a low-grade fever, which makes the child appear drunk. The tongue has a yellow-brown coating, and the edges are dark red. They child may lie on one side, curled up tightly. The child is quite ill, dull, confused, and restless. They may have delusions that they are doubled or scattered in pieces, or that their limbs are not connected to their body. They may have nightmares.

Worse from: Around 6 PM, swallowing solids, open air, cold, heat and humidity, and pressure on waking. **Better from:** Drinking liquids.

Belladonna: Sudden onset with severe symptoms after getting chilled or overheated. The child may feel fine in the morning, but by 3 PM they have a high fever with a sore, bright-red throat. The throat feels burning, dry, hot, raw, constricted, and tender to the slightest touch. Even the muscles involved in swallowing are sensitive. It is hard to swallow, but there is a constant desire to do so. Pains are severe, needle-like, and worse on the right side. The glands in the neck and throat are usually swollen. There may be a sensation of a lump or scraping in the throat. The child only wants cold water or lemonade in sips, and is usually not thirsty. They will hold the head forward and take sips of liquids in order to help them swallow solid food. The child's tongue may look like a strawberry. (For this symptom, please refer to the "Supportive measures" section below.) The child is restless and irritable, and all senses are acute and heightened. They can become agitated to the point of biting, screaming, and hitting.

Tonsillitis: The tonsils are swollen, quite enlarged, hot, and bright red. The right tonsil is usually worse, and may have red streaks. Other glands may also be affected.

Worse from: Swallowing liquids, cold air, touch, noise, odors, jarring, light, turning the head, sudden motion, and around 3 PM. **Better from:** Rest, light covers, sitting semi-erect, low lights, and quiet.

Calc Carb:

Tonsillitis (only): Onset is from changes in the weather. The throat feels very dry, with needle-like pains and difficulty swallowing. There is much swelling of the tonsils, with yellow and white ulcerations. The uvula and soft palate are swollen. The child will hawk up salty-tasting mucus. There may be burning pain at the tip of the tongue. They do not like to talk, and hoarseness is not unusual. They are very thirsty. The child is sluggish, stubborn, sensitive, and tearful.

Worse from: Cold, damp, drafts, morning, exertion, fresh air, tight clothes, and milk. **Better from:** Heat, rest, and loose clothing.

Ferrum Phos: The onset is slow for this type of sore throat. This remedy may be given at the first sign of a sore throat with nonspecific or few symptoms. The throat is scratchy and slightly sore, with a feeling of rawness. Swallowing is painful. There may be symptoms, but if there is nothing distinctive about them, this is the remedy to use. It is also a remedy for general inflammations. This is most useful in the early stages of a sore throat, and may even completely abort this condition. The child doesn't feel well, but can't tell you much more than that. You will notice that a baby is just "off." They are weak, chilly, and thirsty for cold drinks. The face alternates between being pale and being flushed. The eyes can be a little bloodshot, and burn. The child may need another remedy if the symptoms worsen or do not improve. If this happens, reassess the case. This child is talkative, excited, irritable, and averse to company.

Tonsillitis: When there is swelling and redness of the tonsils.

Worse from: Nighttime and from 4–6 AM, on the right side, and from touch, motion, and jarring. **Better from:** Cold applications on the head, and lying down.

Hepar Sulph: Slow onset, from getting too cold or from a cold wind. Severe, sharp, splinter-like pains that shoot up into the ear on swallowing or yawning. The child may have a sensation of a plug or fishbone stuck in their throat. The right side is usually most painful, but both sides can be affected. Glands are swollen, and solid food is hard to swallow. Swollen tonsils can also diminish the child's hearing. The child is chilly, with smelly sweat. Their breath may smell like old, ripe cheese. They hawk up smelly, yellow mucus. They have a lack of appetite, but may crave vinegar or sour foods. This child is extremely irritable, hypersensitive, easily angered, and does not want to be examined or looked at. This is a child to be kept indoors and warm.

Laryngitis: When there is hoarseness and a distorted voice, with thick, yellow mucus, or when a child loses their voice completely. The child has the sensation of a plug in the throat on swallowing.

Tonsillitis: When there are pus-filled abscesses on the tonsils.

Worse from: Touch, being uncovered, exertion, cold drafts, winter, solid food, cold dry air, exertion, and at night. **Better from:** Warm drinks, moist heat, being wrapped up, and damp weather.

Kali Mur:

Tonsillitis (only): The throat is grey, with white spots. There is much mucus. The child can hardly breathe because the tonsils are so swollen. The tongue has a greyish-white coating. There is hoarseness or loss of voice. Swallowing is extremely painful. The child hawks up cheesy, thick, white mucus. The ears are usually blocked up with mucus. The child is irritable, angry, and discontent.

Worse from: Open air, drafts, night, dampness, motion, lying down, fats, and rich foods. **Better from:** Cold drinks, and being kept warm.

Lachesis: Onset of this type of sore throat is usually in cloudy weather during spring. It begins on the left side, sometimes spreading to the middle or right side of throat. There are tearing pains extending to the ear, and sensations of constriction, choking, and a lump in the throat going up and down when swallowing. The constriction causes a constant desire to swallow. The throat feels very swollen, and is dark red or purple. The child has sticky mucus, which they try to hawk up. The tongue is red, dry, burning, and may be swollen, cracked at the tip, or trembly when protruded. The child wants any clothes or blankets around the neck to be very loose. They are anxious, nervous, excitable, very talkative, rambling on and on, and sensitive to touch and pain.

Laryngitis: Loss of voice, with larynx painful to the touch.

Tonsillitis: The tonsils are swollen, and purplish or dark red.

Worse from: Pressure from anything around the neck or from the slightest touch; upon waking, lying down, at night, on falling asleep, on the left side, heat, and swallowing hot drinks or saliva. **Better from:** Open air, cold drinks, swallowing solids, eating—especially fruits, and loose clothing, especially around the neck.

Lycopodium: Onset from wet weather. This sore throat begins on the right and then moves to the left. The throat is inflamed, dry, burning, and constricted, with needle-like pains. It may feel as if there is a hard ball in the esophagus. The tonsils are swollen and ulcerated. The child swallows a lot, but there is no thirst. They are very likely to be gassy and bloated. They are weak and chilly, but crave air. They are sensitive to noise and strong smells. These children are irritable and temperamental, kicking, screaming, and throwing tantrums. They are difficult to deal with, especially if contradicted.

Worse from: Between 4–8 (both AM and PM), on falling asleep, lying on the back, cold drinks, cold food, wet weather, warm rooms, going downhill, and after naps or on waking in the morning. **Better from:** Warm drinks and food, motion, early afternoon, burping, and cool (not cold) applications.

Mercurius Iodatus Flavus: Onset is from a cold draft while sweating. This is a right-sided sore throat that can move to the left side. There is a sensation of a lump in the throat, causing a constant desire to swallow. There is a thick, cheesy mucus, and foul-smelling breath. The tongue has a thick, yellow coating at the base and tip, and the edges may be red and imprinted by the teeth. The glands are very swollen, and may be hard. The child may have sudden sharp pains in the ears. There is nausea at the sight of food. The child tends to be lively and talkative.

Tonsillitis: The right tonsil is dark red, and more swollen than the left.

Worse from: Warm drinks, warm rooms, odors, cold damp weather, and spring. **Better from:** Open air, lying on the right side, and cold drinks.

Mercurius Iodatus Ruber: Onset from weather changes, or getting wet. This is a left-sided sore throat. The throat is dark red, and swallowing is painful. Tonsils and throat glands are very swollen and painful, and the glands may feel hard. The muscles of the neck and throat are usually stiff. There is mucus in the nose and throat, which the child tries to hawk up, and profuse saliva to the point of drooling. The tongue may feel scalded and painful to move. There may be the sensation of a lump in the throat. The ears may pop. The child is irritable and weepy.

Tonsillitis: The left tonsil is dark red, and more swollen than the right.

Worse from: After sleep or getting wet, touch, pressure, cold air, afternoon and evening, and swallowing food. **Better from:** Open air if not too cold, and being warmly dressed.

Mercurius Viv (also known as Mercurius Sol): Onset is from getting chilled, which brings on a sore throat at every change in the weather. The throat feels sore, swollen, raw, and burning, and looks red or bluish-red with a white or yellow coating. The pains are needle-like, and shoot into the ear or neck on swallowing. The right side is usually the sorest. Glands in the neck are usually swollen and tender. The child will drool clear saliva onto their pillow. They hawk up lumpy mucus. There is a constant desire to swallow. The breath smells bad, and there is usually a putrid or metallic taste. The tongue may have a white or grey coating and show imprints of the teeth. Like a thermometer, the child is sensitive to heat and cold, and the temperature can be unstable. They are usually quite sweaty. The child is very thirsty for cold water, but it does not satisfy the thirst. They may be hoarse, or lose their voice. The child is weary and may tremble. They are restless, nervous, and constantly changing their mind.

Tonsillitis: The tonsils are very swollen, deep, dark red or bluish-red, with ulcers that drain white pus. They may also have a yellow coating.

Worse from: Evening, drafts, damp weather, sweating, too much cold or heat, lying on the right side, a warm bed, and warm drinks. **Better from:** Moderate, even temperatures, rest, lying on the stomach, and in the morning.

Nitric Acid: Onset from loss of sleep and getting run-down. Sticking pains, as if there are sharp splinters in the throat. The pain is cutting and severe, and can shoot into the ears. Swallowing is difficult. The sweat, urine, and stools have a very offensive odor. The child is chilly. Their eyes may water. They are very irritable, headstrong, pessimistic, sad, and can become despondent. They may get so angry that they tremble. The older child or teen may use vulgar or profane language. They have a lot of self-pity. They are sensitive to noise.

Laryngitis: With hoarseness and tickling.

Tonsillitis: The tonsils are red, swollen, and uneven in size, with patches of small, white ulcers.

Worse from: Swallowing, touch, noise, jarring, motion, after eating, both cold and hot weather, at changes in weather, evening and nighttime, and loss of sleep. **Better from:** Gliding motions, mild weather, plenty of sleep, being kept cool if it is hot, wrapping up if it is cold, and steady, even pressure.

Phytolacca: Onset from exposure to cold, damp weather. The throat is dark red or bluish-red, and feels hot, burning, too narrow, and raw. There is much achiness at the root of the tongue and in the soft palate (back part of the roof of the mouth). Pain comes and goes on the right, and shoots into the ear on swallowing. There is a sensation of a lump or red-hot ball in the throat. There is thick, choking, stringy, greyish-white or yellow mucus that causes much hawking and clearing of the throat. The child cannot swallow anything hot. The tip of the tongue is fiery-red, and may have a yellow patch down the center. Glands are swollen in the neck and under the ear near the jaw joint. The child usually refuses food. They can feel faint on rising. The child may moan a lot, and has very little interest in anything. They are sensitive and restless.

Tonsillitis: The tonsils are swollen and dark blue or dark red. There is pain in the right tonsil, with much burning.

Worse from: Cold damp weather, changes in weather, hot drinks, touch, and pressure. **Better from:** Warmth, cold drinks, rest, and lying on the stomach or left side.

Rhus Tox: The onset is from getting wet, sitting on damp ground, overexertion, or getting overheated after being chilled. The throat is red and puffy. The sore throat starts on the left and may stay there, or move to the right side. There is usually itching of the soft palate. There is a sticking, stinging pain upon swallowing, especially of solids. The tonsils are swollen and appear to be covered with a yellow membrane. The tip of the tongue may be red. The glands are swollen and hot. The child has a dry mouth and throat and is intensely thirsty for small sips of water. They feel stiff after resting, and may complain of joint pain. They are exhausted. This child is anxious, weepy, helpless, mildly delirious, and extremely restless. They cannot get comfortable, and they toss and turn all night.

Laryngitis: For loss of voice after straining it (often occurring in teachers and singers), with yellow mucus, and stiffness of the neck and limbs. Even after resting it, the voice is still lost or very strained, but eventually returns with continued gentle and limited use.

Worse from: Cold damp weather, autumn, cold food or drinks, being uncovered, drafts, lying still, on first movement after resting, and at night. **Better from:** Warm drinks and food, constant gentle motion, stretching, warmth, changing positions, and massage.

Sabadilla: Onset is from getting chilled in cold air. The child cannot stick their tongue out because the throat is so sore. The sore throat starts on the left side and moves to right. There is the sensation of a lump or thread in the throat, with a constant desire to swallow, although this is very painful. The saliva is jelly-like and tastes sweet. There may be itching in the soft palate. The child has no thirst except after a chill. The head and face are hot, and the feet cold. Tip of the tongue is sore, with a pricking sensation. The child feels very chilly. They are extremely sensitive to odors. The child is miserable. Any effort, even thinking, is overwhelming. They are nervous, easily startled, and obsessed that their condition is really dangerous.

Worse from: Cold air, cold applications, any pressure on the larynx, any odors, especially flowers or garlic. **Better from:** Heat, warm food and drinks, open air, eating, calm, and being wrapped up.

Sulphur: Onset from getting chilled. The pains are burning, raw and needle-like. The mucus is so hot that it burns the throat and makes it sore. The throat is red, very dry, and hot. The tonsils are swollen. There may be sensations of choking, or that there is a lump, hair, or splinter in the throat. The whole throat hurts, but the left side is worse. They may have a deep, hoarse voice in the morning. The external throat, lips, nose, ears, eyelids, or skin in spots may be red. The room is likely to smell noticeably stale and sour. Frequent loose stools may accompany this sore throat. You may notice that the child is sleeping with their feet out from under the covers. They drink a lot, but eat little. The child is irritable, sluggish, quarrelsome, and restless.

Note: Sulphur is used in the later stages of an acute illness, where other remedies helped initially but are no longer working. This is true especially after **Mercurius Vivus** or **Lycopodium.** Make sure the symptoms fit the remedy description. **Sulphur** should not be overused. If the child does not improve after giving this remedy, consult your healthcare practitioner.

Worse from: Bathing, a warm bed, standing, overexertion, around 11 AM, and at the full moon. **Better from:** Dry, warm weather, open air, gentle motion, and sweating.

More remedies for laryngitis:

Causticum: For laryngitis with an onset from cold drafts, or during the later stages of a cold. There is a sore, raw, scraping, and burning dryness in the throat. It feels too narrow, which produces a constant desire to swallow. It is difficult to get mucus up. The vocal cords feel paralyzed, which makes the voice hoarse, husky, weak, and cracking. The throat and larynx are very tender to the touch. The least thing makes the child cry. They are sensitive, anxious, and irritable, do not want to go to bed alone, and may be fearful of the dark or ghosts.

Worse from: Voice strain, inhaling cold dry air, coughing, talking, from 3–4 AM and 6–8 PM, stooping, exertion, and darkness. **Better from:** Moist air, sipping cold water, damp wet weather, pressure on the chest, a warm bed, and gentle motion.

Kali Bich: Onset from getting chilled. The throat is red and inflamed, with dryness, burning, roughness, constriction, and tickling. The larynx is sore and raw, with a burning that extends up to the nostrils and sometimes down into the stomach. The voice is very hoarse or completely lost due to the thick mucus around the vocal cords. The tonsils are swollen, which can diminish the child's hearing. They clear their throat a lot. If they can hawk up the mucus, it is profuse, thick, and comes out in strings. Glands are swollen. The child may feel as if there is a hair on their tongue or in their nostrils. The child is very weak. They are ill-humored, low-spirited, indifferent, and lazy.

Worse from: Cold, damp, spring, autumn, undressing, evening and morning after sleep, talking, and laughing. **Better from:** Warmth, being wrapped up, pressure, and motion as tolerated.

Phosphorus: Onset from getting drenched in rain. The throat is raw, dry, burning, and constricted, and very painful, with violent tickling when talking. The tonsils and uvula are swollen. The larynx is very painful, with needle-like and tearing pain, and the voice is low, squeaky, and hoarse. The child hawks up thick mucus. They are thirsty for ice-cold drinks and food, but feel chilly. They may have a tickling cough as well. This child needs attention, consolation, and massage, which will make them feel much better. The child is affectionate, fearful, easily upset, and irritable.

Worse from: Changes in weather, wind, cold thunderstorms, odors, light, lying on the left side, exertion, talking, morning, evening, and laughing. **Better from:** Sleep, sympathy, low lights or darkness, eating and drinking cold things, cool applications, open air, and sitting.

Spongia Tosta: Onset can be from dry, cold winds, or too much excitement. There is burning and stinging in the throat, and hoarseness and constriction while talking or singing. The voice often gives way. The tonsils are swollen. The chin and outside front of the throat may be swollen. Everything is dry—the mucous membranes, tongue, throat, and all air passages. The child may grasp at the throat when swallowing. There is soreness, burning, constriction, dryness, bruised pain, and the feeling of a plug in the larynx. The larynx is sensitive to touch. The child has a bitter taste in their mouth, and constantly clears their throat. They like to have the throat covered. This child has much anxiety, exhaustion, and a feeling of heaviness. They are easily excitable.

Worse from: Warm rooms, dry cold wind, after sleep, touch, singing, too much excitement, during the day, swallowing, talking, cold drinks, sweets, and the full moon. **Better from:** Warm drinks, eating a little warm food, calm, quiet, lying on the back, moist heat, and keeping the throat covered.

Dosage: If the onset is fast, give 2 pellets every 15 minutes for four doses, then hourly until there is improvement. If there is no improvement after seven doses, choose a new remedy. If the onset has been slow, give the remedy every 1–2 hours for six doses. Repeat the remedy only if there is a return of the same symptoms. Repeat only as necessary. You may need to repeat the remedy 2–3 times per day for a few days.

If you get no result within twenty-four hours, then reassess the symptoms. You may not have been wrong with your initial choice of remedy, but the child may have moved on to needing a different one. Change the remedy if you have followed the above guidelines with no results, or if the symptoms clearly change. For instance, **Mercurius Viv** may be needed initially but, as hours or days go by, symptoms may change and indicate that **Sulphur** is now needed.

Supportive Measures:

Push fluids, especially if there is a fever, to prevent dehydration. Discontinue or keep dairy products to a minimum, because they cause excess mucus and raise the level of acidity in the system. Goat's milk or products made from it may be substituted for cow's milk and products containing it. Use organic dairy. The older child can gargle with one teaspoon of Calendula Tincture in one cup of warm water, three times a day.

In children over three years old, you can use lozenges that do *not* contain camphor, menthol, or eucalyptus. Blackcurrant pastilles or lemon drops do not have these nullifying products in them. Humidify the room if your home has forced-air heat. If warm drinks feel better to the child, you can give them hot water with lemon and honey. This can be very soothing to a sore throat. If your child feels better from cold drinks, fresh carrot juice is soothing to a sore throat.

Call your healthcare practitioner if:

- Your baby is under three months old, and has any rise in temperature.
- Your child is over three months old, and has a temperature over 103 degrees.
- Your child is under two years of age, and has had a fever for more than twenty-four hours.
- Your child is over two years of age, and has had a fever for more than three days.

Call your healthcare practitioner if (cont):

- Your child has a lack of reaction, trouble breathing, convulsions, or is listless or limp.
- A rash appears on the body at the same time as the child has influenza.
- There is stiffness and pain in the neck along with fever.
- There is great difficulty swallowing, with severe pain.
- Your child's tongue looks like a strawberry; this can indicate scarlet fever.
- There is difficulty breathing.
- Your child has had laryngitis for longer than seven days.
- There is a high fever and rapid swelling in the larynx. You will notice the child excessively drooling on the pillow because they are unable to swallow from the swelling. This can be indicative of a condition called epiglottitis, which can be fatal if the swelling closes the airway completely. The swelling initially causes a croupy-sounding cough, and can rapidly start to block the breathing. Inhaling causes a raspy, noisy sound. There is pain, and the child will lean forward to relieve it. This condition affects children from two to six years of age. It is a rare condition, but very dangerous; if you suspect epiglottitis, take your child to the emergency immediately.
- Tonsillitis is extremely severe. It can produce thickened membranes in the throat and difficulty breathing because of severely swollen and enlarged tonsils. This can indicate presence of a streptococcal infection known as "quinsy." If you suspect this, call your healthcare practitioner, and if they cannot be reached, go to the nearest urgent-care center or emergency room. Quinsy requires close and immediate attention.

THE SEVEN MOST COMMON REMEDIES FOR SORE THROATS

	Aconitum	Apis	Belladonna	Hepar Sulph	Lachesis	Mercurius Viv	Phytolacca
Onset	Sudden high fever after being exposed to icy winds, fright, or shock.	Onset can be from anger, fright, or grief.	Sudden onset, with severe symptoms, after getting chilled or overheated.	Slow onset, from getting too cold or being in a cold wind.	Onset in spring and cloudy weather. Pain begins on left side but may move to middle or right side.	Onset from getting chilled, which brings on a sore throat at every change in the weather.	Getting chilled from dry, cold winds, or from getting over-excited. Onset from exposure to cold, damp weather.
Symptoms	The throat feels constricted. It is red, dry, and hot. Burning and needle-like pains that can shoot into the ears. Difficulty swallowing.	Swollen, dry, constricted, and inflamed throat. Sensation of a splinter in throat. Stinging and burning pains. Tongue, uvula, and throat are swollen.	Child is fine in the morning, but by 3 PM they have a high fever with a sore, bright-red throat that is burning, dry, hot, raw, tender, and constricted.	Severe, sharp splinter-like pains that shoot up into ear on swallowing or yawning. The right side is the most painful, but both sides can be affected.	Tearing pains extending into the ear. Sensation of constriction and choking. Feels like a lump is moving up and down in the throat, which causes a constant desire to swallow.	The throat feels sore, swollen, raw, and burning. It is red or bluish-red, with a white or yellow coating. Needle-like pains shoot into the ear or neck on swallowing.	Throat is dark red or bluish-red. Feels hot, too narrow, raw, and burning. Root of tongue and soft palate aches. Pain comes and goes on the right, and shoots into the ear.
Mood	Child is restless, fearful, and anxious. An older child may have a fear of death. May have nightmares.	Restless, sleepy, and very irritable when disturbed. They may be weepy, but do not want to be touched.	The child is restless and irritable. They can become agitated to the point of biting, screaming, and hitting.	This child is extremely irritable, hypersensitive, easily angered, and does not want to be examined or looked at.	The child is anxious, nervous, excitable, and very talkative, rambling on and on. Sensitive to touch and pain.	The child is weary and may tremble. They are restless, constantly changing their mind, and nervous.	Child may moan a lot. They have very little interest in anything. They are sensitive and restless.
Indications	Tonsils are swollen and feel dry. It feels like something is stuck in the throat. Strong thirst for cold drinks.	Right side is worse. Tongue is fiery-red and raw. Mouth is dry. Throat is red or purple. Skin feels sore and sensitive. The child wants cold water to soothe the throat, but is not thirsty.	Throat muscles are sensitive, making it hard to swallow, but there is a constant desire to do so. Pains are severe, needle-like, and worse on the right side. Glands are usually swollen.	Sensation of a plug or fishbone stuck in the throat. Glands are swollen. Solid food is hard to swallow. Very chilly, with smelly sweat and breath.	Throat is swollen, dark red, or purple. Sticky mucus, which they try to hawk up. The tongue burns, swells, and trembles when protruded.	Right side is usually sorest. Child drools clear saliva on the pillow. Hawks up lumpy mucus. Constant desire to swallow. Breath smells bad.	Sensation of lump or red-hot ball in the throat. Thick and choking greyish-white or yellow mucus. Cannot swallow hot things. Swollen glands in the neck and under the ear.
Worse	Nighttime around midnight, or midday, noise, and pressure.	From 3–5 PM. Warmth, touch, heavy blankets, pressure, swallowing solids, and hot or sour food.	Around 3 PM. Swallowing liquids, cold air, touch, noise, jarring, light, turning the head, and sudden motion.	Touch, uncovering, exertion, cold drafts, winter, solid food, cold dry air, and at night.	Slightest touch on the front of the neck, on waking, lying down, nighttime, on falling asleep, swallowing hot drinks, on the left side, and heat.	Evening, drafts, damp weather, sweating, too much cold or heat, lying on the right side, warmth in bed, and warm drinks.	Cold damp weather, changes in weather, hot drinks, touch, and pressure.
Better	Fresh air, rest, sweating, and hot applications.	Cool applications, cold liquids, air, and being uncovered or lightly covered.	Rest, light covers, sitting semi-erect, low light, and quiet.	Warm drinks, moist heat, being wrapped up, and damp weather.	Open air, cold drinks, swallowing solids, eating, especially fruits, and loose clothing, especially around the neck.	Moderate, even temperatures, rest, lying on the stomach, and morning.	Warmth, cold drinks, rest, and lying on the stomach or left side.
Also For	Laryngitis	Tonsillitis	Tonsillitis	Laryngitis, tonsillitis	Laryngitis, tonsillitis	Tonsillitis	Tonsillitis

PART THREE

First Aid and Travel

Note: It is strongly recommended that you take a first-aid course and learn how to administer CPR (cardio-pulmonary resuscitation) and the Heimlich maneuver for choking. It is also strongly recommended that you purchase a first-aid kit, with sterile dressings for cuts, etc., and that you purchase a bottle of Calendula Tincture to put on cuts, to discourage bacterial growth and slow the bleeding. This can be purchased from a health-food store or natural pharmacy. Keep a bottle of spring water on hand to dilute the tincture: Place 5 drops of the tincture in a quarter-cup of bottled spring water, or fresh water that has been boiled and cooled. Do not put Calendula Tincture on any wound that has not been thoroughly cleaned and disinfected.

YOUR FIRST ASSESSMENT (VERY IMPORTANT!)

In any traumatic situation, it is important to know what remedy to give if the child is in shock. There are two specific remedies for shock—**Aconitum** or **Arnica**—and they are used in different situations, so please familiarize yourself with the specific indications for each remedy:

Aconitum: The child is very fearful, anxious, extremely reactive to pain, and inconsolable, with glassy eyes or dilated pupils; they are likely to be screaming, crying out, and trembling with terror and pain.

Arnica: The child is stunned, irritable when offered help, exhausted, and uncooperative; they say they are fine, and don't want to be touched. They may complain of pain, but will maintain that not much is wrong with them.

Dosage: Give 2 pellets of Aconitum or Arnica every 15 minutes until improvement. After the shock has cleared, you can then give the appropriate remedy.

ALLERGIC REACTIONS

Allergic reactions can be mild (the child may sneeze for a few minutes) to severe (anaphylactic shock and potentially fatal respiratory arrest). An allergic reaction is the body's response to an allergen—any substance that the body tries to defend itself against. This response can trigger a release of histamines into the tissues, causing inflammation and other symptoms.

Typical allergic responses to an allergen include: sneezing, runny nose, eyes that are swollen, puffy, red, watering, or excessively dry, swelling and itching in other parts of the body, inflammations, hives (itchy, stinging welts on the skin), rashes, vomiting, or diarrhea. Hives can also be produced by an emotional upset.

Extreme allergic responses to an allergen include: paleness, swelling of lymph glands, swelling of the tongue or throat, which blocks the air passages and constricts breathing; extreme itching, extreme sweating, rapid pulse, shallow and/or irregular breathing, confusion, collapse, or unconsciousness.

Asthma responses to an allergen include: mild to severe wheezing, shortness of breath, coughing, chest tightness, rattling, increased mucus in the bronchi (the main tubes into the lungs), and sometimes sneezing. Coughing can lead to retching and sometimes vomiting. The underlying cause of asthma needs to be addressed by your healthcare practitioner. *If the child's breathing is obstructed in any way, take them to the hospital immediately.*

Hay fever is a common allergic response to various plants or trees that are in bloom throughout the seasons. The underlying cause to this overactive response needs to be addressed by your healthcare practitioner.

Remedies for allergies from the most common allergens (excluding hay-fever allergens):

Animal Dander: Arsenicum
Car Fumes: Carbo Veg, Petroleum
Cold: Rhus Tox
Dust: Arsenicum
Pesticides: Arsenicum
Poisonous Plants: Arsenicum, Rhus Tox
Pollution: Carbo Veg
Shellfish: Arsenicum, Urtica Urens

Remedies for hives:

Apis, Arsenicum, Carbolic Acid, Rhus Tox, Urtica Urens

The most commonly used remedies for (non-hay fever) allergic reactions:

Apis: For hives accompanied by the following symptoms:

Eyes: Swollen, puffy, red eyelids. Burning, stinging, and shooting pains. Hot, burning tears. Whites of eyes are bloodshot.

Face: Swelling, redness, and puffiness, especially of the eyelids, lips, nose, mouth, and throat.

Lungs: Panting breathing; the child feels they cannot get enough air, or cannot take another breath.

Skin: Swelling, itchy, puffy, sensitive, sore, hot, and a shiny, rosy-red color. Sensations of constriction and stiffness. Large masses of hives, with burning, stinging, and itching that is especially intense at night. Very sensitive to touch. Swelling is rapid. No thirst. The child can be drowsy, and is constantly whining, weepy, restless, anxious, irritable, fidgety, tired, and wanting to lie down.

Note: Do not use this remedy in combination with **Rhus Tox.**

Worse from: Heat in any form, touch, late afternoon, nighttime, pressure, after sleep, when lying down, and on the right side. **Better from:** Cold applications, cool air, cool baths, sitting up, cool drinks, and being uncovered.

Arsenicum: For hives from eating shellfish, or reactions to dust, smoke, pesticides, poisonous plants, or animal dander.

Eyes: Burning, with extreme sensitivity to light.

Face: Pale, with an anxious or pinched look, swelling, and sometimes covered with a cold sweat.

Hands and feet: Swelling.

Lungs: Wheezing, shortness of breath, whistling breath, burning in chest, and difficulty coughing up frothy mucus.

Nose: Sneezing with a thin, clear, burning discharge, and itching.

Skin: Burning, itching, sensitivity to touch, swelling; transparent bumps that are dry, rough, scaly, and itchy. Scratching makes itching worse. The child may have sensations of crawling or tickling.

The child has many burning symptoms; however, they are very chilly and feel better with warmth. They may have heart palpitations. They have frequent thirst for small amounts of water. They do not want to lie down for fear of suffocation. The child is weak and exhausted, but may be restless in bed. They are anxious, irritable, oversensitive, needy, and demanding. The older child may fear they are dying or will not get better.

Worse from: Physical exertion, after midnight, anything cold, and lying down. **Better from:** Warmth, hot compresses, warm drinks, sitting at a forty-five-degree angle, fresh air, and company.

Carbo Veg: For reactions to pollution or car fumes.

Eyes: Heavy, droopy look, burning; muscles of eyes are sore, and pupils can be nonreactive to light.

Face: Pale, puffy, covered in cold sweat; may have a bluish tint, especially around the mouth, and nose may be cold.

Lungs: Breathing is shallow, quick and labored. The chest feels heavy, burning, sore, or weak on waking, with wheezing and rattling sounds produced by thick, sticky, yellow mucus. There is gagging and retching while trying to get the mucus up. The breath is cold, but the child feels hot and wants to be fanned. The voice may be deep and raspy.

Skin: Burning, hot sweat that can develop into a moist, burning, itchy rash that is worse at night.

If the child is having a reaction to pollution or car fumes, the head becomes hot and they have an intense pain at the base of the skull. They feel weak, sick, and exhausted to the point of showing very little reactivity. The breathing may become quickened. The body and breath are cold, but they want to be fanned, and crave fresh air. Internally there is a general coldness throughout the body, or in specific spots. The child is thirsty. This child is low in vitality, and weak to the point of collapse. They are exhausted by even the slightest exertion.

The child will be indifferent to everything, a bit confused, irritable, and very sluggish. May exhibit fear of dark and ghosts. May complain of numbness in limbs.

Worse from: Warmth and warm rooms, on waking, evening times, walking, eating, talking, and changes of temperature.
Better from: Being fanned vigorously, elevating the feet, cool air, belching, and rest.

Carbolic Acid: For hives.

Face: There is paleness around the nose and mouth, but the rest of the face is a dusky-red color, which may be subtle. The face, ears, tongue, and throat may become swollen. If swallowing or breathing becomes difficult, *call 911! Give 2 pellets of this remedy immediately, and repeat every 15 minutes.*

Skin: Inflamed, burning, and itchy, with sensations of tingling and numbness. Hives that severely sting, burn, and itch. The hives may spread over the entire body.

The affected part will be weak, with severe burning, pricking and intensely itching pains that come and go. One symptom strongly indicating this remedy is that the sense of smell becomes very acute. The child may have cold hands and feet, and may break out into a cold, clammy sweat or tremble. They rapidly loose vitality and strength, which may bring about collapse. The least amount of physical or mental exertion leaves them exhausted.

Worse from: Warm rooms, cold drafts, jarring, and reading.
Better from: Tepid temperatures, rest, strong green or black tea, and scratching that temporarily relieves itching.

Petroleum: For reactions to pollution or car fumes.

Face: Pale or yellow.

Child has nausea, with or without vomiting, from every movement of a boat, train, or car. Profuse salivation while nauseated, with a dizzy, heavy feeling. The nausea may be relieved by constantly eating; the appetite can become ravenous. There is pain with a cold, empty sensation in the stomach, and there may be heartburn. The child may have a dull, heavy headache. Their sleep is restless, with frightening dreams. The child is disoriented, irritable, and quarrelsome.

Worse from: The smell of gas or diesel, fresh air, especially if it is cold, and closing the eyes. **Better from:** Warm air, lying, and head elevated.

Rhus Tox: For rashes from poison ivy, poison oak, or other plants that may cause allergic reactions; hives, including those from an allergic response to cold water or air.

Hives: Intense itchiness and redness, with fluid-filled blisters that can become infected.

Skin: Hot, inflamed, dry, burning, swollen, with a red rash. Water-filled blisters or hives that itch intensely. Sensitivity to cold air. The skin may become scaly.

The glands, joints, or muscles around the affected area may become stiff and achy. There is a loss of appetite, and sometimes nausea. The child can have a headache at the base of the skull or across the forehead. The head feels heavy, and the scalp is sensitive. There may be a bitter or metallic taste in the mouth. The tip of the tongue may be red in the form of a triangle. Even though the child feels worse with cold, they do crave cold drinks. The child has extreme mental and physical restlessness and irritability. They cannot get comfortable. They are anxious, and may become confused and/or weepy.

Note: *Do not use this remedy in combination with **Apis.***

Worse from: Cold, damp, cold applications on skin, scratching, beginning to move after resting or sitting, and nighttime. **Better from:** Movement, limbering up, warm applications, and heat.

Urtica Urens: For hives, stinging-nettle rash, or allergic reactions to eating shellfish.

Face, hands, and feet: Swelling, stinging, redness, burning.

Hives: Burning, stinging, intense itching, possibly pains in the joints, especially if reaction is to shellfish.

Skin: Itching, with raised, pale welts on a background of red skin. These areas appear in blotches. The itching can be quite severe. The child feels hot in bed at night, with sweating. May experience burning in throat. The child is very restless, and wants to rub the affected area.

Worse from: Cold water, cool moist air, touch, nighttime, and strenuous exercise. **Better from:** Lying down (but not on the affected parts), and rubbing the affected area.

Dosage: To administer a remedy if a child's breathing is severely compromised, or if they are unconscious (although it has been said not to touch the remedies in normal circumstances), put the remedy into a half-glass of water, and dab it with your finger onto the child's lips, or onto the wrist where the pulse is beating (just above the thumb).

If the condition is severe, give 2 pellets every 10–30 minutes until there is improvement. If the condition is significant, give 2 pellets hourly until there is improvement. If there has been no improvement after two hours, choose a new remedy. Repeat the remedy only if there is a return of the same symptoms. Repeat only as necessary. You may need to repeat the remedy 2–3 times per day for a few days. Change the remedy if you have followed the above guidelines and have had no results, or if the symptoms clearly change.

Supportive Measures:

Baking soda or oatmeal baths and poultices can be soothing for the swelling and itching. For a bath, use one cup of baking soda in a bathtub full of warm (not hot) water. For a poultice, mix one teaspoon of bottled spring water, or fresh water that has been boiled and cooled, with one teaspoon of baking soda or oatmeal, and put the paste on the affected area. Lightly cover the area with sterile gauze. Remove gauze and rinse with cool water when the itching has subsided and the swelling has gone down.

You can use cold compresses if it makes the child feel better. Have the child drink lots of water to flush out the histamine. Give vitamin C, or foods rich in vitamin C, to continue the flushing out.

Call your healthcare practitioner if:

- *Your child is experiencing an extreme allergic response.* Anaphylactic shock is a condition where the body releases large amounts of histamine into the bloodstream. This causes dilation of the blood vessels and constriction of the airways. It can come on quickly, causing heat and difficulty in breathing due to closing of the air passages. The blood pressure can drop dramatically, causing faintness and irregular heart palpitations that can set off extreme panic in a child. *In the case of severe allergic responses, the child should be taken to an emergency room immediately. If you are not close to a hospital, call 911.* **Apis** can save a life if there is an extreme allergic reaction. Give every 15 minutes, *even while waiting at the hospital.*
- Your child keeps having acute asthma attacks.
- *Call the hospital or local poison control center* if you suspect that your child has eaten a poisonous plant. There are some plants for which you would want to induce vomiting, and others you would *not* want the child to vomit.

BITES AND STINGS

With any bite or sting, first, assess whether your child is in shock. See "Your First Assessment" at the beginning of this section (page 229).

Note: You do not need to give a remedy for a bee, wasp, mosquito, flea, or nonpoisonous spider bite unless the child is in great discomfort or has been stung repeatedly.

Remedies for specific animal bites
(see details on specific remedies below):

Cats: Arsenicum, Hypericum, Lachesis, or Ledum. These bites are puncture wounds. The flesh may also be torn by claws. (See "Wounds" section, p. 347)

Dogs: Arnica or Bellis Perennis, for deeply bruised wounds when a child has been nipped by a dog. If the bite has actually drawn blood, you may also need Apis, Arsenicum, Hypericum, Lachesis, or Ledum.

Horses: Arnica or Bellis Perennis, for deeply bruised wounds when they have been nipped by a horse. If the bite has actually drawn blood, you may also need Arsenicum, Hypericum, Lachesis, or Ledum.

Infected bites: Hepar Sulph, Pyrogenium.

Rodents: Arsenicum, Hypericum, Lachesis, or Ledum. These bites are puncture wounds. The flesh may also be torn by claws. (See "Wounds" section, p. 347.)

Snakes: Snakebites are puncture wounds, and may be poisonous. Immediately give a dose of Aconitum to reduce anxiety, therefore reducing the spread of venom. Repeat if the anxiety returns. Next, within 3 minutes, give 2 pellets of Ledum to further restrict the spread of venom. Then choose the appropriate remedy from the following: Apis, Arsenicum, Carbolic Acid, Crotalus, Lachesis, or Ledum. Alternating Ledum and Lachesis every hour is very effective, if the symptom picture fits.

Trauma after a bite: Being bitten by an animal, especially a family pet, can be quite traumatic. If the child feels abused by the animal and can no longer trust it, **Staphysagria** will resolve the trauma. If the child is extremely afraid of the animal, give 3 **Aconitum** pellets every 2 hours, for three doses.

Remedies for specific insect and other bites or
stings (see details for specific remedies below):

Ant: Apis, Lachesis
Bedbug: Lachesis

Bee: Apis, Hypericum, Ledum, Urtica Urens
Flea: Apis, Ledum
Hornet: Apis, Hypericum, Ledum
Horsefly: Hypericum, Ledum
Jellyfish: Medusa, Urtica Urens
Mosquito: Apis, Ledum
Scorpion: Carbolic Acid, Crotalus, Lachesis
Sea Urchin: Silicea
Spider: Carbolic Acid, Crotalus,
Hypericum, Lachesis
Wasp: Apis, Hypericum, Ledum

The most commonly used remedies for bites and stings:

Apis: This remedy is used for puncture wounds with rapid swelling. The skin is puffy, rosy-colored, and very sensitive to touch, with burning, hot, piercing, stinging pains. The child is not thirsty. They are constantly whining, weepy, restless, anxious, irritable, fidgety, tired, and wanting to lie down. They can become scared of being alone.

Worse from: Heat in any form, touch, late afternoon, lying down, pressure, after sleeping, and on the right side. **Better from:** Cold applications, cool air, cool bathing, sitting up, cool drinks, and being uncovered.

Arnica: For bruising and swelling from a bite that has not broken the skin. The pain is sore, aching, and bruised-feeling. The skin is black-and-blue. There may be tingling, and the child may be sleepy. They do not want to be touched, approached by anyone, or fussed over. They will say they are OK, just so they will be left alone.

Worse from: Touch, jarring, and motion. **Better from:** Lying stretched out or with head low, and not talking.

Arsenicum: For puncture wounds with burning symptoms. Swelling with burning pain. The skin is dry, rough, scaly, sensitive to touch, and may have sensations of crawling and/or tickling. If the wound becomes infected, it oozes foul, yellow pus. The child may have heart palpitations. They have frequent thirst for small amounts of water. They are very chilly and feel better with warmth, even though most of the symptoms are of a burning nature. They do not want to lie down for fear of suffocation. The face is pale, with an anxious or pinched look, and may be covered in cold sweat. The child is weak and exhausted, but may be restless in bed. They are anxious, irritable, oversensitive, needy, and demanding. The older child may fear they are dying or will not get better.

Worse from: Physical exertion, after midnight, anything cold, and lying down. **Better from:** Warmth, hot compresses, warm drinks, sitting at a forty-five-degree angle, fresh air, and company.

Bellis Perennis: For bruising from a bite that has not broken the skin. Use this remedy for a dog or horse bite that has damaged an area of soft flesh. This is a very important remedy for bites to the breast. The pains are achy and throbbing; there is intense soreness and sensitivity to touch. There is much swelling, sometimes long after the trauma occurs. Nearby glands can swell as well. Pains are throbbing, aching, and squeezing. There may also be a sensation of coldness in the wound. The child is restless, and may wake at 3 AM. They can also be detached and confused.

Worse from: Touch, cold or hot bathing, getting chilled after being overheated, and immobility. **Better from:** Continued motion, rubbing, and cool compresses.

Carbolic Acid: Remedy for scorpion and spider bites. The part affected will be weak, with severe, burning, pricking pains that come and go. A strong indicator for this remedy is that the sense of smell becomes very acute. There is inflammation and burning, with sensations of tingling and numbness. Bites may form blisters with smelly, clear fluid, which intensely itch and burn. The child may have cold hands and feet. They may break out into a cold, clammy sweat. They may tremble. They rapidly loose vitality and strength, to the point of collapse. The least amount of physical or mental exertion leaves them exhausted.

Worse from: Warm rooms, cold drafts, jarring, and reading.
Better from: Tepid temperatures, rest, strong green or black tea, and scratching, which gives temporary relief.

Crotalus: Remedy for rattlesnake bites. Rapid onset with burning. The breath smells moldy. The tongue is scarlet-red, and it is difficult to swallow. There is sensitivity of skin on the right side of the body. The perspiration is hot, with high fever and delirium, but the skin is cold and dry. Profound nervous shock, with trembling and prostration. The area around the bite can become discolored with a dark or bluish tint. There is much swelling. If the bite becomes infected, there is a putrid, moldy smell. The wound oozes dark, unclotted blood. The child has a haggard expression. The head can feel as though there has been a blow to the base of the skull. There is sensitivity to light. The child is irritable, forgetful, trembling, weepy, emotionally sensitive, and easily tired by even the slightest exertion.

Worse from: Jarring, lying on the right side, waking and falling asleep, damp, and wet. **Better from:** Light, rest, gentle motion, and cool.

Hepar Sulph: For bites that have become infected and are not healing; this remedy can keep the infection from spreading. The pains are sore, splinter-like, and sharp. The bite area is hard, with much heat. The skin around the area is dry. The wound may ooze pus, or look abscessed. The pus may smell like old, rotten cheese. The child is chilly and sensitive to cold drafts. It is not unusual to have a low-grade fever with much sweating. The child is touchy, irritable, easily dissatisfied, and overly sensitive to pain, cold, noise, and odors.

Worse from: Touch, cold, cold drafts, loud noise, and night. **Better from:** Warmth, moist heat, and quiet.

Hypericum: Effective for bites in nerve-rich areas such as fingers, toes, eyes, or lips. Bites in these areas are very painful, tender, and inflamed, with burning heat in the skin; wounds are tenderer than they would be elsewhere. Severe, tearing pains that shoot upward along the nerve pathways. Nerve pains are sharp and intense. There is usually swelling. There is a heightened sense of pain, smell, and hearing. The child may experience numbness and tingling. They have a great thirst. They can become nervous and depressed, and may seem confused, forgetful, and have a wild, staring look on their face. They are constantly drowsy.

Worse from: Pressure, touch, cold, and damp. **Better from:** Lying on the face, rubbing, and bending the head back.

Lachesis: For snakebites that are especially slow to heal. The wound is dark red, bluish, or purplish. There is much burning, throbbing, or shooting pain. The wound is swollen, feels tense, tight, and very full. It feels like it is going to burst open. The onset is rapid, and they go down fast. The skin is cold and clammy. There is great sensitivity of the affected area, because the nerves become very sensitive. The wound from the bite may profusely bleed thin, dark-red blood. The child is tense, nervous, excitable, and very talkative, jumping from one topic to another. They may fear going to sleep.

Worse from: Touch, nighttime, heat, constriction, pressure, tight clothing, especially around the neck or waist, and on awakening. **Better from:** Allowing the wound to freely discharge, open air, and cold drinks.

Ledum: This remedy is effective for bites on the fingers, toes, or face, and if there are a lot of puncture lacerations from any bite. The site is puffy, tender, and very dark-red or purple. There may be a spotty rash. The skin feels cold to the touch; however, it feels better with cold applications. There may be twitching around the site of the bite. Pains are throbbing, shooting, and pricking, and may shoot up an arm or leg. There is usually weakness and numbness of the affected part. If the wound becomes infected, the pus is foul-smelling. Repeat the remedy only if the pain returns, or if the child complains that the bite feels cold. The child is angry, dissatisfied, and wants to be left alone. They may be anxious.

Worse from: Heat, warmth, touch, pressure, motion, and nighttime. **Better from:** Cold applications and rest.

Medusa: Medusa is specifically for jellyfish stings in the Mediterranean Sea or tropical waters. Repeat this remedy often, because this sting is quite painful. The eyes, ears, nose, and face are puffy and swollen. There are numbness, burning, pricking heat, a rash, and fluid-filled blisters. The child may experience retention of urine. They are extremely anxious, and may have difficulty talking.

Worse from: Touch and pressure. **Better from:** Rest.

Pyrogenium: For bites that have become infected. The bite site is dark-red or purple, with much swelling and inflammation. The site is very painful, with much burning internally. The skin at the edge of the site is pale, dry, and cold. There is a feeling of soreness and aching in the limbs, as if they are coming down with the flu. A fever may be present. This remedy is indicated for swollen wounds that ooze foul-smelling pus or if, after the wound is healed, there remains a state of lethargy, depression, achiness, and soreness. The child's bed feels too hard. They are restless, sensitive, anxious, confused, and talk a lot. They are also lethargic with no energy in the morning.

This type of wound should be followed up with your healthcare practitioner. If the fever becomes high, take the child to the hospital.

Worse from: Cold, damp, morning, prolonged motion, and prolonged sitting. **Better from:** Heat, hot drinks, stretching, rocking, pressure, changing positions, and short walks.

Silicea: For stings from the spines of a sea urchin. The site becomes inflamed and produces a discharge of smelly, creamy-colored pus. The area may be slow to heal, and this remedy will help complete the healing process. The child is extremely chilly, but also sweaty, with a sour smell, especially around the head. They have cold hands and feet. They tire easily and lack stamina. This child is subdued, shy, anxious, nervous, and overly sensitive, especially to all senses and pain. However, they can also be stubborn and uncooperative.

Worse from: The left side, cold air and drafts, being uncovered, morning, damp, being consoled, loud noises, and the full moon. **Better from:** Warmth, being wrapped up, urination, yawning, and swallowing.

Urtica Urens: For jellyfish and bee stings. Repeat often for a jellyfish sting, because it is quite painful. This remedy is for when there is much itching, with raised, pale welts on a background of red skin. These areas appear in blotches. There is burning, swelling, and stinging. The itching can be quite severe. The child feels hot in bed at night, and sweats. They may experience burning in the throat, or pains in the joints. They want to rub the affected area. This child is very restless.

Worse from: Cold water, cool moist air, touch, night, and strenuous exercise. **Better from:** Lying down (but not on the affected parts), and rubbing (but not scratching) the stings.

Dosage: If the condition is severe, give 2 pellets every 10–30 minutes until there is improvement. Otherwise, give 2 pellets hourly until there is improvement. If there has been no improvement after two hours, choose a new remedy. Repeat the remedy only if there is a return of the same symptoms. Repeat only as necessary. You may need to repeat the remedy 2–3 times per day for a few days. Change the remedy if you have had no results, or if the symptoms clearly change.

Supportive Measures
(after you have given a first dose of the remedy):

Note: Some bite wounds may take quite a bit of time to heal.

Insect stings: Remove a bee stinger (wasps do not leave stingers behind) by scraping a sterilized needle across the skin as soon as possible. Do not pull the stinger out with fingers or tweezers, as this can squeeze more venom into the puncture. Clean the wound. A paste of baking soda

Supportive Measures (cont):

and water feels best on the sting. Use an ice pack to reduce swelling and prevent the venom from spreading to surrounding tissues. You can crush a few pellets of **Apis** in half an ounce of bottled spring water, or water that has been boiled and cooled, and apply directly onto the sting. If your child is extremely reactive to bee stings or anything else, ask your homeopath for a higher (1M) potency of **Apis** or go to www.hchild.com and link onto Natural Health Supply to order a higher potency; carry this with you at all times. Remember to keep remedies away from cellphones.

Jellyfish stings: Rinse the sting with seawater. (Fresh water will increase the pain.) Do not apply ice packs, or rub the area. Apply 5% acetic acid (white vinegar) or isopropyl alcohol (except in the eye area). Flush eye-area stings with one gallon of bottled spring water, or fresh water that has been boiled and cooled. Use 1 part vinegar to 4 parts of water for mouth-area stings. However, do not use vinegar if there is any swelling in the mouth or throat, or difficulty swallowing. Carefully remove any tentacles with tweezers while wearing gloves. Apply a paste of baking soda, mud, or shaving cream to the injury, and then shave any hair from the area with a knife or razor, and reapply the vinegar or alcohol. (The paste will absorb any additional toxin discharge during the shaving.) You can crush a few pellets of **Medusa** in half an ounce of spring water and apply directly to the sting site.

Sea-urchin stings: Remove any spines carefully with tweezers while wearing gloves. You probably can't get the entire spine out, so get out what you can. Do not dig too deeply. Do this as soon as possible, to reduce pain and

Supportive Measures (cont):

start the healing process. Cover the area immediately with a clean cloth soaked in white vinegar with 5% acetic acid, and leave it on for as long as possible. Have the child soak the affected area in the hottest water they can tolerate for 20–40 minutes. This eases the pain, and will help to alleviate soreness on the following day. Soak the area with the vinegar cloth again, all night if possible. Watch for infection. There may be a dark discoloration immediately after the sting. Any stingers that are not removed will dissolve on their own; giving a small extra dose of vitamin D can speed this process. All sea urchins are poisonous to varying degrees, but there are a few deadly varieties. *If you suspect your child has been stung by a deadly one, seek immediate medical help.*

Snakebite: A snakebite causes swelling, intense pain, and redness or blueness of the skin that looks like a bad bruise. There may be a fever, with muscle or abdominal cramping. Sometimes there are burning pains or sensations throughout the body, or in certain parts. Apply an ice pack to keep the venom from spreading, keep the area immobilized, and give the appropriate remedies on the way to the hospital. It is important to follow up with your healthcare practitioner, because chronic symptoms can appear long after the bite has occurred.

Spider bites cause both swelling and pain. All spiders are poisonous to varying degrees. The bite can be anything from a tiny red welt to a very toxic reaction. Apply an ice pack to keep the poison from spreading. There are usually two puncture wounds if the bite is from a spider. *Seek medical help if you suspect the spider was a dangerous variety.*

Supportive Measures (cont):

Use a natural insect repellent. Avoid using chemical-
-based insect repellents. There are good repellents in
health-food stores that have been tested in tropical jungles. Apply the lotion or spray to any exposed areas, and
reapply as needed. You can also purchase natural lotions
that relieve stinging sensations from bites.

*Do not use bug spray to kill insects, because it is toxic
and can be harmful to a child if inhaled.*

Baking soda or oatmeal baths can soothe the swelling and itching. Use one cup of baking soda in a bathtub full of warm (not hot) water. Externally apply creams
that contain calendula, or apply a few drops of Hypercal
to bites and stings from mosquitoes, bees, wasps, hor-
nets, and fleas. Hypercal is a combination of Hypericum
Tincture, which heals damaged nerves, and Calendula
Tincture, which repairs damaged skin. This combination
is invaluable when applied topically, as it not only brings
about rapid healing but also helps to prevent scarring.
Some health-food stores or natural pharmacies may
have this product. If it is not available, you can obtain
each of these tinctures and make your own solution:
Put 5 drops of each tincture in a quarter-cup of bottled
spring water, or fresh water that has been boiled and
cooled. Apply to the skin with a sterile cloth or cotton
ball on an as-needed basis until healed. This solution
stings at first, but then takes the pain and stinging away.
*The skin must be clean and disinfected before applying
this solution.*

Supportive Measures (cont):

Clean all wounds by washing the area with mild soap and running water. If running water is not available, use a sterile cloth with soap and water. Wipe away from the wound, not into it. Keep all wounds clean and dry. If the wound does not have any redness, you can apply sterile gauze soaked in 5 drops of Calendula Tincture (found in health-food stores or natural pharmacies) to a quarter-cup of bottled spring water, or fresh water that has been boiled and cooled. Apply a new dressing once a day. If the area is inflamed and not healing, see **Hepar Sulph** or **Pyrogenium,** above. Follow the guidelines below.

Call your healthcare practitioner if:

- There are *red streaks running up or outwards* from the wound. This requires *immediate* attention! Take your child to the hospital.
- You have any suspicion that the animal may have rabies.
- Your child has a swollen throat, difficulty swallowing or breathing, and/or a puffy face. This may indicate *anaphylactic shock,* a condition where the body releases large amounts of histamine into the bloodstream. This causes dilation of blood vessels and constriction of airways. It can come on quickly, causing heat and difficulty in breathing due to closed-off air passages. The blood pressure can drop dramatically, causing faintness and irregular heart palpitations, and this can set off extreme panic in a child. *In cases of severe allergic response, the child should be*

Call your healthcare practitioner if (cont):

taken to an emergency room immediately. If you are not close to a hospital, call 911. **Apis** can save a life if there is an extreme allergic reaction: Give 2 pellets every 10 minutes, even while waiting at the hospital.

- The site of the bite becomes inflamed, bright-red, or purple.
- The child has a high fever and/or is delirious.
- The wound starts oozing foul-smelling pus; this can indicate a bacterial infection.
- A child has been stung in the mouth or throat; airways can swell and obstruct breathing. Give 2 pellets of **Apis** every ten minutes, ice to suck on, and take your child to an urgent-care center or emergency room.
- You suspect your child has been bitten by a poisonous snake. The poisonous snakes in the U.S. are rattlesnakes, copperheads, water moccasins, and coral snakes. Spring is the time of year when the venom of the snake is strongest. The wound must be dealt with as soon as possible in order to avoid nasty symptoms. *If you know your child has been bitten by a poisonous snake, OR if you are not sure whether the snake is poisonous, immediately take your child to the hospital.* If a young child has been bitten by a snake, breathing can become difficult, because the throat can close off. Place the child horizontally on their side with the chin slightly tipped up to keep the air passages open. Apply an ice pack to keep the venom from spreading, keep the area immobilized, and give the appropriate remedies on the way to the hospital. It is important to later follow up with your healthcare practitioner.

Call your healthcare practitioner if (cont):

- You think your child has been bitten by a poisonous spider. The most poisonous spiders in the U.S. are the black widow, brown recluse, and tarantula, although not all tarantula bites are dangerous. *If you know that your child has been bitten by a poisonous spider, immediately take them to the hospital.* Apply an ice pack to keep the venom from spreading, and give the appropriate remedies on the way to the hospital. It is important to later follow up with your healthcare practitioner.
- A baby or young child has been stung by a scorpion. *Take your child to the emergency room.* The poison can easily overwhelm a young child's body. Give 2 pellets of **Carbolic Acid** every 10 minutes on the way to the hospital. Stop when there is relief.
- There is any severe reaction to a sting, which includes the following symptoms:
  - Swelling is severe and spreads rapidly.
  - Pain is severe.
  - Lips, tongue, or joints are swollen or extremely painful.
  - The child is confused, feeling faint, or losing consciousness.
  - There is difficulty breathing. *This requires immediate action, and the child needs to be taken to the emergency room.* Whatever remedy you give, and whatever the response, take the child to the emergency room anyway so that they can be examined. Take no chances, because the child could collapse and go into anaphylactic shock.

BURNS

There are various types of burns to be considered: from a hot object, steam, an exhaust pipe, chemicals, live electric wires, scalding-hot liquids, and sunburn.

In a **first-degree burn,** e.g., a sunburn or minor scald, the upper layer of the skin has intense heat, swelling, pain, and redness.

In a **second-degree burn,** the first and second layers of the skin are burned; there is much pain, redness, swelling, and blisters that may ooze fluids. Blisters should *not* be popped open.

In a **third-degree burn,** the first and second layers of the skin are blackened, charred, or deathly white, with damage to the nerves and underlying tissue. There is usually no pain on the site of the burn, where nerve endings have been destroyed. However, the outlying skin burns and is very painful.

If the burn is severe, the child can go into shock. The combination of a deep burn and shock is dangerous—take the child immediately to the nearest hospital, or call 911 if there is no hospital nearby.

It is important to know which remedy to give if the child is in shock. There are two specific remedies for shock—**Aconitum** or **Arnica**—and they are used in different situations, so please familiarize yourself with the specific indications for each remedy:

Aconitum: The child is very fearful, anxious, extremely reactive to pain, and inconsolable, with glassy eyes or dilated pupils; they are likely to be screaming, crying out, and trembling with terror and pain.

Arnica: The child is stunned, irritable when offered help, exhausted, and uncooperative; they say they are fine, and don't want to be touched. They may complain of pain, but will maintain that not much is wrong with them.

Dosage: Give 2 pellets of Aconitum or Arnica every 15 minutes until improvement.

The most common remedies for burns are
(see individual remedy descriptions below):

First-degree or minor burns: Urtica Urens
Second-degree burns: Causticum
Third-degree burns: Cantharis (If given immediately, this remedy can prevent blistering.)

Remedies for specific types of burns
(whether first-, second-, or third-degree):

Burns over a large area: Carbolic Acid
Chemical burns: Cantharis, Causticum
Chemical burns to the eyes: Apis, Cantharis
Electrical burns: Cantharis, Phosphorus
Grease or oil burns: Arsenicum, Cantharis
Radiation burns: Phosphorus
Scalds: Cantharis, Causticum, Urtica Urens
Sunburns: Apis, Belladonna, Urtica Urens
Tailpipe burns: Causticum, Cantharis
Tongue burns: Apis, Arsenicum, Cantharis, Causticum, Urtica Urens

The following are the most commonly indicated
remedies for burns:

Apis: For sunburn, minor burns, and burns on the tongue.

The skin is sensitive, very swollen, puffy, and either reddened or pale. The pains are intense, burning, and prickling, with intense stinging. The child is thirstless, and may be sweaty. The child is constantly whining, weepy, restless, anxious, irritable, fidgety, tired, and wanting to lie down. They may become scared of being alone, or become dull, absentminded, clumsy, liable to drop things, and apathetic.

Worse from: Heat in any form, touch, late afternoon, sleeping, lying down, pressure, and the right side. **Better from:** Cool applications, cool air, cool bathing, sitting up, cool drinks, and being uncovered.

Arsenicum: Burns from oil or grease; tongue burns, any severe burns.

The skin burns like fire, but the child does not want anything cool on the burned area. This remedy is for burns that have formed blisters. The blisters may ooze a foul discharge, or become bloody. For burns where the skin has turned bluish or black. The child is anxious, agitated, restless, chilly, and weak.

Worse from: Cold applications, cold drinks, and night. **Better from:** Warm (not hot) applications, and warm (not hot) baths.

Belladonna: Sunburn.

The skin is bright red. The pains are of a burning nature, and there may be throbbing. There is much heat with burns helped by this remedy. If the sunburn is severe, the eyes may be glassy and sparkling, with a wild look and dilated pupils. The child may have a throbbing headache. They usually have a craving for very cold water or lemonade. The child's senses are very acute to noise, light, touch, and motion. They are easily excited. They may bite and hit others.

Worse from: Getting overheated or chilled, touch, noise, jarring, light, the sun's heat, and around 3 PM. **Better from:** Rest, light covers, sitting semi-erect, low lights, and quiet.

Cantharis: Serious burns, electrical burns, chemical burns, chemical burns to the eyes, severe sunburns, and scalds to the mouth.

The pains are sharp, needle-like, and burning. The skin feels raw, smarting, stinging, itchy, and inflamed. If there are blisters, touching them produces a burning sensation. The blisters with this remedy tend to ooze fluid. They start out bright-red, and later may start turning black. The child cannot stand to have the cool applications removed for even a few seconds. They are extremely thirsty—but do not give them iced drinks. The child is irritable, restless, and moaning. They are extremely aggravated by the pain, and complain loudly.

Worse from: Touch, scratching, coffee, and iced drinks. **Better from:** Cool applications, lying down, rest, and quiet.

Carbolic Acid: Burns that cover a large area of the body.

The pains are severe, coming and going, and with much burning and pricking like pins and needles. There may also be sensations of tingling and numbness. This is a remedy to use if other remedies are unable to relieve the symptoms within a few days. The blisters burn and itch, and tend to ulcerate and ooze blood. A strong symptom indicating this remedy is that the sense of smell becomes very acute. The child may have cold hands and feet. They may break out into a cold clammy sweat, or tremble. They rapidly loose vitality and strength, which may bring about collapse. The least amount of physical or mental exertion leaves them exhausted.

Worse from: Warm rooms, cold drafts, being jarred, and reading. **Better from:** Tepid temperatures, rest, strong green or black tea, and gentle rubbing, which provides temporary relief.

Causticum: Burns of the tongue, caustic chemicals that have been swallowed, severe burns, and chemical burns.

The pains are burning, with intense soreness. The skin feels raw, stiff, and tight. This remedy is for burns that are very slow to heal, old burn scars that are still painful, burns with painful or tender blisters, burns that keep breaking open and bleeding, or for a child who has never been well since a burn. If this remedy has not helped with blister pain, call your healthcare practitioner. The least little thing will make this child cry. They are sensitive, anxious, very restless, and irritable. They do not want to go to bed alone, and may be fearful of the dark or ghosts.

Worse from: 3–4 AM and 6–8 PM, cold drafts, stooping, motion, and darkness. **Better from:** Sipping cold water, warmth, damp wet weather, and gentle motion.

Phosphorus: Electrical burns and radiation burns.

This remedy should be given first for electrical burns, because it will take care of the shock from electricity as well as the burn. These pains are some of the most intense of all burns. The pains are of a violent burning nature. There is much heat. They can have twitching and numbness at the site of the burn. It can feel as though there is something crawling under the skin. There is usually a dryness of the mouth, lips, and throat. They have a very strong craving for ice cold water, which they can vomit if it is consumed in great quantities or too fast. They are very sensitive to light, sound, odors, touch, and electrical changes, like a thunderstorm. These children are irritable, a bit fearful, and sluggish. They need sympathy, touch, and attention.

Worse from: Change of weather, cold air, cold wind, cold thunderstorms, evening, exertion, and lying on the left side. **Better from:** Sleep, warmth, sympathy, company, low lights or dark, eating, drinking cold things slowly, cool applications, and sitting.

Urtica Urens: Sunburns, scalds, and minor burns.

This remedy is useful both as a tincture and an internal homeopathic remedy. It is indicated for skin that feels sore, raw, intensely itching, stinging, and burning. There is usually swelling. The skin may be raised in red blotches, or have tiny, clear fluid-filled blisters. This remedy can be used for old burns that itch and sting, and sunburns with much itching. The child usually wants to rub the affected area. They look tired and pale. It is good for them to rest, but gentle movement is encouraged to rebuild stamina. The child is very restless.

Worse from: Cold water, after sleeping, cool moist air, cool baths, touch, night, and strenuous exercise. **Better from:** Lying down (but not on the affected parts), and gentle movement.

Dosage: If the condition is severe, give 2 pellets every 10-30 minutes until there is improvement. You may have to repeat every ten minutes for quite a few doses. If the condition is significant, give 2 pellets hourly until there is improvement. If there has been no improvement at all after two hours, choose a new remedy. If there is some improvement, keep repeating for another two hours. Repeat the remedy only if there is a return of the same symptoms, and only as necessary.

You may need to repeat the remedy 2–3 times per day for a few days. If you get no result within twenty-four hours, then reassess the condition. You may not have been wrong with your choice; the child may just have moved on to needing a related remedy. Change the remedy if you have followed the above guidelines with no results, or if the symptoms clearly change.

Supportive Measures:

Do not put any creams, oils, butter, or ointments on a newly burned area. This holds the heat in and can cause more burning. Then the oil or creams may have to be removed, which causes more trauma to the skin and child. *Do not puncture burn blisters.* It is important to keep the child's fluid intake up, in order to prevent dehydration. If there is clothing on top of the burn, gently remove what is loose and easily removable. If the clothing cannot be easily removed and is sticking to the burn, cut around it and take your child to your healthcare practitioner or hospital, depending on its severity.

Burns do better if they are lightly covered with *sterile* gauze that allows the maximum amount of air to circulate. Using herbal tincture of Calendula, which prevents scarring and infection, tincture of Urtica Urens, which prevents burning pain, and tincture of Hypericum, which prevents infection and severe nerve pains from a burn, topically in solution can considerably reduce the chances of an infection and ease the pains. Cover with a *sterile* piece of gauze dampened with a weakened solution of the three tinctures: Place 5 drops of each tincture in a quarter-cup of bottled spring water, or fresh water that has been boiled and cooled. (Anything stronger can cause painful stinging at first.) It is important to keep the gauze moist to prevent it from sticking to the burn. This solution can also be sprayed onto a sunburn.

Do not put creams, oils, or ointments on the skin until the blisters have healed and the burning is gone. Calendula cream may be used at that point. No kitchen should be without an aloe vera plant; its gel provides immediate relief and healing for first-degree and minor second-degree burns. *Do not put aloe vera on open blisters.* With clean hands, cut one leaf off at the base of the plant. Cut the leaf open lengthwise, scrape out the gel, and apply it to the burn. Or you may apply commercially prepared organic aloe vera juice or gel.

Treating specific types of burns:

Chemical burns: Give the appropriate remedy, and flush with cool water for five minutes.

Electrical burns: There may be deeper damage than appears on the skin. Treat as a severe burn. Do not attempt to touch the child. *Break the contact from the source of electricity with a stick, a chair, or anything that does not contain metal. Call 911 if the child is unresponsive, and give CPR.*

Large-area burns: These burns need to be closely and constantly checked for infection.

Scalds: Thousands of children are scalded by hot water from the tap. If you have young children in the house, your hot water heater should not be turned any higher than 125 degrees F. Most of these burns occur when a child is left in the bathtub and they turn on the hot water. A scald can happen in less than five seconds. *Never leave a child unattended in a tub.* Keep all hot liquids away from the dining table and pushed back from the edges of counters, especially your coffee or teapot. Keep all handles of pans on the stove turned inward to prevent the child from reaching up and pulling a pan of hot liquid onto themselves.

Sunburns: Use a natural sunscreen. Keep babies and young children out of strong sun, or covered appropriately. Cloudy days and reflection from water or snow can produce a sunburn. Because there is a cool breeze on a sunny day, you may not think about the child getting a sunburn, and they may not feel it. Apply cool compresses (not cold, or ice). When the child has a sunburn, keep them out of the sun until the skin has healed and is no longer red. See information about creating a spray made from Calendula, Hypericum, and Urtica Urens Tinctures in "Supportive measures," above.

Call your healthcare practitioner if:

- *The burned area is large—you must take the child to the hospital.* Cover the child with a clean sheet. Give the appropriate remedy on the way to the hospital. Homeopathic remedies will not interfere with anything the doctors may have to do.
- Your child has a third-degree burn.
- Your child has had a chemical burn, because an antidote to that chemical may be needed.
- The burn is becoming infected, i.e., with redness, severe swelling, or oozing pus, or if there is a high fever.
- *There are red streaks running up or outwards from the burn. This requires immediate attention! Take your child to the hospital.*
- Your child, especially if young, has a severe sunburn.
- You suspect that your child has heatstroke or sunstroke with a sunburn.
- The child has a fever, a fast pulse, confusion, lethargy, or nausea. They may be suffering from sunstroke. *This requires immediate professional attention.*

EMOTIONAL TRAUMAS AND FEARS

Your First Assessment

Is the child in shock? If the trauma is severe, the child can go into shock.

It is important to know which remedy to give if the child is in shock. There are two specific remedies for shock—**Aconitum** or **Arnica**—and they are used in different situations, so please familiarize yourself with the specific indications for each remedy:

257

Aconitum: The child is very fearful, anxious, extremely reactive to pain, and inconsolable, with glassy eyes or dilated pupils; they are likely to be screaming, crying out, and trembling with terror and pain.

Arnica: The child is stunned, irritable when offered help, exhausted, and uncooperative; they say they are fine, and don't want to be touched. They may complain of pain, but will maintain that not much is wrong with them.

Dosage: Give 2 pellets of Aconitum or Arnica every 15 minutes until improvement.

A Note about Rescue Remedy

Rescue Remedy (Bach Flower Essences) is found in health-food stores next to the homeopathic remedies. It is a liquid made up of five different flower essences preserved in an alcohol-water solution. This flower essence was invented by an English homeopath by the name of Dr. Edward Bach. It has calming and comforting properties to reduce stress and shock when there has been a crisis, emergency or accident, and is completely safe. If your child or any member of your family is experiencing any of the above conditions, you can administer it in the following way: Add 3 drops to a glass of water, and have the child sip it frequently until you see progress; then every 15 minutes, then every 30 minutes, repeating as long as needed. Stop when emotional stability has returned. (See symptom details below.)

A Note about Stress

If a child is under stress, their body will begin producing symptoms of illness. If your child is unhappy at school, they may develop headaches, stomachaches, anxiety, or sleep difficulties. It is important to not let this situation become chronic. Encourage the child to talk to you about it. If necessary, intervene by speaking with teachers, coaches, school counselors, etc. Children can be the victims of bullying. Do not hesitate to speak with other parents to remedy the situation. In our society, there are some children who have no downtime, or are being forced to participate in too many sports, dance, or academic activities. Your son may not want to play football or be on the debate team. Your daughter may not want to play basketball or take dance lessons. Listen to them.

Make sure your child is not eating junk food, playing too many video games, spending long periods of time on the computer, watching too much TV, or getting inadequate sleep. If your child is not responding to remedies, stress could be an obstacle to cure. Any child or teen who has suffered a great emotional shock such as divorce or death will more than likely need professional psychological help as well as a professional homeopath for support.

Note: *If your child keeps re-living a trauma,* give them **Stramonium**. The child keeps reexperiencing the initial fright and may exhibit hysteria, talkativeness, rage, loud laughter, or a fear that they are going to die. The child needing this remedy may become afraid of the dark and not want to sleep alone. They can also wake screaming from nightmares. Give every 15 minutes until improvement.

See in-depth explanation of specific remedies below.

Fears

Acute fears will be addressed here. Phobias, which are deep-seated, chronically ingrained fears, need to be dealt with by a professional. Hypnosis is probably the most effective modality for phobias. Any of the following may develop into a phobia.

Fear of seeing the doctor or dentist, or going to the hospital: Aconitum, Argentum Nit, Gelsemium

Fear of flying in airplanes: Aconitum, Argentum Nit, Gelsemium, Rhus Tox

Fear and anxiety before performances, tests, etc.: Argentum Nit, Gelsemium

Fear with trembling: Arsenicum, Gelsemium, Pulsatilla, Rescue Remedy

Fright

Fright is a sudden emotion that arises from being threatened or attacked. It can bring about feelings of terror, fear, anxiety, panic, or dread. It can even cause a histamine reaction that produces welts on the skin, or hives. It is important to keep your children from viewing movies or TV programs with scary, grotesque, or violent images. This causes frightful imagery in your child's mind—which they do not need—and can cause nightmares in younger children. If they see a scary movie or TV show, look to the following remedies.

The most common remedies for fright are: **Apis, Ignatia, Gelsemium, Pulsatilla,** and **Rescue Remedy.**

Grief

Grief is an emotional state caused by the loss of family members, friends, a pet, a home, etc. Some children are so sensitive that a movie or TV program can evoke this emotion. A teenager may need one of these remedies if they have broken up with their girlfriend or boyfriend. Grief can be manifested by uncontrollable crying, hysterical sobbing, long bouts of weeping or wailing, fear of being alone, much sighing, withdrawing, or depression.

The most common remedies for grief are: **Ignatia, Natrum Mur, Pulsatilla,** and **Rescue Remedy.**

Humiliation

Humiliation from severe criticism, name-calling, or being bullied will damage a child's dignity, pride, and self-esteem. It brings up feelings of shame, disgrace, embarrassment, and dishonor. It is very important that you not ignore your child, thinking that they have to find their own way or toughen up. The child will feel further victimized if the parents do not step in and support them. It may be necessary to take further steps with the school or other parents to remedy the situation. Remember that your child may be the victim of humiliation not only from other children; look also to how they are treated by siblings, coaches, babysitters, teachers, or other family members. Besides giving a remedy, it is important to teach the child coping skills. Professional help may be needed. This kind of situation should not be allowed to continue, because the child may develop unhealthy emotional patterns, and be affected by long-term stress.

The most common remedies for humiliation are: **Ignatia** or **Staphysagria.**

Rage

Rage is a powerful, intense emotion expressed in sudden and extreme anger. The child is usually in a state of fury, frenzy, and wrath, brought on by frustration, pain, overwhelm, grief, loss, low blood sugar, poor diet, or hormone fluctuations. It can even cause a histamine reaction that produces welts on the skin, or hives. It is not unusual for two-year-olds or teenagers to throw temper tantrums. This is a normal stage of development. A fit of rage can be quite distressing, but should not be suppressed. However, rudeness, verbal abuse, or violence should always be addressed and not tolerated. Your teen may need help from a professional, or a class in anger management, if the rage becomes chronic.

The most common remedies for rage are: **Apis, Arnica, Arsenicum, Ignatia, Nux Vomica,** and **Staphysagria.**

The following are the most commonly indicated remedies for intense negative emotions:

Aconitum: For fear of flying on airplanes, or nightmares from scary movies or stories, which can lead to fear of the dark and/ or ghosts, or aftereffects from fright. There is sheer terror! There is a rapid pulse, and profuse perspiration. The child is very fearful, anxious, panicked, restless, extremely reactive to pain, and inconsolable, with dilated pupils, and likely to be screaming and crying out with terror and pain. They are afraid of crowds and death, because they are sure they are going to die, and are easily startled.

Apis: If any strong fright or rage has caused a sudden histamine reaction, this remedy will help. It is also used if there is an intense reaction of jealousy. The arrival of a new baby in the family can cause an older child to feel jealous, making them difficult, irritable, hypersensitive, and hyperactive. If there is a histamine reaction, the skin becomes puffy, red, swollen, hot, and itchy. The child is constantly whining, hard to please, fidgety, fussy, jealous, and suspicious. They are awkward, and usually drop things a lot. They can be listless, but become irritable if disturbed. However, they do not want to be left alone. If in pain, they cry out with piercing, shrill screams. Teenage girls at puberty can become hysterical.

Argentum Nit: Fear of flying—the child fears heights, and fears being unable to escape once the door is closed on the plane; claustrophobia, fear of failure because they think they can't do anything right, of being alone, of losing control, or of going to the doctor because they fear disease. This child is anxious, nervous, easily excitable, trembling, timid, and impulsive. They have a sense that time is going too slowly and they want everybody to hurry up, and they may pace up and down in a panic. They may become so anxious that they get diarrhea that is frequent, watery, and smelly. They may talk fast, in a childish way. There is usually a great desire for sweets.

Arnica: For a bout of rage after which the child looks battered, with a sunken, pale, or red face. The child is stunned, irritable when offered help, exhausted, uncooperative, adamant that they are fine, and do not want to be touched. They will say that nothing is wrong because they are afraid and do not want anyone approaching them. They feel beaten-up, sore, and bruised emotionally. They act like a wounded animal wanting to go to a corner, be left alone, and lick their wounds. It is best to give the remedy and then leave them alone until it has had a chance to relieve the symptoms.

Arsenicum: For anxiety after a bout of rage, attacks of fear for no apparent reason, or fear of being alone. The whole body, or parts of it, trembles. They are irritable, restless, oversensitive, anxious, impatient, demanding, critical, and forgetful. The toddler will want to be carried briskly. They may want mom, then dad, then mom again. The older child may have a fear of dying. They get upset about disorder, and want to have their bedroom or surroundings orderly and neat.

Gelsemium: Fear of doctors and dentists, because the child wants to be left alone and not examined; fear of public performance, crowds, or flying (because they anticipate mechanical problems with the plane, the pilot, etc.). Even though they are anxious and afraid, the child's reactions become slow, with great weakness, confusion, exhaustion, and trembling, which makes them want to be held. They become dull, heavy, sluggish, and sometimes dizzy. They may stutter. This state can also occur if the child has become overexcited. They may get diarrhea. The head may ache at the forehead and/or the back of the head. The eyelids are droopy. The child looks drowsy. It is helpful to have them bend forward while sitting, or lie down with their head slightly elevated. They need fresh air. The older child may completely freeze up mentally and physically in a public-performance situation. The teenager may need this remedy before taking their driver's license test or college entrance exams.

Ignatia: For anxiety after a bout of rage, grief, fright, or humiliation. This child is very sensitive, especially to pain, nervous, excitable, introspective, easily frustrated, moody, and weepy. They sigh a lot, yawn, grieve quietly, do not want sympathy, and may become antisocial. This child may complain of a lump in their throat, a sore throat, tightness in the chest, cramping of muscles, numbness or tingling of the nerves, spasms, or a stomachache. They may have strange sensations anywhere in the body. This condition comes on after the trauma of grief, fright, shock, reprimand, humiliation, or if they are homesick. They can have unpredictable reactions—they can be hysterically crying one moment, laughing the next, furious the next, distant the next, anxious the next, and restless the next. They may try to hold the tears back, but end up sobbing. There is often a loss of appetite.

Natrum Mur: This is a major remedy for grief. It is also for a child who has a fear of being rejected or hurt, and is very sensitive to being teased. They may have a sore throat that aches even when they are not swallowing. The pain is needle-like, and can extend into the ears. The throat feels better if they eat solid food. The child is irritable, angry, serious, anxious, abrupt, absentminded, and confused, and cries at the least little thing. However, they do not want consolation, and desire to be alone. The older child is emotionally sensitive but withdraws, and finds it hard to cry in front of others. They tend to hold grudges. Teenagers will be depressed, discontented with life, withdrawn, and irritable.

Nux Vomica: For crying and/or anxiety after a bout of rage. These children are oversensitive, especially to noise, odors, and light, and are easily offended. They can be angry, spiteful, impatient, jealous, stubborn, irritable, mischievous, and very competitive. The older child pouts when they do not get their way, and makes life quite difficult for those around them. The teenager does not want any restrictions, and can be very quarrelsome.

Pulsatilla: For fright from movies or TV, especially if an animal has been hurt or killed, or any disturbing impressions such as witnessing a bad car accident; for grief with lots of weeping, and fear of crowds or narrow places. The child is mild, timid, clingy, tearful, whiny, weepy, and fretful, but affectionate and craving attention. This child needs attention and gentleness. They can be quite pitiful. Your older son might be described as feeling sorry for himself. They need to be gently encouraged out of their self-pity and not allowed to wallow in it for too long. They may say, "It's not fair!" They will feel better after a good cry. They have very changeable moods, like being on an emotional roller coaster, especially at puberty. This is a very important remedy for teenage girls whose emotions are all over the place after an emotional trauma.

Rescue Remedy: For fright, shock, emotional trauma, grief, and fearfulness that causes a loss of energy. This remedy will restore a sense of balance, calm, and harmony. It reduces the effects of shock, trauma, panic, fear, and sadness. The child needing this remedy may feel faint, tremble, or become hysterical or speechless. This is a very gentle yet effective remedy to keep the ill effects of the above conditions from imprinting on the child mentally and emotionally. Obtain this remedy at your local health-food store.

Rhus Tox: The child fears flying because of the lack of fresh air, and cannot sit still for long periods of time. They are very restless and apprehensive, and this is worse at night. They may burst into tears, but not be able to tell you why they are crying. This is a good remedy for a child that cannot get negative pictures from a trauma out of their head, e.g., after a bad car accident. Mentally and emotionally, they become stiff, cloudy, confused, and forgetful.

Staphysagria: For trauma from humiliation, shame, or anger. The child feels disempowered, downtrodden, inadequate, and indignant they have sadness with crying, constant seething anger, and trembling. It is not unusual for them to throw or smash things. This can bring about headaches that make them want to lean their head against something hard, menstrual cramps, cessation of periods, or bladder infections after rage. The child is touchy and sensitive, especially to rude treatment. It is not good for this child to suppress their emotions. They will fume inside, but then have an inappropriate outburst or become sick, shaky, unable to sleep, and exhausted.

Dosage: If the condition is severe, give 2 pellets every 10–30 minutes until there is improvement. If the condition is significant, give 2 pellets hourly until there is improvement. If there is no improvement after two hours, choose a new remedy. Repeat the remedy only if there is a return of the same symptoms, and repeat only as necessary. You may need to repeat the remedy 2–3 times per day for a few days. If you get no result within twenty-four hours, then reassess the symptoms. Change the remedy if you have followed the above guidelines with no results, or if the symptoms clearly change.

Supportive Measures:

The quickest way to get a child to calm down is to establish eye contact and have them take slow, deep, rhythmical breaths into their belly. Keep the focus on the breath. Listen to your child, and talk it out with them. Try to understand without judgment or criticism. Do not minimize the child's fears or feelings. Do not force your child to talk if they are not ready. Keep an open ear. It can be helpful for the older child to write or draw pictures about what they are experiencing.

Call your healthcare practitioner if:

- Your child becomes withdrawn, irritable, rude, arrogant, dictatorial, bullying, or violent. The child may have an unexpressed emotional conflict that they do not know how to deal with.
- Temper tantrums persist, or become destructive or violent.
- Your child has not responded to the above remedies—there may be a deeper-seated problem that needs to be addressed. Or a higher dose of the above remedies may be needed. If either of these is the case, contact your homeopath.
- Do not allow depression or anger to become chronic. Seek psychological counseling.

FAINTING AND COLLAPSE

Fainting is a temporary loss of consciousness from a lack of blood flow that inhibits oxygen getting to the brain. Fainting can result from a strong fright, an extreme emotional upset, shock, poor ventilation, overheating, severe pain, loss of bodily fluids, exhaustion, hyperventilation, or dehydration. It can also result from a drop in blood pressure or in blood sugar from going too long without food. Fainting is nature's way of quickly making a body horizontal— a favorable position for restoring blood flow to the brain.

Any of the fainting remedies below can be placed on the inside of the cheek in order to bring the child back to consciousness. Put 2 small pellets, or 1 large one, between the gum and cheek. *Never* put your fingers inside a child's mouth if they are experiencing a seizure, and do not attempt to give any remedies until the seizure has passed.

The following are the most commonly indicated remedies for fainting and collapse:

Aconitum: Fainting from fright, severe anxiety, shock, or fear. The symptoms come on suddenly. The child experiences heavy perspiration, rapid pulse, heart palpitations, and a hot, burning heaviness in the head. This remedy is useful after a fright, or if the breathing was severely restricted from an asthma attack. The child is extremely anxious, restless, and fearful that they are going to die. They need rest, fresh air, and cool drinks after regaining consciousness.

Arnica: Fainting from shock, physical trauma, or blood loss. The child feels sore, beat up, and bruised. They are stunned, irritable when offered help, exhausted, and uncooperative, saying they are fine and not wanting to be touched. They will say that nothing is wrong because they are afraid and do not want anyone approaching them. They need to lie down with their head lowered, not be touched, be somewhere away from people, and allowed to rest.

Carbo Veg: Fainting from exhaustion, or weakness with breathing difficulties. This is usually due to a loss of body fluids from bleeding, vomiting, or diarrhea. The child may be gasping for breath. The face is pale, with a bluish tint. They greatly need fresh air, and may ask you to fan them. The child will be indifferent to everything, a bit confused, irritable, and very sluggish. They need to be fanned vigorously with fresh air if possible, have their feet elevated, cool air, and rest. Belching also makes them feel better.

Cinchona (also known as **China Officinalis**): Fainting from loss of fluids, as in hemorrhage or diarrhea. The child gasps for breath. They may complain of ringing in the ears, or blurred vision. They are very weak, with much sweating. They are irritable, oversensitive, nervous, and may have problems sleeping. They need much quiet rest, firm pressure, bending double, warmth, and fresh air.

Coffea: Fainting from sudden joy, shock or excitement. The child may tremble. Their mind becomes overactive, and it is hard for them to unwind. They are hypersensitive to pain, noise, strong smells, and emotions. They may be wide-awake at 3 AM—in which case, repeat the remedy. They need to sleep and be kept warm.

Gelsemium: Fainting from fear, e.g., stage fright. The child may tremble. They will often get frequent diarrhea. The head may ache at the forehead and/or the back of the head. The eyelids are droopy. The child looks drowsy and may complain of dizziness. Even though they are anxious and afraid, they are confused, dull, and weak. It is helpful to have them bend forward while sitting, or lie down with their head slightly elevated. They need fresh air.

Ignatia: Fainting from grief, sudden bad news, loss, or a major disappointment. The child may complain of a lump in their throat, a sore throat, tightness in the chest, cramping in their muscles, numbness or tingling of the nerves, or a stomachache. This child is very sensitive, especially to pain, nervous, excitable, introspective, easily frustrated, moody, weepy, sighing a lot, and yawning. They can have unpredictable reactions; they can be hysterically crying one moment, laughing the next, and then furious the next. There is often a loss of appetite. Remind the child to take slow, deep, rhythmical breaths into the belly to calm themselves down. Remain calm for your child.

Pulsatilla: Fainting from being in a hot, stuffy, crowded room, or because of dehydration. The child's mouth feels dry, but they are not thirsty. They may be chilly, but want the window open for fresh air. The child is clingy, tearful, whiny, weepy, and fretful, and has changeable moods but is affectionate and craves attention. This child needs attention and gentleness. They will feel better in fresh air, cool applications, and motion once any dizziness or faintness has passed. Be sure your child is well hydrated.

Veratrum: Fainting after strong emotions, extreme vomiting, and/or diarrhea. The least exertion can make the child feel faint. They are nauseous, sweaty, and very weak. The face has a bluish color, and the forehead, hands, feet, and abdomen are icy cold. The breath can even feel cold. The child has a huge thirst for great quantities of cold water. They are restless. They need warmth, covering-up, hot drinks, and lying down.

Dosage: After the child has regained consciousness, give 2 pellets every 10–30 minutes until there is improvement. Repeat the remedy only if the child is feeling faint again. Change the remedy if you have followed the above guidelines with no results, or if the symptoms clearly change.

Supportive Measures:

Place the child on their back and loosen any tight clothing, especially around the neck. Keep onlookers at a distance, for optimum ventilation. Put a cool compress on the forehead. When the child tries to stand up, make sure they are supported, in case they are dizzy. If your child is dehydrated, push liquids slowly and steadily. If they have fainted from lack of food, give them a nutritious, high-carbohydrate snack. Observe the child closely for the next twenty-four hours.

Call your healthcare practitioner if:

- Fainting begins to occur repeatedly.
- The child has not regained consciousness after a few minutes—keep the child warm, and take them to the hospital.
- The child has fainted after falling and hitting their head or receiving a serious blow. Do not move the child. Keep the child warm. If they are seriously hurt, *call 911.*
- You suspect there is internal bleeding—*call 911.*
- The child is having trouble breathing—*call 911.*
- Your child is diabetic and has fainted.

HEAT EXHAUSTION AND SUNSTROKE

Keep all babies and small children out of strong sun. Be sure to keep the whole family well hydrated. Sugary or caffeinated drinks are not good beverage choices—water is best.

Heat exhaustion

This is a response to excessive exposure to or exertion in the sun. It can happen quite quickly if the humidity is high. Dehydration causes an electrolyte imbalance through a loss of the body's salt in sweat. This then affects brain function. The child becomes weak, nauseous, fatigued, and usually has a headache. Sweating is profuse. Their skin becomes pale, cool, and clammy. They may be anxious and irritable. They may feel dizzy or faint, or have blurry vision. Their pulse is weak, and the blood pressure drops.

The following are the most commonly indicated remedies for heat exhaustion:

Bryonia: This remedy is for the child who has a severe, splitting headache with a bursting and heavy sensation. It hurts to even move their eyes. Many times they are nauseous. The key to identifying when to use this remedy is that they do not want to move. They are grumpy, like a bear, and want to be left alone. They are very thirsty for cold drinks. They may complain about their mouth and throat being dry.

Cinchona (also known as **China Officinalis**): The child is completely drained, very weak, trembling, and gasping for breath. They may complain of ringing in the ears, or blurred vision. There is much sweating. This remedy is especially helpful when there is severe dehydration. The child is irritable, sensitive, and cannot think straight.

Gelsemium: This child looks as though they are drunk, with droopy and heavy eyes. The face is flushed, but not bright red. They are drowsy, and cannot think straight. If they have a headache, it is at the nape of the neck. The skin is dry and hot, but the hands and feet are cold. They may complain of chills going up and down their spine.

Pulsatilla: This child is very sensitive to heat and the sun. This child suffers from air hunger, and is always taking deep breaths.

They are weak and can feel faint. They are weepy, clingy, dependent, and feeling sorry for themselves. They tend to not be thirsty, so it is important to have this child constantly sip fluids to get rehydrated.

Sunstroke

This condition is a much more serious condition than heatstroke and *may require a trip to the emergency room.* The child can become so overheated that their body can no longer sweat and cool itself. Perspiration is not as profuse as with heat exhaustion. The skin is dry and hot, and the child has a fever of 104° or above. This can happen quite quickly if the humidity is high. The child is dizzy, weak, fatigued, and nauseous. They have a very intense headache, with rapid pulse and breathing. They may vomit, become delirious, or have a seizure. Your child will be vulnerable in the future to getting overheated, and react poorly to heat and sun exposure. Take extra precautions.

The following are the most commonly indicated remedies for sunstroke (these can be given on the way to the hospital):

Belladonna: This remedy is for symptoms that come on fast and furious. There is intense heat radiating from the body. The face is bright-red and hot. The skin is burning, hot, and dry. The child has a throbbing headache that is worse on the right side, and better from bending the head backward. The eyes may be glassy and sparkling, with a wild look and dilated pupils. They usually have a craving for very cold water or lemonade. The child's senses are very acute to noise, light, touch, and motion. If the child has a high fever, they may be confused and delirious. They can become agitated to the point of biting, screaming, and hitting. They will feel better with rest, light coverings, sitting semi-erect, low lights, and quiet.

Glonoinum: This remedy is for when sunstroke symptoms come on rapidly and violently: The child has a throbbing and bursting headache, with a feeling that the eyes and head are expanded; the pounding pain comes in waves, causing the child to shudder. There is a strong sensation of heat and blood rushing into the head. They cannot bear to have anything hot around the head, or tight clothing. The skin may be sweaty. The veins in the temples of the head protrude and can be seen pulsing. The child may clench their jaw. They are confused, very irritable, and weepy. The child will need to be still with their head elevated, stay in cool, fresh air if possible, and have cool applications and drinks. They will benefit from a long sleep after the crisis has passed. Give this remedy until the throbbing stops, and repeat only if it begins again.

Dosage: Give 2 pellets every 10 minutes until there is improvement. Repeat the remedy only if there is a return of the same symptoms. Change the remedy if you have followed the above guidelines with no results, or if the symptoms clearly change.

Supportive Measures:

Get the child to a shaded or cool area. If your child has any of the above symptoms, keep them out of the sun. Cool the child off as quickly as possible by pouring or sponging liberal amounts of tepid (not cold) water over the body. You can wrap the child in a sheet that has been wetted in tepid water. Put a cool compress on the head. Have the child slowly sip many glasses of cool saltwater (½-teaspoon of salt in 8 ounces of spring water). Have the child lie down and rest.

Call your healthcare practitioner if:

- Do not hesitate to take your child to the hospital or call an ambulance if you suspect your child has sunstroke.
- The body temperature is rapidly rising, or the child has had a seizure—*call 911.*
- The child is delirious for longer than forty minutes.
- Your child does not respond to any of the remedies within an hour.

INJURIES

Blows and Bruises

A blow to any part of the body will cause blood vessels under the skin to burst and release blood into the surrounding soft tissue. The affected area then turns deep purple and/or blue. Later it turns yellow, before eventually disappearing. Homeopathic remedies can help to reduce swelling, bruising, infection, and pain. They will also speed up the healing process. Look at the "Supportive measures" section below for further care of the following injuries.

Blows to the Back

In cases of blows to the back, you need to check the kidney area for trauma. The kidneys are located on either side of the spine, just below the rib cage. If there is pain around the kidney area, call your healthcare practitioner at once. In the meantime, give **Bellis Perennis** every 30 minutes until the pain subsides or until you talk with your healthcare practitioner. Give this remedy at least six hours before bed, because this remedy can interrupt sleep. However, it is better to give the remedy, if it is needed, than to be concerned about disrupted sleep.

Arnica: Give 2 pellets immediately if the child has had the wind knocked out of them in a fall. This will help with shock, and release spasms in the diaphragm, which tenses upon impact. Repeat if the tenseness returns. The pain produces a sore and bruised feeling; the child feels beaten-up. This remedy will also help if a child falls on the length of their back awkwardly, causing a twist. Follow up as soon as possible afterward with a cranial-sacral osteopath. Give 2 pellets 3 times a day, for three days.

Hypericum: For trauma to the spine. The pains are intense, violent, and shooting upwards from the point of impact. The pains appear suddenly, and then disappear gradually. The area is very tender and sore. There may be tingling, twitching, trembling, or numbness. The back feels weak. Give 2 pellets every 15 minutes until there is relief. Repeat only if symptoms return.

Nux Vomica: This remedy will relieve intense muscle spasms where there is also great sensitivity to pain. Give 2 pellets every 15 minutes until there is relief. Repeat only if symptoms return.

Blows to the Breasts

Blows to the breasts can damage the ducts, lymph nodes, mammary glands, or fatty tissue. A severe blow can have long-lasting and serious consequences, including pain and swelling.

Arnica: Give 2 pellets at once. If the blow was severe, call your homeopath immediately. *Always* follow with **Bellis Perennis,** give 2 pellets 3 times a day for three days. Give this remedy at least six hours before bed, because it can disrupt sleep. However, it is best to give the remedy if needed rather than be concerned about sleep. If pains are achy, squeezing, and throbbing, give 2 pellets every 2 hours until relieved.

Staphysagria: If the blow was the result of anger or physical abuse, then give 2 pellets for emotional healing.

Blows to the Coccyx (Tailbone)

A blow to the tailbone can send a shock wave all the way up to the head, and have long-term consequences. The blow can tense the pelvic floor, negatively affecting the bowels, uterus, sacrum, sciatic nerve, bladder, or lower-back area. In the mid-back area, the lungs, heart, and digestive processes can also be negatively affected. The shock can even trigger excess mucus production in the ethmoid sinuses, above the bridge of the nose. For this injury, it is imperative to see a cranial-sacral osteopath as soon as possible.

Arnica: Give 2 pellets immediately for the shock to the spine.

Hypericum: This remedy acts as a tonic for injured nerves. It is for pain in nerve-rich areas such as the tailbone. The area is very tender and sore. The child feels pressure, and the pains are intense, violent, and shooting upwards. The pains appear suddenly and then disappear gradually. There may be tingling, twitching, trembling, or numbness. Give 2 pellets every 15 minutes until there is relief. Repeat only if symptoms return.

Note: Sometimes it is necessary to alternate these two remedies every 15 minutes until the child becomes more comfortable. Then continue with the **Hypericum** only, on an as-needed basis if symptoms return.

Blows to the Eyes

A black eye affects the flesh and orbital bone (the bony structure around the eye).

Two black eyes at the same time can indicate a fracture at the base of the skull. Have this checked out at a hospital or urgent-care facility.

Arnica ensures that all the bruising comes out to the surface, which is what needs to happen. It helps heal the soft tissue in the eye socket. Take 2 pellets every hour until symptoms are relieved. If there is no response, read on to see if other remedies are needed.

Hamamelis is needed if the eye feels painfully weak. The child has a sensation that the eye is trying to force itself out, and it feels good to gently press their finger on the eyelid. There is much inflammation, and the eyes may be bloodshot. This remedy will help absorption of any bleeding inside the eyeball. Give 2 pellets every hour until symptoms are relieved.

Hypericum is needed if there is severe pain. This remedy is especially helpful for a superficial scratch on the cornea. Give 2 pellets every 15 minutes until improvement.

Ledum is for treating a black eye where the tissue around the eye feels cold. Cold compresses will feel particularly good. There is much swelling around the eye, with tender, purple tissue. **Ledum** will absorb serum and blood clots. It will also help if there is pain in the orbital bone. After **Arnica,** if indicated, give **Ledum** twice a day for three days.

Symphytum is for a black eye with pain in the eyeball. It will also heal any trauma to the orbital bone around the eye. It is particularly helpful for a blow to the eye from a ball or fist, or for pain that continues after the bruising is gone. After the **Arnica,** if indicated, give **Symphytum** twice per day until the pain is gone. This is a good remedy if the black eye resulted from a fistfight.

Blows to the Head

Be sure to read about head injuries in the "Supportive measures" section below. An injury to a baby's head most often happens from accidentally dropping the child. Do not panic. The baby's skull is still soft, and can sometimes withstand a blow better than an adult's. Bumps on a child's head swell quickly, and appear far worse than they actually are. A child will often develop a swelling that looks like an egg is protruding from the skull.

Keep a close watch on a child with a head bump: Look out for drowsiness, sleepiness, and especially vomiting. These are signs that something may be wrong and needs attention. Make sure the pupils of the eyes are the same size. If your child has been knocked unconscious, call your healthcare practitioner. For any major injuries to the head, always contact your healthcare practitioner even if you have given remedies or been to the hospital.

All of the following remedies will help resolve head injuries, including concussions:

Aconitum: Give this remedy if the child has hit their head quite hard on a sharp corner or a hard surface. The resulting fear, shock, and insecurity call for a dose of this remedy immediately. A child needing this remedy will have a deer-in-the-headlights look in their eyes; they are quite scared. Give 2 pellets and repeat every 10 minutes until the shock and fear have subsided. Then look to **Arnica** if there is any swelling. Repeat if there is a return of symptoms.

Arnica: This remedy can often bring out the bruising very quickly, which is a good sign. It will also help with any swelling, internal or external. If a child has been knocked unconscious, put 2 pellets of **Arnica** on the inside of the cheek; this will usually bring them back to consciousness. The child will have a blank, dazed, no-one-home look on their face. They may not even remember the accident. They will say that they are OK but only because they are anxious and don't want to be touched, just left alone.

Note: If the child is having nightmares or reliving an accident, give 2 pellets of **Arnica** each night before bed for three nights. If they are still reliving the accident after that, give the same dosage of **Stramonium**.

Hypericum: This can be given to reduce shock to the brain or spinal nerves. The child is experiencing dizziness, headaches, upward-shooting pains, numbness, and tingling. The head feels heavy, and as though there is an icy-cold hand resting on it. The headache can shoot pains into the cheek, and make the eyes feel sore. If you are having a hard time choosing between **Arnica** and **Hypericum**, they can be alternated every 15 minutes until there is an improvement of symptoms. After the injury, if the child seems forgetful or dull, give 2 pellets of **Hypericum** three times a week for three weeks, or until there is improvement. If any symptoms linger, consult your healthcare practitioner. It is always a good idea to follow up with a cranial-sacral osteopath if possible.

Natrum Sulph: For head injuries, especially to the back of the head. The child may be dizzy, have headaches in the back of the head, sensitivity to light, or visual disturbances. If the child is experiencing these symptoms after **Arnica** has been given, a dose or two of this remedy will follow **Arnica** well. If symptoms persist after three doses one hour apart, call your healthcare practitioner immediately. This remedy can be given long after a head injury if there is an inability to think or perform mental tasks. It can undo the lingering effects of a concussion. Music makes the child feel sad; the scalp is sensitive, the top of head feels hot, the brain feels loose when stooping, the head jerks to the right side, or they may have piercing pains in the ears. They may also have digestive problems, especially recurrent diarrhea. The child is oversensitive to criticism or scolding, and overly concerned about family members. Give 2 pellets three times a week, for three weeks or until there is improvement. If any of these symptoms linger, consult your healthcare practitioner. It is always a good idea to follow up with a cranial-sacral osteopath, if possible.

Blows to the Jaw, Lips, Mouth, and Teeth

Arnica relieves soreness and bruising after a blow to the teeth. Give 2 pellets 2–3 times per day for three days or until soreness is gone.

Hypericum is a good remedy for blows to the mouth because the lips are rich in nerves, and this remedy helps relieve nerve pain. Give every 15 minutes until there is relief. It is also for nerve pains in injured teeth, when the teeth are excessively tender and sensitive. Give 2–3 times a day for three days or until the sensitivity is gone. A broken tooth will need both remedies as well as a trip to the dentist.

Chamomilla will relieve unbearable pains from a broken or injured tooth. Give every 15 minutes for four doses, and then hourly until relieved. See the "Supportive measures" section below if the pain is severe and **Chamomilla** has not helped.

Note: These three remedies are complementary to each other. Use the indicated remedy until you can see your dentist, healthcare practitioner, or homeopath. For a blow to the teeth, alternate **Arnica** and **Ruta Grav** every two hours until the pain has subsided. Repeat only if pain returns. If it is not resolving, consult your dentist.

Blows to Muscles

Arnica: This is the first remedy to give for blows followed by bruising. The muscle feels very sore and beat-up. Give 2 pellets every 3–4 hours, or more frequently if the pain is severe.

Rhus Tox: This is the most common remedy for inflammation, stiffness, and tearing pains after an injury to the muscle, which usually leads to inflammation of the muscle tissue. The keynotes for choosing this remedy are: The area feels better from massage, hot applications, and sustained movement, and worse on the first movement after resting. Give 2 pellets every 3–4 hours, and soak in a hot bath. Repeat as necessary.

Blows to the Nose

Trauma to the nose can cause the blood vessels to rupture. Also, please refer to the "Supportive measures" section below. **Arnica:** This is the first remedy to use if the nose bleeds after a blow. It will also help with pain and swelling. Give every 10 minutes until there is relief.

Millefolium: Will be needed if the nose continues to bleed bright-red blood profusely after being given **Arnica**. Keep the child resting and quiet. Give every 10 minutes until the bleeding has stopped.

Blows to Organs and Soft Tissue Areas

Bellis Perennis is for damage to soft tissue of the abdominal area (housing the stomach, liver, and spleen), the kidneys (located on either side of the spine just below the rib cage), or the pelvic area (housing the intestines, bladder, and reproductive organs). You should be in touch with your practitioner if your child has received a blow to any of the above areas to ensure that the whole picture is assessed. Give 2 pellets every 2 hours for at least three doses. Give this remedy at least six hours before bed, because this remedy can interrupt sleep; however, it is better to give the remedy if needed rather than be concerned about disrupted sleep. Further doses should be on the advice of your practitioner. *If there is pain located around the kidney area, call your healthcare practitioner at once.*

Blows to the Testicles

Give one dose of **Arnica** immediately; fifteen minutes later give a dose of **Staphysagria** and continue on an as needed basis up to every fifteen minutes for four doses. If the pain is subsiding after an hour, use only if there is a return of pain or swelling.

Call your healthcare practitioner if:

- There is difficulty urinating or blood in their urine.
- The injury penetrated the scrotum.

Call your healthcare practitioner if (cont):

- Pain is not lessening after an hour.
- They continue to feel nauseous and are vomiting.
- There is bruising, swelling or fluid filling the scrotum.
- They develop a fever.

Bone Injuries and Dislocations

Bone Injuries

If the bone pains do not respond to **Arnica, Eupatorium,** or **Ruta Grav,** have the limb checked in case there is a fracture to a bone or growth plate. Simple or hairline fractures will cause persistent, nagging pain, and can sometimes go unnoticed. If the pain is not subsiding, there is severe pain on using the limb, or there is pain from rotating the limb, keep the limb immobile, and call your healthcare practitioner or go an urgent-care facility. A bone fracture may also affect the periosteum, a fibrous, dense covering on the bone where tendons and muscles attach.

For helping the bone to knit quickly, you can use **Symphytum** *only* if the fracture is simple, or if it is well set and no further surgery is needed. **Symphytum** should not be used until the bones are set in the right place, because of its rapid-healing properties. Give **Symphytum** twice a week for bone bruises and daily for a break until the cast or immobilization device is removed. In addition to helping the bones to mend completely and quickly, this remedy alleviates soreness, tenderness, pain, and bruising.

Note: Do not use for a collarbone break unless you have consulted your homeopath.

If the break is slow to heal, you can give **Calc Phos** once a week in addition to **Symphytum**, to assist with healing. Children needing this remedy will be moody, restless, and irritable.

The following remedies can be used to reduce pain and swelling from a bone bruise or fracture:

Arnica: Start with this remedy, whether or not you suspect a break. It will help with shock, pain, swelling, and bruising, and can speed the healing time. Give 2 pellets every 15 minutes for the first hour, then every 2–4 hours for the first twenty-four hours.

Bryonia: This remedy may be needed after the shock has worn off. The child does not want to move the injured part. Any motion brings much pain. The child is irritable, grumpy, and wants to be left alone.

Eupatorium: This remedy will help with pain. The child complains of bone-breaking pain, or intense aching deep in the bone. The child moans a lot, and is restless. They may be nauseous from the pain. The skin can feel quite sore around the bruised bone. Give hourly until relieved, then on an as-needed basis.

Ledum: This remedy will help with bruising and swelling. The tissue around the injury is swollen, purple, and tender. The affected part feels cold to the touch. Pains travel upward.

Ruta Grav: Give this remedy if the bone is bruised and there is inflammation of the periosteum. The pains are intense, sore, and aching. The affected part feels weary. The child is restless. Give hourly until relieved, then on an as-needed basis. If this remedy fails to relieve the pain after twenty-four hours, move on to **Symphytum** using the same dosage guidelines. **Symphytum** has a deeper action.

Symphytum: This can be a helpful remedy for pricking and stitching pain for any injury to a bone. The child tends to be irritable. Give hourly, then on an as-needed basis.

For specific bone fractures:

Face, jaw, fingers, toes, spine, or tailbone: Give **Hypericum** every 2–4 hours until relieved, then on an as-needed basis.

Jawbone: Alternate **Bryonia** and **Rhus Tox** every hour until there is relief.

Near a joint, or for a severely bruised jawbone, or severely bruised or broken shinbones: Give **Ruta Grav** every 2–4 hours until relieved, then on an as-needed basis.

Ribs: Give **Bryonia** every 2–4 hours until relieved, then on an as-needed basis. Often the muscles between the injured ribs go into spasm. For severe spasms, you can give **Phosphorus** every 15 minutes until relieved, and then on an as-needed basis.

Dislocations

Arnica can be given hourly until the pain is relieved. Repeat only if there is a return of pain. Once the dislocation has been corrected, give 2 pellets of **Arnica** in the morning and 2 pellets of **Rhus Tox** in the afternoon, for three days.

Note: A dislocation should be immobilized, and x-rays taken as soon as possible.

Dislocation of the elbow: Arnica 3 times a day until relieved, or for three days.

Dislocation of the jaw: Arnica, 2 pellets at first, followed by Rhus Tox 3 times a day for three days or until relieved.

Nerve Injuries

Arsenicum is useful for pains that burn like fire, with a sensation of hot needles, though it feels better with warm applications. The skin is sensitive to the touch. The child is restless, anxious, and demanding. This remedy is usually needed more at night. It can be given every 15 minutes until there is relief. Repeat it only when the benefit of the last dose wears off. If there are no results after six doses, choose a different remedy.

Coffea is useful for pain from nerve-tissue injuries that is intense, intolerable, and triggered by the least motion or noise. The pain can keep the child awake and in a heightened state of awareness of the injury. They are hysterical, hypersensitive to everything, screaming, and weepy. This can be given every 15 minutes until there is relief. Repeat only when the benefit of the last dose wears off. If there are no results after six doses, choose a different remedy.

Hypericum acts as a tonic for injured nerves. It is for pain in nerve-rich areas such as the fingertips, toes, knees, coccyx, elbows, and parts of the face, lips, and mouth. It is particularly useful if the area has been crushed. There is pressure, and the pains are intense, violent, and shooting upwards. The pains appear suddenly, and then disappear gradually. The area is very tender and sore. There may be tingling, twitching, trembling, or numbness. This remedy can be given every 15 minutes until there is relief. Repeat only when the benefit of the last dose wears off. If there are no results after six doses, choose a different remedy.

Sprains and Strains of Ligaments and Tendons

Ligaments attach bone to bone, or organs to structural tissue. Tendons join muscles to bone. This section addresses sprains and deep strains of ankles, knees, hips, wrists, elbows, shoulders, and backs. If there is severe pain and no response to remedies, an x-ray may be needed to rule out dislocation or bone fracture.

The following are the most commonly indicated remedies for sprains and strains:

Arnica: This is the first remedy to give for sprains and strains, to reduce bruising, swelling, and pain. It is useful for shin splints, *overuse of muscles,* or when overstretching a joint leads to a strain. The muscles feel sore, bruised, and beat-up. This can leave the child feeling exhausted, but they are restless. They feel better with cold applications.

Bellis Perennis: For sprains and *deep strains* where there is much swelling and bruising around a joint. This remedy resembles **Arnica**, but its action goes deeper. The sprain or strain may or may not feel cold. This remedy is useful for deep trauma with achy, squeezing, and throbbing pains. The area will feel better with gentle rubbing and motion. Give this remedy at least six hours before bed, because it can interrupt sleep; but it is better to give the remedy if needed than to be concerned about disrupted sleep.

Bryonia: This is a good remedy for a *twisted or strained knee,* and for sprains where there is much inflammation, swelling, redness, and heat around a joint. The child does not want to move, because any motion sets off the pain. The pains are tearing and needle-like. The child is grumpy like a bear, and does not want to be disturbed. They will feel better with pressure, firm bandaging, rest, quiet, and hot applications after the first twenty-four to forty-eight hours, depending on the degree of swelling.

Ledum: This is a remedy for sprains with bruising where the *joint feels cold.* Even though the joint feels cold, they want cold compresses—the colder the better.

Rhus Tox: This remedy is most useful for sprains and strains from overexertion, over-lifting, or being in a *twisted position* while lifting a heavy load, or for *an arm, back or shoulder strain* caused by stretching upwards or outwards for something out of reach. The strained part is stiff, and gets worse if kept still for too long. It will hurt on first movement, especially in the morning on waking, but then the pain subsides with continued gentle movement. The area is weak, and trembles after exertion. The pains are tearing, shooting, and needle-like, and will be worse at night. The child will feel better with gentle rubbing, stretching, flexing, warm applications, or a hot bath. Straining the back can set up chronic patterns that can result in many painful symptoms and may affect other body systems. For instance, digestion may become compromised from a lower-back strain, or breathing and circulation problems may occur from an upper-back strain. It is imperative to see a cranial-sacral osteopath as soon as possible after such a strain has occurred.

Ruta Grav: This is the main remedy for inflammation of cartilage, joints, tendons, and the protective sheath resulting from a strain or sprain. It is useful for *strains and sprains of ankles, hips, lower back, neck, wrists, and elbows.* It is also helpful for *tennis elbow.* There will be bruised-feeling, sore, deeply aching pains that can be quite intense. There are sensations of heaviness and weariness. The affected area can be quite lame. The child will feel better from lying on their back, warm applications, and gentle rubbing. They also crave iced drinks. Lower-back strains feel better from gentle motion and pressure.

Strontium Carb: Look to this remedy if **Rhus Tox** and **Ruta Grav** fail to relieve the symptoms of a sprain. This remedy has an affinity for *sprains that are not healing, with swelling that is not going down, and on the right side.* It is helpful for ankles, knees, hips, wrists, shoulders, neck, and back. There are deep, tearing, and burning bone pains, which increase and decrease gradually. The injured area feels better from being kept wrapped up and warm. The legs feel weak, and the muscles may cramp or twitch. The pain is worse in the evening and night. The ankle retains a buildup of excess serous fluid between the tissue cells. This is a remedy for *an ankle that remains swollen long after the sprain has healed.* In this case, give the remedy three times a week for three weeks.

Dosage for Sprains: Give 2 pellets every 1–2 hours for six doses, then 2–4 times a day for two or three days, depending on the pain. Discontinue once the sprain feels better.

Whiplash

Your first assessment: Is the child in shock?

It is important to know which remedy to give if the child is in shock. There are two specific remedies for shock—Aconitum or Arnica—and they are used in different situations, so please familiarize yourself with the specific indications for each remedy: **Aconitum:** The child is very fearful, anxious, extremely reactive to pain, and inconsolable, with glassy eyes or dilated pupils; they are likely to be screaming, crying out, and trembling with terror and pain.

Arnica: The child is stunned, irritable when offered help, exhausted, and uncooperative; they say they are fine, and don't want to be touched. They may complain of pain, but will maintain that not much is wrong with them.

Dosage: Give 2 pellets of Aconitum or Arnica every 15 minutes until improvement.

Remedies for whiplash:

The effect of a forward/backward/forward jolt to the upper spine can be deeply shocking to the system. If hit from the side, the jolt is side-to-side, which also deeply shocks the brain and the entire system. Watch for dizziness, nausea, faintness, numbness, tingling in the arms, breathing difficulties, disorientation, lethargy, or pains in the neck or shoulder area. It is imperative to see a cranial-sacral osteopath as soon as possible after this injury.

Rhus Tox: The neck is stiff with painful tension, and worse from keeping still for too long. It will hurt on first movement, especially in the morning on waking, but then the pain subsides as gentle movement is continued. The neck feels weak, and the child may have a sensation that they cannot hold their head up.

The pains are tearing, shooting, needle-like, and worse at night. The child will feel better with gentle rubbing, warm applications, or a hot bath.

Ruta Grav: There will be bruised and sore pains, with a deep aching. The pain can be quite intense. There are sensations of heaviness and weariness. The child will feel better lying on their back with the neck supported, and from warm applications, pressure, and gentle rubbing.

Dosage: Unless otherwise directed as above, give 2 pellets every 3–4 hours. If the pain is severe, you may repeat the dose every 15 minutes for four doses, and then hourly for the first twenty-four hours. Discontinue the remedy as soon as there is improvement. Repeat only if necessary.

Supportive Measures:

Note that pain is a necessary communication from the body that there is something wrong. Although you may give a remedy to make your child more comfortable, it is very important to also give an injury rest and proper support measures to insure complete healing. For instance, **Ruta Grav** can almost take the pain away of a strained ankle—however, it is still imperative to rest the ankle and not let the child run or play sports until fully healed. Pain is a warning to stop. If it is not heeded, further damage can result.

Back injuries: Follow up as soon as possible with a cranial-sacral osteopath.

Eye injuries: In most cases, a cold compress will feel best.

Head injuries: Keep the child in a quiet, stress-free environment. Apply a cold compress to the injured area, if there is no bleeding. Watch for signs of concussion. Give clear liquids with no caffeine or high sugar content. Do not give liquids or solids if the child is vomiting.

Supportive Measures (cont):

Nose injuries: Apply pressure by firmly pinching the nose together between the thumb and forefinger for two to five minutes. Allow at least fifteen minutes before encouraging the child to gently blow the clot out, so the nose does not start bleeding again. Apply a cold compress to the nose.

Sprains and strains: Keep the affected part elevated. An ice pack over a thin cloth placed on the affected area, applied for twenty minutes at a time, with an hour between applications, in the first twenty-four hours, will reduce swelling. Continue icing as needed to reduce swelling. Some sprains will feel better if heat is applied after the first twenty-four hours, but ice is best to keep the swelling down. Wrists, ankles, knees, and elbows can be supported by wrapping them firmly with an Ace™ bandage. Give the sprain plenty of rest. Do not let the child run or play sports after the injury until you are sure that the healing is complete.

Tailbone injuries: Go to a pharmacy and purchase a blow-up donut for the child to sit on. This will relieve pressure on the tailbone, and make the child more comfortable.

Call your healthcare practitioner if:

- Your child is prone to having accidents, their clumsiness results in frequently hurting themselves, or they are always dropping things. This may indicate the need for a deep constitutional treatment from your homeopath.

Call your healthcare practitioner if (cont):

- There is any vision disturbance, bleeding, persistent headaches, severe pain, or two black eyes after a blow to the head. Two black eyes at the same time can indicate a fracture at the base of the skull.
- Your child has broken a tooth—immediately call your dentist. Your young daughter has a severe blow to the breast; this includes being hit with a hard ball, or hitting the breast on a steering wheel in a car accident. This injury can make her susceptible to a future lump or tumor, because of bleeding-out in the breast. An ultrasound or thermogram is a noninvasive way of checking the damage.
- Your child lost consciousness, had a seizure, is unable to move or feel any part of the body, cannot recognize familiar people or surroundings, has balance, speech, or vision problems, has drainage of clear fluid (cerebral-spinal fluid) from the nose or mouth, has severe headaches, is vomiting, falls asleep right after hitting their head, or if you suspect there is a skull fracture. *Take them to the emergency room or urgent-care center immediately.* If the child has fallen and has the above symptoms, do not move them—call 911. In the meantime, keep the child warm. You can still give the appropriate remedies. If you are in doubt about any symptom, if your child just does not seem right, or if they are is drowsy for more than six hours, take them to the emergency room or urgent-care facility. *Do not ever worry about wasting someone's time with overreacting;* you are being responsible by making sure that your child is OK. In dealing with a head injury, you must make sure that everything has been checked out. Make sure the pupils of the eyes

Call your healthcare practitioner if (cont):

are the same size. Sometimes one pupil may seem more dilated than the other, or both may be dilated. *This symptom alone is reason enough to go to the emergency room immediately.*

- Your child is having nightmares (even after taking **Arnica**), keeps reliving a traumatic event, e.g., a car accident (even after taking **Stramonium**), or is depressed long after an injury.
- There has been a blow to the back. Check the kidney area for trauma—either side of the spine, just below the rib cage. If there is pain around the kidney area, call your healthcare practitioner at once. In the meantime, give **Bellis Perennis** every 30 minutes until the pain subsides, or talk with your healthcare practitioner.
- There is any blood in the urine after a blow to the back—go to the emergency room.
- Your child has suffered a severe fall or received a hard blow on their back—go to the emergency room.
- You believe a blow has severely traumatized a vital organ, such as the kidneys, spleen, stomach, liver, or lungs. This must be checked out to ensure that the whole picture is assessed and that there is no internal bleeding.
- Your child has an injury to the tailbone, because this can have long-term consequences. It is best to see a cranial-sacral osteopath as soon as possible.
- You suspect that a joint is dislocated. Immediately immobilize the child, and get x-rays taken as soon as possible.
- You suspect a fracture. Look for the following symptoms: severe pain or swelling, deformity, weakness, inability to bear weight, shortening of a limb,

Call your healthcare practitioner if (cont):

or extreme tenderness; or if a crushed finger or toe does not respond to the remedies given.

- You suspect that your child has broken their collar-bone. This bone cannot be put into a cast, and this kind of fracture can puncture the adjacent lung, so immobilize the arm and keep the child as still as possible. Only prescribe **Aconitum** and/or **Arnica** until your healthcare provider or emergency-room physician has assessed whether there is a fracture.

- You suspect that your child has a broken rib. Immediately give 2 pellets of **Bryonia.** This kind of fracture can puncture the adjacent lung. Keep the child as still as possible and seek immediate medical attention.

- If your child has had a concussion, it is important to remove them from any situation where they could hit their head again, e.g., by making them take a leave of absence from the football team. Multiple concussions can have long-term negative effects on your child's future.

POISONING

Ninety percent of all accidental poisonings happen to children under five years old. It is imperative that you keep all medicines, household cleaning products, industrial chemicals, and poisonous plants out of reach. If any chemicals are corrosive, they should be locked up and inaccessible to the child. Parents should make sure any plants in the home are not poisonous. Any corrosive chemical can severely damage a child's esophagus. It is also important never to refer to any medicine or homeopathic remedy as candy.

Post the phone number of your local poison control center on your refrigerator or near the phone so it is readily accessible. If the child has ingested poison and is fearful, give 2 pellets of **Aconitum** for two doses, 15 minutes apart. Some poisons cause internal symptoms, and others cause skin reactions. Identify the source of the poison. The more you can tell the physician or 911 operator about the poison, the better they will be able to assess and help your child.

Note: To administer a remedy if a child's breathing is severely compromised or if they are unconscious, dissolve the remedy in a half-glass of water and dab it with your finger onto the lips or wrist where the pulse is beating (on the wrist just above the thumb).

Most conventional children's clothing is coated with toxic chemicals added for stain-, fire-, and wrinkle-resistance. Non-organic cotton is laden with several toxic insecticides and pesticides. Conventional dyes can be full of carcinogenic heavy metals such as chrome, copper, and zinc. It is important to buy toxin-free and sustainable fibers in any fabric that will touch the delicate skin of your child. The safest fibers for your child are: organic cotton, industrial hemp, silk, bamboo, wool, and recycled polyester. See "Resources" section at the end of the book for places to buy toxin-free clothing.

Remedies for poisonings (these will not interfere with any emergency treatment, and can be given afterward to ease symptoms and speed recovery):

Alcohol Poisoning

See "Poisoning/Alcohol" section (page 103) under "Teenage Discomforts."

Carbon Monoxide Poisoning

After sitting in a traffic jam for a long period of time on a hot day with no wind, your child may react to the exhaust fumes.

Carbo Veg: The head becomes hot, and they have an intense pain at the base of the skull. They feel weak, sick, and exhausted to the point of very little reaction. The breathing may become quickened. The body and breath are cold, but they want to be fanned, and crave fresh air. The face may be red. They are thirsty. This child is low in vitality, and weak to the point of collapse. They are exhausted by even the slightest exertion. The child will be indifferent to everything, a bit confused, irritable, and very sluggish. Their extremities are cold, and so is the breath; however, they feel hot inside, weak, nauseous, and heavy-headed. Give this remedy every 15 minutes until there is improvement. If the child has inhaled carbon monoxide *in a closed space,* immediately *dial 911.* This requires immediate medical treatment. However, until help arrives, give 2 pellets every 15 minutes.

Chemical Poisoning

The toxic chemicals available in most households include ammonia, bleach, detergents, glue, solvents, and pesticides.

Arsenicum: The child needing this remedy has burning pains in the throat, esophagus, or abdominal area. Their mouth and throat may be dry, and they are thirsty for sips of cold water. There can be severe vomiting and retching. If a chemical has come in contact with the skin, there is itching, burning, and swelling. Blisters can form. They are extremely exhausted, but anxious with great restlessness. Even though there is much burning, they feel better with warm applications, because they are usually chilly.

Phosphorus: This remedy is also indicated where there are burning pains. It is for an oversensitive reaction to industrial chemicals, or food containing monosodium glutamate. There is oppressive breathing, with anxiety and palpitations. The lungs are congested and tight, feeling as though there is a heavy weight pressing on the chest. There is a sensation of rawness and burning from the throat to the bottom of the rib cage. There might also be palpitations or an elevated heartbeat, and labored breathing from the least exertion. There is a thirst for ice-cold drinks. The skin reactions are mild itching, burning, and swelling. Blisters can form and easily bleed. The child is weak and can become listless. These children are irritable, lightheaded, oversensitive, disoriented, a bit fearful, and sluggish.

Dosage: Give 2 pellets every 15 minutes for four doses, then hourly until improvement. If there has been no improvement after a total of eight doses, choose a new remedy. As soon as there is improvement, repeat the remedy only if there is a return of any symptoms.

Supportive Measures:

In the case of chemical or drug poisoning, determine whether the substance swallowed is likely to cause more damage if vomited. In the case of poisonings, except for corrosive or petroleum chemicals, and *only with professional advice*, you may induce vomiting by giving 1 tablespoon of pure ipecac syrup in one cup of water and having your child drink the entire amount. If the child has not vomited in fifteen minutes, repeat the dose. Have the child lie on their side so that the tongue cannot drop back, which can cause choking or inhibit the passage of air. If the child is cold, cover them with a blanket. If a chemical has burned the skin, look to the section on "Burns," above, and give the appropriate remedies.

Call your healthcare practitioner if:

- Your child has swallowed a corrosive material such as oven cleaner, lye, drain opener, kerosene, paint

Call your healthcare practitioner if (cont):

- thinner, or gasoline. *Do not induce vomiting;* these materials can do more damage by coming up than by being swallowed. *Dial 911*—the operator will put you through to someone who will can talk you through what you need to do.
- Your child has swallowed a prescription, over-the-counter, or hallucinogenic drug. It is absolutely imperative to seek expert help. *Take the child to the emergency room and call your healthcare practitioner as soon as you can!*

Drug Poisoning

See "Poisoning/Drugs and Glue-Sniffing" section (page 105) under "Teenage Discomforts."

Food Poisoning

This condition occurs when the child has consumed contaminated meat or fish, impure water, or overripe fruit. It usually comes on violently anywhere from 2–8 hours after ingestion of the offending food or drink. Various viruses and bacteria can be associated with the symptoms of severe diarrhea, nausea, and vomiting. A low-grade fever and/or headache may also be present. These incidents are usually over in six hours, but leave a residual weakness. Whether the food poisoning is from salmonella, E. coli, or another pathogen, it is helpful to know what contaminated food or water was ingested. Vomiting and diarrhea are the body's way of getting the offending poison out. Homeopathy will not repress or stop this necessary response, but it will lessen the duration and severity. Also see the section on "Diarrhea, Nausea, and Vomiting" on page 30, as other remedies may apply.

The following is an overview of remedies for food poisoning from eating specific foods:

Beef: Arsenicum, Carbo Veg, Cinchona (China Officinalis)
Chicken: Arsenicum, Carbo Veg
Fish: Arsenicum, Carbo Veg, Cinchona (China Officinalis), Pulsatilla
Fruit—spoiled: Arsenicum, Cinchona (China Officinalis), Zingiber
Fruit—too much: Bryonia, Cinchona (China Officinalis), Ipecacuanha
Fruit—unripe: Ipecacuanha
Pork: Ipecacuanha, Pulsatilla
Shellfish: Arsenicum, Urtica Urens

The following are the most commonly indicated remedies for food poisoning:

Arsenicum: After eating spoiled chicken, beef, shellfish, fish, or fruit.

Nausea and vomiting: Retching after eating or drinking ice-cold water, anxiety, burning, and rawness in the pit of the stomach. Vomiting and diarrhea, which give temporary relief and may be simultaneous. Vomit burns the throat. Abdomen is sensitive to the touch. The child will only want small amounts of food, often after the vomiting has subsided.

Diarrhea: Very watery, burning, slimy, brown, yellow, or black stools that may contain undigested food; foul-smelling stools in small quantities, which burn the anus; and cramping in the abdomen. Great weakness follows the stool. The child is chilly, but wants sips of cold water to wet the mouth, or might refuse water for fear of vomiting. They can't bear the thought of food. The child is anxious, restless, can't lie still, and is exhausted but has energy enough to be demanding. The older child may have a fear that they are going to die.

Worse from: Midnight to 2 AM, cold food or drinks, getting chilled, and cold. **Better from:** Heat, and warm applications to the abdomen.

Bryonia: For distress after eating too much fruit, or drinking ice-cold drinks after getting overheated.

Nausea and vomiting: Nausea and faintness on rising. Vomits solid food, bile, and water.

Diarrhea: The stools are loose, yellow, and mushy. The area around the anus burns. There is usually little or no cramping. The diarrhea is worse in the morning after getting up and moving around. The stomach is sensitive to touch. The child is very grumpy, irritable, does not want to move, and wants to be left alone.

Worse from: Movement, morning, hot weather, and eating cabbage. **Better from:** Pressure, rest, being quiet and left alone, and cool drinks.

Carbo Veg: From eating spoiled chicken, beef, or fish. Any food at all disagrees with the digestive tract. Extreme burning pains.

Nausea: Nausea with sour belching, restricted breathing, and faintness. The child cannot bear the sight or thought of food. Severe bloating makes the skin feel stretched tight, and they cannot bear anything tight around the waist; their belly is very tender. They have bad breath, and a pale face that sometimes has a bluish tint. They feel faint on arising, and have low vitality, exhaustion with chilliness or cold sweats, and a feeble pulse. They may be bent over from the pain. They want fresh air, although they are cold to the touch and have cold sweats. They have a strong desire to be fanned.

Diarrhea: Lots of gas and burning in the anus when passing acidic, foul-smelling stools. This child is anxious, confused, indifferent, irritable, and sluggish.

Worse from: Drinking ice water, loss of fluids, butter, fats, milk, and lying down. **Better from:** Cool, fresh air, being fanned, elevating their feet, passing gas, and burping.

Cinchona (also known as **China Officinalis**): For food poisoning from eating spoiled beef, fish, or fruit, or too much fruit.

Vomiting: Frequent vomiting of undigested food, sour-smelling vomit, very swollen, painful abdomen with lots of gas, and belching that gives no relief. There is a sore and cold feeling in the stomach, hiccups, and abdominal rumbling with thirst for cold water.

Diarrhea: Pale stools are acidic and profuse, have undigested food, and look frothy. The diarrhea is painless, but they do have gas pains that can make them bend double. The diarrhea may be involuntary. This is a remedy to give if your child is dehydrated from diarrhea and vomiting—they are weak with much sweating, may feel faint, and/or have ringing in the ears. Dehydration may cause a feeling of weakness to persist after the child is no longer vomiting or passing diarrhea. The child is weak, irritable, and oversensitive to touch and drafts. They are nervous, and may have problems sleeping. Rehydrate this child.

Worse from: Drafts, noise, tea, nighttime, and eating. **Better from:** Much quiet rest, hydration, firm pressure, bending double, warmth, and gently moving the limbs.

Ipecacuanha: From eating unripe fruit, too much fruit, or spoiled pork.

Nausea and vomiting: Constant, unyielding nausea. The child may want to vomit, but can't. If they vomit, it does not relieve the nausea. They vomit food, bile, green mucus, and/or bright-red blood. They usually have a headache, increased salivation, horrible cutting and cramping pains, and sometimes dark circles around the eyes. The face is pale. The child cannot stand the smell of food. They sometimes twitch, and may have hiccups. They may have an odd sensation that the stomach is too relaxed and is hanging down. There may be violent itching of the skin.

Diarrhea: Stools are yellow or green, streaked with blood, and very offensive-smelling. The stools are bright-green if the cause is from overeating. These children get angry when they don't get their way. They complain, scream, and howl a lot, and nothing pleases them.

Worse from: Eating ice cream, rich foods, pastries, sweets, and berries; stooping, heat, motion, and overeating. **Better from:** Open air, rest, and closing the eyes.

Pulsatilla: From eating spoiled pork or fish.

Vomiting: The child vomits food long after it was eaten. It feels as if there is a stone lodged in the stomach just below the ribs. Can still taste the food that caused the problem. Gas and belching.

Diarrhea: Watery, green stools, but the child does not pass as much as they would like to. No two stools look alike; there is rumbling in the gut, and low appetite, and the child is rarely thirsty. They are tearful and moody, weep easily, and want lots of sympathy and company. Boys will feel sorry for themselves.

Worse from: Heat, after fright, twilight, warm stuffy rooms, rich food, fats, and ice cream. **Better from:** Cool, fresh air, hydration, and being carried slowly and gently.

Urtica Urens: For hives caused by eating spoiled shellfish. The hives are burning, stinging, and very itchy, with possible pains in the joints. The itching can be quite severe. The skin has raised, pale welts on a red background. These areas appear in blotches.

Nausea: With burning in the throat.

Diarrhea: After passing greenish-brown stool, the urge persists but with little effect. The anus may feel raw or burning. There may be swelling, stinging, redness, and burning in the face, hands, and feet. The child is hot in bed at night, with sweatiness. The child is very restless, and wants to rub the hives.

Worse from: Cold water, cool moist air, touch, night, and strenuous exercise. **Better from:** Lying down (but not on the affected parts), and rubbing the affected area.

Zingiber: From eating spoiled melons or impure water.

Nausea: Stomach feels heavy and also empty, with rumbling, gas, and acidity. The taste of any food remains for a long time afterward. The child has a dry mouth and much thirst.

Diarrhea: From drinking impure water, or eating overripe or rotten melons. The diarrhea is accompanied by lots of gas and belching. The pains are cutting. There is a feeling that the anus is loose, and hot, with much soreness. The stools are extremely loose. The child will feel exhausted and weak. The face is red and hot. They may feel hot and chilly at the same time. The child is confused, irritable in the evening, nervous, and fidgety.

Worse from: After eating, especially bread; touch, lying down, evenings and 3 AM, and cold, damp air. **Better from:** Sitting, standing, and being covered.

Dosage: Give 2 pellets every 15 minutes for four doses, then hourly until improvement. If there has been no improvement after a total of eight doses, choose a new remedy. As soon as there is improvement, repeat the remedy only if there is a return of any symptoms.

Supportive Measures:

It is imperative that the child is kept hydrated with good water. You can make a homemade fluid replacement with a fifty-fifty mix of apple (or any clear, pulp-free) juice and water. Fresh, pulp-free watermelon juice and water is one of the most quick and natural ways to replenish their electrolytes. Even if the child is vomiting, encourage them to drink small sips frequently. Giving a child bananas, applesauce, white toast, and white rice will give binding power to the intestines and slow the diarrhea. These foods can be slowly reintroduced after vomiting. It is better for the child to eat small amounts frequently. Cut out all dairy products and fruit, with the exception of bananas or applesauce. Use organic foods when possible. Have the child get plenty of rest.

After a heavy loss of fluids from vomiting and diarrhea, expect improvement to be gradual. Do not overtax the system by reintroducing any rich or fatty foods too quickly. If the child has no appetite, encourage them to eat just a little. Some young children want to stop eating for fear of vomiting, if the symptoms have been severe. **Cinchona** (China Officinalis) may be needed if the child is weak, exhausted, and can't seem to get their energy back. Give this every 2 hours until improvement. If there is no improvement after twenty-four hours, call your healthcare practitioner.

Call your healthcare practitioner if:

- There has been no improvement in twenty-four hours.
- The skin shows no rebound effect, that is, if pressed on the shinbone, it does not spring back.
- There is severe abdominal pain that worsens or has not responded to remedies.
- Your baby under three months old has any rise in temperature.
- Your child over three months old has a temperature over 103 degrees.
- Your child under two years of age has had a fever for more than twenty-four hours.
- Your child over two years of age has had a fever for more than three days.
- Your child is nonreactive, has trouble breathing, has convulsions, or is listless or limp.
- Blood repeatedly appears in the stools or vomit.
- Your child cannot stop vomiting.
- There is unexplained vomiting, with severe pain around the navel or in the extreme lower-right pelvic area; this may indicate appendicitis in an older child.
- Your child is refusing to drink. You must ask for professional help, as shock and collapse with dehydration can cause severe damage to brain cells.
- You suspect that your child has a parasite.
- Your child is depleted, in pain, or becoming dehydrated, you need to see a doctor. Then you can follow up with your homeopath.

SHOCK

Shock is a condition where there is a lack of circulation to the brain, central nervous system, organs, or tissues. This reduces the supply of oxygen and therefore produces a state of shock.

To administer a remedy if a child's breathing is severely compromised, or if they are unconscious, put the remedy into a half-glassful of water and dab it onto the lips or wrist where the pulse is beating (on the wrist below the thumb.)

It is important to know which remedy to give if the child is in shock. There are two specific remedies for shock—**Aconitum** or **Arnica**—and they are used in different situations, so please familiarize yourself with the specific indications for each remedy:

Aconitum: The child is very fearful, anxious, extremely reactive to pain, and inconsolable, with glassy eyes or dilated pupils; they are likely to be screaming, crying out, and trembling with terror and pain.

Arnica: The child is stunned, irritable when offered help, exhausted, and uncooperative; they say they are fine, and don't want to be touched. They may complain of pain, but will maintain that not much is wrong with them.

Dosage: Give Aconitum or Arnica every 15 minutes until improvement.

Rescue Remedy: This remedy reduces the effects of fright, shock, emotional trauma, grief, panic, hysteria, and fearfulness that cause trembling and loss of energy. It will restore a sense of balance, calm, and harmony. The child may feel faint, and may be speechless. **Rescue Remedy** is a very gentle yet effective remedy to keep the ill effects of shock from imprinting themselves on the child mentally and emotionally. **Rescue Remedy** is found in health-food stores, usually next to the homeopathic remedies. It is a liquid made up of five different flower essences preserved in an alcohol/water solution, invented by an English homeopath by the name of Dr. Bach. It is completely safe.

Dosage: Add 3 drops to a glass of spring water, and have the child sip it frequently until you see progress; then give every 15 minutes, then every 30 minutes, repeating as long as needed. Stop when emotional stability has returned.

Anaphylactic Shock

A child with anaphylactic shock should be taken to an emergency room immediately, if close by. If you are not close to a hospital, call 911. Do not delay, because time is of the essence, especially if the hives have come on quickly and/or the throat is swelling. Give **Apis** or **Carbolic Acid** on the way to the hospital if you can grab it quickly, or give it while waiting for the ambulance. Anaphylactic shock is a condition where the body releases large amounts of histamine into the bloodstream. This causes dilation of blood vessels, and constriction of the airways. It can come on quickly, causing heat and difficulty in from closed-off air passages. The child may also experience flushing, numbness, itching, hives, swelling, or sneezing. The blood pressure can drop dramatically, causing faintness and irregular heart palpitations, which can set off extreme panic and/or agitation in a child.

Apis: This remedy can save a life if there is an extreme allergic reaction. Swelling is rapid, the child has no thirst, and they are panting, feeling as if they cannot get enough air, or cannot take another breath. The child is constantly whining, weepy, restless, anxious, irritable, and fidgety. However, they are also tired and want to lie down. Give the remedy every 5–15 minutes, even while waiting at the hospital. Repeat when symptoms return.

Carbolic Acid: For shock following an insect sting. The part affected will be weak, with severe burning and pricking pains that come and go with intense itching. A strong indicator for this remedy is that the sense of smell becomes very acute. The child may have cold hands and feet, and may break into a cold, clammy sweat. The child may tremble. They rapidly loose vitality and strength, which may bring about collapse. Give every

5–15 minutes, even while waiting at the hospital. Repeat when symptoms return.

Clinical Shock

Shock can be caused by a large loss of body fluid from bleeding, surgery, vomiting, diarrhea, or sweating to the point of sunstroke, or from a head injury. The symptoms of clinical shock are: skin that is cold, clammy, either pale or a bluish color, rapid and weak pulse, difficulty breathing, or hyperventilating, debility, disorientation, sleepiness, or restlessness. If the child is not responding to remedies for shock, take them to the emergency room immediately! *If they become unresponsive, call 911.*

Carbo Veg: For acute shock with breathing difficulties. This is usually due to a loss of body fluids from bleeding, vomiting, or diarrhea. The face is pale, with a bluish tint. The child may be gasping for breath. Because they have a great need for fresh air, they may ask to be fanned. The child will be indifferent to everything, weak, exhausted, a bit confused, and irritable, if they have enough vitality. They are cold externally, but do not want to be covered because they are burning up internally. They need to be fanned rapidly and closely, with fresh air if possible. Keep their feet elevated, keep the air cool, and give them lots of rest.

Cinchona (also known as **China Officinalis**): For shock from loss of bodily fluids, especially blood, or from vomiting, sunstroke, or diarrhea. The child is completely drained, very weak, and trembling. They gasp for breath, and may complain of ringing in the ears or blurred vision. There is much sweating. This remedy is especially helpful when there is *severe dehydration:* The child is irritable, sensitive, and cannot think straight.

Veratrum: For shock from loss of bodily fluids, especially from vomiting and diarrhea. The child experiences intense chills, cold sweats, and beads of sweat on the forehead. They go down quickly. The forehead, hands, feet, and abdomen are cold and clammy.

The skin has a bluish tint. They have a huge thirst for great quantities of cold water. The pulse is feeble, but the child is restless.

Dosage: Give the remedy every 10 minutes until improvement, for up to eight doses. Repeat only if there is a return of symptoms.

Electrical Shock

Electrical shock is caused by contacting a live electrical wire, or being struck by lightning. The shock may be a mild jolt, or quite severe. If the shock is severe, the child may lose consciousness, experience severe muscle contractions, heart palpitations, and/or difficulty or cessation of breathing. Check for electrical burns on the skin. After assessing the shock picture and giving 2 pellets of **Aconitum** or **Arnica**, the remedy for electric shock is **Phosphorus**. Give this remedy as soon as possible.

Always follow up with your healthcare practitioner to monitor any after effects. Refer to the "Burns" section if the child's skin is burned. Look at the "Supportive measures" section, below.

Dosage: Give the remedy every 10 minutes until improvement, for up to eight doses. Repeat only if there is a return of symptoms.

Emotional Shock

See section on "Emotional Trauma and Fears" (page 257).

Septic or Toxic Shock

These conditions are caused by an overwhelming bacterial infection. The symptoms include: diarrhea, headaches, high fever, with or without chills, low blood pressure, muscle aches, nausea, vomiting, seizures, redness of the eyes, mouth, or throat, or a widespread rash that is red like a sunburn.

Note: Do not try to treat either of these conditions. *Take your child to an emergency room.*

Septic shock is a serious condition that usually occurs from a wound infection after surgery. Look for red streaks traveling outwards from the wound toward the heart.

Toxic shock syndrome is a serious condition that can be caused by leaving a tampon inserted for too long, especially during menstruation.

Supportive Measures:

Take a deep breath, and be reassuring to your child. Place the child on their back, unless you think there is trauma to the spine or neck. Loosen any tight clothing. Check to be sure the child's airway is clear, and that they are breathing. Keep the child warm (not hot, to avoid sweating and further loss of fluids). Unless there is a head injury, raise the legs slightly above the head. In case of a head injury, slightly elevate the head above the feet. If the child is going to vomit, turn the head so the airway is clear to prevent choking. If they ask for a drink, avoid cold liquids. If there is a wound, apply pressure to stop the bleeding.

Call your healthcare practitioner if:

- There is loss of consciousness, or a persistent state of shock with confusion—take the child to an emergency room immediately, if close by. If you are not close to a hospital, call 911.
- Your baby is under three months old and has any rise in temperature.
- Your child is over three months old and has a temperature over 103 degrees.

Call your healthcare practitioner if (cont):

- Your child is under two years of age and has had a fever for more than twenty-four hours.
- Your child is over two years of age and has had a fever for more than three days.
- Your child is nonreactive, has trouble breathing, has convulsions, or is listless or limp.
- If the child has stopped breathing, start CPR (cardio-pulmonary resuscitation), and have someone call 911 immediately.
- A wound has red streaks in different directions or traveling toward the heart—go to an emergency room immediately!
- If you suspect your teen daughter has toxic shock syndrome, take her to the emergency room immediately!

SPLINTERS

Wood, thorn, fishbone, and glass splinters:

These splinters cause puncture wounds and bleed very little, or not at all. The body is capable of causing foreign objects to be expelled naturally; it surrounds the object with white blood cells, forming a pocket of pus. The area around the splinter swells, and eventually the body ejects both the splinter and the pus. This may take days, or even weeks.

Remedies for different types of splinters:

Fishbone splinter **in the throat**: Silicea
Splinters or thorns **under fingernails**: Ledum

Splinter or thorn sites **that are very sensitive and painful**: Hypericum

Splinters **of wood or glass**: Silicea

Hypericum: For tearing pain that shoots upward along the nerve pathways. Nerve pains are sharp and intense. This is especially effective for splinters in nerve-rich areas such as fingers or toes. The splinter area is very painful, tender, and inflamed, with burning heat of the skin. There is usually swelling. The child may experience numbness and tingling. This remedy can be alternated with any of the splinter remedies.

Ledum: This is a good remedy if there are a lot of puncture lacerations. The site is puffy, tender, and very dark-red or purple. The skin feels cold to the touch, but feels better with cold applications. Pains are throbbing, shooting, pricking, and biting. Repeat up to four times a day, only if the pain returns or the child is complaining that the site feels cold.

Silicea (also known as **Silica Terra**): This is the most useful remedy to help expel foreign objects from the body. It promotes the painless expulsion of any foreign object, including fish bones caught in the throat. For minor punctures, it will expel the object without producing pus at the puncture site. For a deeper splinter, pus will form that is a creamy color.

For puncture areas that have become infected, use **Hepar Sulph** twice a day until resolved; it will keep the infection from spreading. The area becomes swollen, red, hot, sometimes hard, and extremely sensitive. The skin around the area is dry. The pains are sore, splinter-like, and sharp. The wound may be bloody, look abscessed, or ooze pus that is yellow or green and tends to smell like old, rotten cheese.

Dosage: Use twice a day until the problem is resolved. Hypericum can be used every 4 hours if the site is extremely painful; then use on an as-needed basis.

Supportive Measures:

If your child has a glass splinter, it can be hard to see and also to remove all of it, because it can so easily break off. If the splinter or thorn is not too deep, use a sterilized needle and tweezers to remove it. Always allow a shallow wound to bleed for a short time. This is very cleansing for the wound, and activates lymphocytes, the immune cells that produce antibodies.

Then cleanse the area with a Hypercal solution. This is a combination of Hypericum Tincture, which heals damaged nerves, and Calendula Tincture, which repairs damaged skin. This combination is invaluable when applied topically, as it brings about rapid healing. Place 5 drops of each tincture in a quarter-cup of bottled spring water, or fresh water that has been boiled and cooled, and apply directly to the site. It will sting for a few seconds, and then give relief. You can obtain these tinctures at any health-food store or natural pharmacy. *The wound must be clean before applying this solution.* Be sure to watch for infections afterward.

Remember that the sight of blood can be quite disturbing to a child. Remind them to take slow, deep, rhythmical breaths.

Call your healthcare practitioner if:

- Your child develops a fever.
- A large splinter or shard of glass has gone too deep to be removed.

Call your healthcare practitioner if:

- A large fishbone is caught in the throat, and/or the child is choking. *Call 911.*
- The puncture site is very red, swollen, hot, and there are red streaks going up from the affected area. The child may or may not have a fever. *Take your child to an urgent-care center or hospital immediately.*

SURGERY

Before Surgery

If your child is afraid, the night before or just before surgery, give them 2 pellets of either **Aconitum, Arsenicum, Coffea, Gelsemium, Glonoinum, Ignatia,** or **Phosphorus,** depending on the following accompanying symptoms:

The child needing **Aconitum** is restless, easily excited, with a fear that they are going to die.

The **Arsenicum** child is restless, chilly, weak, exhausted, trembling, thirsty, and perspiring.

The **Coffea** child will be unable to sleep, because of acute hearing. Every little noise keeps them awake.

The **Gelsemium** child is nervous and trembling, tends to hyperventilate, and may have diarrhea.

The **Glonoinum** child will have high blood pressure because they are so nervous about the operation.

The **Ignatia** child is nervous, sighs a lot, moans, and is inconsolable, with changeable moods and contradictory symptoms.

The **Phosphorus** child is fearful, and wants lots of affection.

The Day of Surgery

Give 2 pellets of **Arnica** just before surgery. (This will not interfere with the protocol of taking nothing by mouth before surgery.) **Arnica** will help to alleviate the effects of shock, control bleeding and swelling, and reduce pain, inflammation, bruising, and soreness.

Just before the dentist performs surgery or dental work, give 2 pellets of **Arnica**, then 15 minutes later give 2 pellets of **Hypericum.**

After Surgery

Remedies for healing from specific types of surgery

Abdominal surgery: Bellis Perennis
Dental surgery: Hypericum
Eye surgery: Calendula
Knee surgery: Bryonia
Laparoscopy: Ledum, Hypericum
Ligament replacement or tears: Ruta Grav
Pain: Chamomilla
Pelvic surgery: Bellis Perennis
Plastic surgery to the face, fingers, or tailbone: Hypericum

Arnica is a major remedy to help recover from an operation. It is best given as soon as possible after the child has awoken from the anesthesia. You can give **Arnica** immediately after an operation, and every four hours, to aid with shock, pain, bruising, and swelling. Discontinue once the soreness is gone.

Bellis Perennis is most helpful for recuperation after **abdominal or pelvic surgery.** There may be swelling of the soft tissue, or around internal organs that have been disturbed by the surgery. There is much soreness, aching, and throbbing. Use twice a day for several days. Can be given every four hours if the symptoms are severe.

Bryonia is most useful when the pains are worse from the slightest movement, even coughing or sneezing. The child does not want anyone to touch any part near the site of the surgery. There are needle-like and cutting pains. This is especially useful after **knee surgery,** and helpful for inflammation after surgery. May be given hourly until improvement.

Calendula *is the first remedy to consider for the healing of surgical wounds.* Give immediately after surgery, then twice a day for up to seven days, if it is a major surgery. For eye surgery, give **Calendula** immediately after the surgery, then twice a day for three days.

Chamomilla is a remedy for pain. It calms nerve irritation. The child is crying, beside themselves with pain, and irritable. The younger child wants to be carried. Not always, but many times, one cheeks is pale and the other is red (this may be subtle); or one cheek is cool, and the other is hot. May be given hourly until improvement.

Euphrasia Tincture: This is a liquid herbal remedy that can support other remedies given internally. You can purchase this from a health-food store or natural pharmacy. It will help relieve irritation and aching in the eye. Put one drop in a quarter-cup of spring water, and use as an eyebath. It is very soothing and healing.

Hypericum is helpful after surgery in **nerve-rich areas such as fingertips, lips, toes, or tailbone.** This is for children who experience much more pain and sensitivity than would be expected. The pains are sharp and shooting. There can also be numbness and tingling. This remedy is also indicated for any **laparoscopic surgery** with the above symptoms. May be given hourly until improvement.

Ledum is indicated for any **laparoscopic surgery,** as well as any incision from surgery. The pain is shooting and pricking in nature. The wound feels cold, but is relieved by cold applications. There is swelling, and the incision looks pale. May be given hourly until improvement.

Ruta Grav is indicated for surgery that has been performed on the **ligaments.** It is complementary to **Arnica,** and can be alternated at a different hour, i.e., give **Ruta Grav** after surgery and then **Arnica** one hour later. Repeat as necessary.

Silicea (also known as **Silica Terra**) helps with infection and post-surgical scarring that is inflamed, painful, and slow to heal. The surgical incision will ooze a cream-colored pus. If there is infection and pain, give every four hours until improvement. Otherwise, give three times a week for three weeks.

Staphysagria is helpful if the wound has become dark-red, or sometimes bluish. There is usually swelling. The incision is very sensitive, and tender to the slightest touch. In many cases it bleeds more than it seems it should. The child cries for many things, and then refuses them when given. They are extremely sensitive, sad, angry, and irritable. They can be quite indignant and angry that they were cut by the surgeon's knife. Give this remedy every four hours until improvement. Consult your healthcare practitioner, if there is no improvement after twenty-four hours. If there is pain in the incised area after it has healed, give 2 pellets three times a week until there is improvement. Consult your healthcare practitioner if there is not improvement after three weeks.

A note about **eye surgery:** If the surgery has left an acute and painful awareness of being cut by a knife, or an acute sense of the eye feeling cut open, give 2 pellets of **Staphysagria.** Repeat if the above sensations return. If your child's eye is not healing well, check to see if this sensation is present. Other remedies may not be able to aid in healing, if this remedy is needed; this means that **Staphysagria** might be the first remedy to give after surgery—but only if this sensation is pronounced.

Strontium Carb is useful for shock after a surgery where there has been much blood loss. There is much soreness; however, there may also be numbness. This remedy will also help reduce the incidence of clots after surgery. The child is irritable and angry. Give every 4 hours until improvement. Call your healthcare practitioner if there is no improvement after twenty-four hours.

Remedies for common conditions following surgery:

Adhesions

Adhesions are bands of fibrous tissue adhering to each other at the site of the surgery. The pulling of this tissue can be quite painful. Give **Calc Fluorica** once a week for six weeks after the surgery to reduce the development of adhesions.

Note: **Calc Fluorica** is not in the emergency kit, if you have one. You will need to purchase it from a health food store or natural pharmacy.

Adverse Reactions to Anesthesia

Phosphorus is an indicated remedy for anesthesia reactions, especially if there is vomiting. The child is fearful and complains a lot, but is sweet-natured and seeks affection. They are thirsty for cold drinks. They have had trouble sleeping since the surgery, and are having nightmares or bad dreams. This remedy can be given before surgery if your child has had a previous surgery and came out of the anesthesia vomiting. You may also want to ask, well in advance of the surgery, whether a less reactive type of anesthetic is available.

Nux Vomica is indicated if the child is violently retching or has constant nausea. They may feel faint, or have a hard time vomiting. They vomit bile, bitter mucus, and/or sour-smelling vomit. The stomach and intestines feel bruised and sore. They experience cramping, gas, sour and bitter belching, and dryness of the mouth. They are chilly. Many times they are constipated. They are sleepy during the day, but have a hard time sleeping at night. These children are angry, irritable, nervous, and spiteful, or very sensitive and easily offended.

Ipecacuanha is indicated for constant and unyielding nausea. They want to vomit, but can't. If they vomit, the nausea is not relieved by vomiting. They vomit food, bile, sometimes green mucus, and/or bright-red blood. They usually have a headache, cannot stand the smell of food, have increased salivation, and experience horrible cutting and cramping pains. The face is pale, and they may have dark circles around the eyes. The child sometimes twitches, and may have hiccups. These children get angry when they don't get their way, and then complain a lot; nothing pleases them, and there may be a lot of screaming and howling.

Bleeding

See "Wounds" section below (page 347).

Catheter Removal Pain

Give 2 pellets of **Staphysagria.** Repeat only if the pain returns.

Difficulty Urinating

Causticum is helpful if the surgery has left the child with difficulties in passing urine. **Causticum** can act as a homeopathic catheter. Give 2 pellets hourly until the child urinates. Repeat only if needed.

Healing Surgical Wounds or Bedsores

Hypercal is a combination of Hypericum Tincture, which heals damaged nerves, and Calendula Tincture, which repairs damaged skin. This combination is invaluable when applied topically; it not only brings about rapid healing but helps prevent scarring and reduce pain. When first applied, it is likely to sting. Then the stinging will subside and it will feel much better. You can obtain these tinctures at any health-food store or natural pharmacy. Make a solution of 5 drops of each tincture to a quarter-cup of spring water. *The wound must be clean before applying this solution.* Vitamin E oil and calendula cream or gel prevent scarring, but use these only after the wound is no longer oozing and has completely scabbed over.

Note: If you suspect that the wound is infected (if it is red, hot, swollen, abnormally painful, or with red streaks), do not use the Hypercal. Contact your healthcare professional.

Oral Surgery

See "Tooth Discomforts" section below (page 321). If there is excessive bleeding, see "Wounds" section below (page 347).

Postoperative Depression or Negativity

Depression after surgery is not uncommon. It can result from the general anesthetic, drugs given to prevent infection, or from pain or slow recuperation. It can also occur if the child has had to endure multiple surgeries. Consult your healthcare provider. **Staphysagria** is able to relieve the child from the trauma of the surgical knife. Give this remedy if the child is acutely aware of the incision, feels indignation toward the surgeon or parents, or has been very angry since the operation. Give 2 pellets. Repeat if the negative emotions return.

Shock

See "Shock" section above (page 304).

Surgical Incisions

See "Wounds" section below (page 347) for care of the incision.

Weakness or Prolonged Prostration

If you feel that your child is not recovering from surgery in a timely manner, consult with the surgeon and then consult with your healthcare provider.

Supportive Measures:

It is always advisable to consult a cranial-sacral osteopath as soon as you can after the surgery. Their work returns all vital organs to their correct situation, and makes sure that lymph drainage is restored. Make sure the child has a balanced diet of easily digested food, and drinks plenty of water to help the kidneys flush the system.

Recommended foods are: fruits for vitamin C, green leafy vegetables, miso soup, and yogurt for good intestinal flora, carrots for vitamin A, and almond butter for vitamin E. Foods to avoid: fat, sugar, eggs (unless boiled), and any highly refined or fast foods. It is important to balance physical activity with rest, achieving a gradual return to their routine as soon as possible. Fresh air, if possible, is very healing. When the operation has been exhausting to the body, nerves, and emotions, it is worth considering using other remedies as well to restore complete health. Consult your homeopath.

Call your healthcare practitioner if:

- The tissue around the surgical wound is bright-red, purple or hot, or the wound is oozing yellow or green pus.
- There are red streaks in different directions from the wound and/ or a fever—take your child to an urgent-care clinic or the hospital immediately.
- Your child cannot urinate, or there is swelling at a catheter site after giving the appropriate remedies.
- Your child is not recovering in a timely manner, either physically or emotionally.

SWIMMING

Diving into Cold Water when Overheated

After swimming, a child may become very chilled.

If they are restless, give them 2 pellets of **Arsenicum**. If they are chilled with much shivering, shaking, and a hot face, give them 2 pellets of **Bellis Perennis.**

With both of these remedies, the child will feel better if they are wrapped up, rubbed to warm them up, and given warm food. Repeat the remedy as needed.

Near-Drowning

If the child is not breathing, or their breath is feeble, try to get help from a lifeguard. If one is not around, *call 911.*

If you suspect that the child may have a neck or spine injury, *avoid turning or bending the neck.* Do not move the child.

Turn the drowning victim's head to the side, and wipe any water that comes up out of the mouth. Return their head to a centered position, and keep the head and neck very still. You can secure the neck by placing rolled towels or other objects on either side of the head. Perform mouth-to-mouth resuscitation if you know how. If the heartbeat is feeble, or has stopped, perform CPR if you know how. If you don't know how to do these, keep the child's airways clear until help arrives.

Follow these additional steps: Keep the victim calm and still. If you do *not* suspect a neck or spinal injury, remove any wet clothes. Otherwise, cover them with something warm so they will not get hypothermia. The victim may cough, expel water from the lungs, and have difficulty breathing. Once breathing restarts, keep reassuring them that everything is all right until medical help arrives.

To administer a remedy if a child's breathing is severely compromised, or if they are unconscious, put the remedy into a half-glass of water and dab it with your finger onto the child's lips, or onto the wrist where the pulse is beating (just above the thumb).

If there is no water, put 2 of the tiny pellets in the cheek, where they will dissolve. As soon as possible, administer 2 pellets of **Antimonium Tart,** and repeat every 15 minutes until there is improvement. Assess for shock and give **Aconitum** or **Arnica.** (See section on "Shock.")

Note: Complications such as pneumonia, infection, or heart failure can arise within forty-eight hours of a drowning incident. Therefore, you should always take a drowning victim to the hospital and have them checked out.

Swimmer's Ear

Turn the head back and forth to utilize the force of gravity to drain water from the ear. Gently pulling the ear in different directions also helps. Using a towel, dry the opening of the ear very carefully, as far in as you can. **Mercurius Dulcis** will clear this condition. You may have to give a few doses. If there is no response after giving three doses, try a few doses of Silicea.

To prevent swimmer's ear, put two drops of rubbing alcohol in the ear before the child goes swimming. Two drops of white vinegar can also prevent the growth of bacteria on the skin in the ear canal.

TOOTH DISCOMFORTS

A good diet will maintain good health in the teeth and oral tissues. A diet free of acidic drinks, refined carbohydrates, laboratory chemicals, and refined sugars is a must.

Loose baby teeth can be a source of pain. There can also be pain from grinding the teeth. Some tooth pain can be referred pain from an infected sinus nearby, but this is rare. These scenarios should be eliminated to determine why the tooth is aching.

Abscess

Unless your child is in poor health and/or undernourished, this is not a common condition. If a tooth is abscessing the pain is intense. There can be swelling and throbbing that comes and goes intermittently. They may have a fever. The area around the tooth is usually red and may be draining pus. Do not delay. Call your dentist in order to keep your child from developing serious complications.

Apprehension About the Dentist

If your child has had a frightening experience at the dentist, choose one of the following remedies based on the previous reaction. Start giving these remedies before the next encounter with the dentist:

Aconitum: Sheer terror! Rapid pulse and profuse perspiration. The child is full of fear, anxiety, panic with restlessness, extremely reactive to pain, and inconsolable. The pupils can be dilated. They are likely to be shrieking and crying out with terror. They are afraid of crowds and death, because they are sure they are going to die. They are easily startled.

Argentum Nit: They are anxious, nervous, easily excitable, trembling, and timid, yet impulsive. They have a sense that time is going too slowly, so they want everybody to hurry up. They may pace up and down in a panic. They can become so *anxious* that they get diarrhea that is frequent, watery, and smelly. They may talk fast, in a childish way.

Chamomilla: Nothing pleases this child. They want to be held, but are only comforted for a short time and then want to be put down again; put them down, and they want to be held again. They scream for something, and when it is handed to them they reject it, or throw it down. They are whiny, restless, irritable, and can be spiteful.

Gelsemium: Even though they are anxious and afraid, their reactions become slow with great weakness, confusion, and exhaustion. Some children tremble, which makes them want to be held. They become dull, heavy, sluggish, and sometimes dizzy. Feeling of weakness in the knees. They may stutter. They may become overexcited. They may get diarrhea. The head may ache at the forehead and/or the back of the head. The eyelids are droopy. The child looks drowsy. It is helpful to have them bend forward while sitting or lying with their head slightly elevated. They need fresh air. The older child may completely freeze up.

Rescue Remedy: This will restore a sense of balance, calm, and harmony. It reduces the effects of shock, trauma, panic, fear, and sadness. The child may feel faint. They can tremble. It can be helpful if the child is becoming hysterical. They may be speechless. Rescue remedy is a very gentle yet effective remedy to keep the ill effects of a trauma from imprinting itself on the child mentally and emotionally. Obtain at your local health-food store. Put 3 drops in 2 ounces of spring water and have your child drink the entire amount. Repeat every 10 minutes until improvement.

Dosage: On the day before visiting the dentist give the appropriate remedy in the morning, and again in the evening. Then give one hour before the appointment. Repeat after the appointment, only if necessary.

Supportive Measures:

Remain calm and composed. The quickest way to get a child to calm down is to establish eye contact, making sure your face is calm and does not have a look of apprehension. Have them take slow, deep, rhythmical breaths into the belly. Keep the focus on the breath. Listen to your child, and talk it out with them. Try to understand without judgment or criticism. Do not minimize the child's fears or feelings. Do not mention anything about a shot unless they bring it up.

Blows to a Tooth

Alternate **Arnica** and **Ruta Grav** every two hours until the pain has subsided. Repeat only on return of pain. If not resolving, consult your dentist, because there may be damage to the root of the tooth. In most cases it takes about ten days for the tooth to tighten itself again. If the tooth is not tightening again, consult your dentist.

Broken Tooth at the Gum Line

Give 2 pellets of **Hypericum** every 15 minutes until the pain subsides and repeat only if the pain returns. Consult your dentist immediately.

Excessive Tooth Decay

Any strong pain, especially set off by hot, cold, or chewing down on hard food, is usually a sign of tooth decay. This requires a trip to the dentist. Some children may have a predisposition to excessive dental decay. If your toddler has a good diet and good oral hygiene, but has cavities, this will require a prescription from a homeopath and a consultation with your dentist. If your water supply does not have fluoride in it, you can give your child 2 pellets of **Calc Fluorica** 6x once a week.

Note: A **6x** potency is a different potency than what is in the kits. You will have to purchase this potency at a health-food store or a natural pharmacy. Do not use toothpaste with sodium fluoride; it is not good for your child's health or central nervous system.

Oral Surgery

If there is excessive bleeding, see the "Wounds" section below (page 347). You may also apply direct, firm pressure with a gauze pad.

Orthodontics

Putting on braces and adjustments to them can be quite painful for days. Obtain a nonsticking, sugarless gum, preferably with a natural sweetener. As soon as your child has the braces put on or gets an adjustment, have them start chewing gum immediately, and chew it as much as possible until bedtime that day. This can work wonders to keep you child from waking up in agony that night or the next day. If they have to be in school all day and cannot, of course, chew gum, you can give them a dose of **Calc Fluorica** three times a day, for up to three days, for the discomfort. It is a good idea to have this remedy on hand in case the gum doesn't help to take the pain away completely.

Note: **Calc Fluorica** is not in the emergency kit, if you have one. You will need to purchase it from a health food store or natural pharmacy.

It is good to have an initial evaluation done by a cranial-sacral osteopath before starting the orthodontic work. Then your child should have follow-up sessions after each orthodontic adjustment.

Toothaches

Mild toothaches can be caused by food getting stuck between teeth, which can irritate the gums, and cause mild swelling and sensitivity in the surrounding tissue. Floss around the tooth thoroughly. Lack of good oral hygiene can also cause these symptoms. Follow up with your dentist.

The following are the most common indicated remedies for tooth discomforts:

Belladonna: The toothache is sudden, with throbbing, sharp, and boring pain. This pain comes on after eating, builds in intensity, and then tapers off. Teeth on the right side are usually the most affected. It is worse from touch or pressure, chewing, or any motion of the jaw. The gum around the tooth and cheek may be swollen.

325

Bryonia: Pains are set off by any movement or pressure. The pains are tearing and needle-like. The child may complain that the tooth feels too long. The molars are the most affected. The cheek can swell on the affected side. Warm food and drink aggravates the pain, but cool water can make it feel better.

Chamomilla: The pains are intolerable. They are sharp and boring. Usually an entire area hurts, not just one tooth. There is usually swelling. They have bad breath and the tongue may be jerky and have a yellow/whitish coat. The toothache is worse from warmth, but not better from cold either. It is also worse at night. This is a very helpful remedy for an irritable teen when the wisdom teeth are descending.

Coffea: The pains are intolerable which makes them have great nervous and emotional excitability. They have over-sensitivity to tastes, noises, and odors. The toothache is worse from heat and feels better if cold water is held in the mouth. The pain returns when the mouth becomes warm again. They may want to bite their teeth together. They are better lying down.

Silicea (also known as **Silica Terra**): This remedy is helpful for children when they are losing a baby tooth. The pains are sharp, boring, and may shoot into the ears, jaw, or cheekbone. Gums are red, sore, and sensitive to cold air and cold water. Sweating of head, neck, hands, and feet. They are worse in the morning and lying on the left side.

The following are the most common remedies for dental procedures:

Arnica is helpful to reduce shock, swelling, bleeding, bruising, and soreness. After the extraction of wisdom teeth, use **Arnica** and then **Hypericum.** Alternate these two remedies, twice a day each, for four days.

Chamomilla: Use this if your child is overly sensitive to pain after a dental procedure. Can be given hourly until the pain subsides. Repeat as needed.

Hypericum: This remedy is helpful to calm nerve pains from drilling, root-canal pains, or pain from tooth extractions, especially wisdom teeth. Can be given hourly until the pain subsides. Repeat as needed.

Ledum: To be used if the injection site is painful and feels cold. The child will feel better from swishing cold liquids over the injection site. Can be given hourly until the pain subsides. Repeat as needed.

Ruta Grav: This remedy will help if there is a deep, achy pain, or for dry sockets. Can be given hourly until the pain subsides. Repeat as needed.

Supportive Measures:

Help your toddler establish good habits by brushing twice daily with natural toothpastes that are free of sugars, fluoride, and laboratory chemicals. Encourage your older child to floss. Do not use toothpaste that has menthol or mint in it. Mint-free toothpastes are available at most health-food stores. A diet free of acidic drinks, refined carbohydrates, laboratory chemicals, and sugars is a must. Calendula Tincture is a liquid herbal remedy given to support other remedies that have been given internally. You can obtain this from a health food store or natural pharmacy. Put a quarter-teaspoon of the tincture in a half-cup of bottled spring water. Have the child use this as a mouthwash three times a day to sooth and promote healing. Do not swallow.

Call your healthcare practitioner if:

- Your child has severe pain in a tooth, and none of the remedies are helping.
- Severe pain is continuing after giving remedies for twenty-four hours.
- Your child has tooth pain accompanied by a fever.
- Pus is draining around a tooth that is hurting.
- Your child has red streaks on their face—*take them to an urgent-care facility or hospital emergency room.*

TRAVEL FIRST AID

A Note about Guarding the Remedies

If you are flying with a homeopathic first-aid kit, cover the remedies with aluminum foil to protect them when your bag gets x-rayed. Put the box in the middle of your suitcase. You can also put any individual remedies that you need during the flight in a purse or carry-on bag. Wrap those remedies in tin foil and put them in the middle of your bag. Remember to keep your remedies away from your cellphone or laptop computer.

Altitude Sickness

This is a condition known as hypoxia, where the oxygen content in the tissues becomes so low that it is unavailable for metabolism. If your child or family member feels nauseated, lightheaded, extremely fatigued, or has a headache, it is best to descend to a lower altitude if possible. Give **Carbo Veg** if there is air hunger, which means that the child keeps taking in deep breaths because the air is so low in oxygen that no amount of it feels satisfying. Breathing is laborious, quick, and short. They may feel faint. They may have a heavy sensation in the body, especially in the eyelids, eyes, or head. They commonly have gas and a bloated abdomen. Two pellets of **Carbo Veg** may be taken on ascending, to prevent altitude sickness.

Note: It is always important to increase water intake to combat the dryness of higher altitudes.

Note: Various cultures of the Andes Mountains have chewed on leaves of the coca plant for thousands of years to ward off the effects of altitude sickness. Drug policy in the U.S. does not allow homeopathic **Coca** use, because the leaves from the coca plant are used to extract cocaine. If you are outside the U.S., you can purchase homeopathic **Coca** for altitude sickness. Its symptoms are the same as **Carbo Veg**, but the **Coca** patient may also have heart palpitations, anxiety, or insomnia.

Worse from: Walking. **Better from:** Descending to lower altitudes, and air blowing in the child's face from wind or being fanned.

Boating

Follow all boating safety rules. Use natural sunscreen. For seasickness on a boat, see remedies for "Motion Sickness" on page 331.

Driving

Always drink plenty of water so you don't get dehydrated. Stop every once and awhile to get the circulation going and prevent sleepiness. Driving nonstop for more than four or five hours is not good for the body.

Have children who suffer from motion sickness look straight ahead, or focus as far away as possible, or lie down, if there is room. Reading or playing a game is the worst thing a child can do if you want to prevent motion sickness. (Also see section on "Motion Sickness" on page 331.)

If you have been sitting in a traffic jam for a long period of time on a hot day with no wind, your child may have a reaction to the exhaust fumes. The head becomes hot, with an intense pain at the base of the skull. They feel weak, sick, and exhausted to the point of very little reactivity. Breathing may become quickened. The body and breath are cold, but they want to be fanned, and crave fresh air. The face may be red. They are thirsty. This child is low in vitality, and weak to the point of collapse. They are exhausted by even the slightest exertion. The child will be indifferent to everything, a bit confused, irritable, and very sluggish. Their extremities are cold, as is their breath, but they feel hot inside, weak, nauseous, and heavy-headed. If this is happens, give 2 pellets of **Carbo Veg** every 15 minutes until there is improvement.

Flying

Air Sickness

Also see "Motion Sickness" on page 331.

Note: Some people suffer ill effects if they have flown over areas heavy in nuclear radiation, such as the Nevada desert or the South Pacific. Ask your homeopath about **Radium Bromide** if this is the case. The best policy is to discuss symptoms with the homeopath in order to select the appropriate remedy.

Ear Pain and Popping in the Ears

Ear pain during takeoff and landing can be excruciating. Be sure to breastfeed or bottle-feed your baby on takeoff and landing, because sucking relieves the pressure. For the toddler, give them a sucker to encourage swallowing. Teach the older child to swallow hard, or yawn. If none of the above works, the main remedy is 2 pellets of Silicea. If this does not help, 2 pellets of **Chamomilla** should relieve the symptoms. Use until there is improvement.

Deep-Vein Thrombosis

For mom or dad: Take 2 pellets of **Hamamelis** before the flight. Stay hydrated, and take a walk up and down the aisle every thirty minutes. A glass of red wine or tomato juice will make your blood thinner.

Fear of Flying

See section on "Emotional Trauma and Fears" (page 257).

Jet Lag

To limit the symptoms, travelers should drink plenty of water. The main remedies for jet lag include:

Arnica, to be taken before and after the flight. Take every 4 hours, and repeat if the flight is longer than four hours.

Belladonna—only if there is a hot, heavy feeling. The face may be flushed. Use on an as-needed basis if symptoms return, depending on how long the flight is.

Gelsemium—only if there is extreme physical tiredness, with a heavy feeling in all the limbs. Take every 4 hours, and repeat if the flight is longer than four hours.

Ill Effects of Air Conditioning

If you sit in a cold draft from the plane's air conditioning system, take 2 pellets of **Causticum**. This can prevent stiff neck and shoulders, earaches, and colds.

Homesickness

Ignatia is given if the child sighs a lot, is disoriented, and seems distressed about everything. Give this remedy 2 hours apart for three doses.

Pulsatilla is given when the child is clingy, whiny, weepy, and feels alone and abandoned. Give this remedy 2 hours apart for three doses.

Motion Sickness

Motion sickness actually originates in the inner ear, bringing about dizziness and nausea. The body's balancing mechanisms are disturbed by rapid acceleration, unusual movement, as on a boat, or confusing visual input, as in a car or boat. Breathing petroleum fumes, smoke, or poor ventilation may aggravate the motion sickness. If the child is at the back of a boat, get them to the front so they are not inhaling the petroleum fumes. If they are down in the hold, bring them above deck.

The motion-sick child is usually sweaty, anxious, and pale. They may have excess saliva, and hyperventilate. They are usually weak and may be lethargic. Encourage slow, deep, and rhythmical breathing. This will bring in much-needed oxygen, and calm the nausea. Giving 2 pellets of **Zingiber** before embarking can act as a preventative for motion sickness. Two pellets of **Tabacum** can also be given as a preventative before getting on a boat. Give 2 pellets of **Bryonia** if your child has had a negative reaction to rides at an **amusement park.**

The most common remedies for motion sickness:

Arsenicum: This remedy may be given after getting off the boat, if the child is still seasick. There is nausea with chilliness, from every movement of a **boat.** There is burning in the stomach, and intense thirst, which makes them crave frequent sips of cold water. However, cold water aggravates the stomach. If you can, encourage warm drinks. The child may have a burning, throbbing headache, and possibly diarrhea. There is great weakness. The child is restlessness, demanding, and anxious. The older child may fear that they are going to die. Anxiety is felt in the pit of the stomach.

Worse from: Cold, exertion, and the sight or smell of food. **Better from:** Open air, being kept warm, warm drinks, and lying down.

Bryonia: This remedy is for motion sickness from upward motion, e.g., in a **plane** when it takes off, or **amusement-park rides.** Also for motion sickness from **cars and boats.** It helps nausea with faintness, shivering, and the feeling of a stone in the stomach. There is usually a strong thirst for cold water. The child may develop a bursting headache. The child will be grumpy, wanting to be absolutely still, not talked to, and left alone.

Worse from: The slightest motion, and cold. **Better from:** Lying still, and pressure on the stomach.

Cocculus: Motion sickness from travel in a **boat, car, or plane.** More than likely the child will experience severe nausea, and/or retching with salivation. There is nausea or vomiting from the sight, smell, or thought of food. There is belching and an "empty, all-gone" feeling in the stomach. They may complain of a metallic taste in the mouth. There is an odd symptom of feeling worse in the open air. They are weak and dizzy. There is an empty feeling in the head, and they cannot watch any moving objects. The child is dazed, confused, and anxious.

Worse from: From raising the head up, standing up, motion, and open air. **Better from:** Keeping the head low, warm rooms, closing the eyes, swallowing, and lying down.

Nux vomica: Motion sickness from **car or plane** travel. There is intense nausea, with a feeling of faintness. The child wants to vomit, but may have a hard time doing so. If they vomit, the retching is painful. They have lots of saliva. They may have a headache over one eye. The child is impatient and irritable. Do not give too much food before the journey.

Worse from: Movement, the thought or smell of food, and tobacco smoke. **Better from:** Lying down, and after vomiting.

Petroleum: Nausea from every movement of a **boat, train, or car.** Profuse salivation while nauseated, empty and sinking sensation, coldness and pain in stomach, heartburn, dizziness, possible vomiting, and sometimes a dull, heavy headache. The nausea is relieved by eating. The child is disoriented, very sensitive, irritable, and quarrelsome.

Worse from: The smell of gas or diesel, cool fresh air, dampness, eating cabbage, and closing the eyes. **Better from:** Warm, dry air, lying down, and having the head elevated.

Tabacum: For **seasickness** with a terrible sinking feeling in the pit of the stomach. Also from motion in a **train or car.** The child feels very faint and dizzy, and becomes covered in a cold sweat.

Intense nausea or violent vomiting. Complete collapse. The child is very pale, almost white, or even green-looking. The child is confused, anxious, restless, gloomy, and miserable.

Worse from: The least motion, the smell of tobacco smoke, pressure, warm stuffy rooms, and stimulants. **Better from:** Uncovering the abdomen, open air, weeping, vomiting, and closing the eyes.

Zingiber: Nausea from movement of a **boat, train, or car.** The stomach feels heavy and empty, with rumbling, gas, and acidity. The taste of any food remains for a long time after eating. The child has a dry mouth, with much thirst. They will feel exhausted and weak. The face is red and hot. They can feel hot and chilly at the same time. They are confused, nervous, fidgety, and irritable in the evening.

Worse from: Eating (especially bread), touch, lying down, evenings, around 3 AM, and cold damp air. **Better from:** Sitting, standing, and being uncovered.

Dosage: Give 2 pellets every 15 minutes for four doses, then hourly until improvement. If there is no improvement after seven doses, choose a new remedy. Repeat the remedy only if there is a return of any symptoms.

Supportive Measures:

Do not get onto a plane or boat with an empty stomach. Give the child a piece of crystallized ginger, ginger snaps, or a fruit bar. Make sure they eat lightly and avoid fatty foods. Encourage them to sip on water. It is best if the child looks straight ahead, or lies down if there is enough space. Reading a book, watching a movie, or playing a game is the *worst* thing for motion sickness. If you are traveling in a car in the mountains, it will be best to have the older child in the front seat. Distract the child by telling them a story,

Supportive Measures (cont):

playing music tapes, or singing. If you are on a boat or plane, sit near the front. If you find a remedy that works for this condition, give it to the child before embarking on the next journey, and repeat at the first sign of any nausea.

Call your healthcare practitioner if:

- Your child is dehydrated, or cannot stop vomiting.
- Your child is having persistent diarrhea that is not responding to remedies.

Travel Abroad

It is very important to be informed about prevalent health conditions in other countries. Before traveling, please check out the website www.tripprep.com.

A Note about Travel Inoculations and Medications

The following information will be helpful if anyone in your family will be traveling abroad. Following the official protocol for travel inoculations could make one feel like a pincushion and, in some cases, very sick. Malaria tablets are recommended by travel doctors for mosquito-infested areas. Unfortunately, antimalarial drugs can be very toxic to the liver. A few years ago, a malarial drug was withdrawn from the market because it seriously undermined liver function; it also appeared to be triggering other severe side effects including first-time mental breakdowns and, in some cases, psychotic breaks.

A yellow-fever inoculation is required for visiting many tropical or developing countries. Sometimes you also may need to have an inoculation if traveling from an infected country. For instance, if you flew from Colombia to Brazil, you might be asked for a certificate showing that you had been inoculated against yellow fever. However, if you went to Brazil from the United States, the yellow-fever shot would not be required. Some insurance companies will insist on certain inoculations before issuing coverage. It is worth getting information from your healthcare practitioner or Internet searches to find out what each country requires. Be informed before your child or any family member embarks on a journey.

There are homeopathic equivalents to the allopathic inoculations. Prescribing potentized (extremely low-concentration) disease material or inoculation material has been found to be effective. Homeopathic remedies for malaria, hepatitis A, typhoid, etc. have been used prophylactically for many years. These remedies do not have any dangerous side effects, but they only last as a prophylactic for a limited amount of time. *Do not attempt to treat yourself or your children prophylactically—contact a homeopath or naturopath.*

If you do get an inoculation, consult with your healthcare practitioner and consider taking **Thuja** in order to detoxify after an inoculation: Take 2 pellets before and after the inoculation. This will not interfere with the efficacy of the inoculation. Immediately after receiving the inoculation, give **Ledum,** which is particularly helpful after receiving a tetanus shot. This remedy will reduce soreness in the puncture site. If there is a severe general reaction, give 2 pellets of **Silicea,** and call your healthcare practitioner at once.

Please make an informed decision on getting inoculations by visiting the following websites: www.tripprep.com, www.vaccines.org, or www.thinktwice.com. A helpful book you may want to purchase is *The World Travellers' Manual of Homeopathy* by Dr. Colin B. Lessell.

Drinking Contaminated Water

Argentum Nit

Vomiting: This remedy is for vomiting preceded by loud belching. The vomit is full of thick mucus, and is sour or bitter. There is burning and constriction in the stomach, with pains radiating into all parts of the abdominal cavity. Severe bloating with gas, and passing gas quite loudly.

Diarrhea: For diarrhea with abdominal rumbling and much bloating. Noisy, watery, green stools that look like they contain chopped spinach or flakes of green. Stools are passed with much gas and an offensive smell. These children are anxious and fidgety.

Worse from: Heat, too much excitement, and eating too much chocolate, sugar, or sweets. **Better from:** Fresh air, motion, passing gas, and burping.

Arsenicum

Nausea and vomiting: Retching after eating or drinking, especially ice-cold water. Burning and rawness in the pit of the stomach. Vomit burns the throat. There may be simultaneous vomiting and diarrhea. The abdomen is sensitive to the touch. The child temporarily feels better after vomiting or diarrhea. After the vomiting has subsided, the child will want small amounts of food often.

Diarrhea: Very watery, burning, slimy, brown, yellow, or black stools that may contain undigested food. They have foul-smelling stools in small quantities that burn the anus. There is cramping in the abdomen. Great weakness follows the stool. The child is chilly, but wants sips of cold water to wet the mouth. They might refuse water for fear of vomiting, and cannot bear the thought of food. This child is anxious, restless, and exhausted, but cannot lie still and has energy enough to be demanding. In the older child, the anxiety may grow into a fear that they are going to die.

Worse from: Midnight, around 2 AM, cold food or drinks, getting chilled, cold, and impure water. **Better from:** Heat and warm applications to the abdomen.

Cinchona (also known as China Officinalis)

Vomiting: Frequent, sour-smelling vomit of undigested food.

Very swollen, painful abdomen with lots of gas and belching, which gives no relief when passed. Sore and cold feeling in stomach, hiccups, abdominal rumbling, and thirst for cold water.

Diarrhea: Pale stools are acidic, profuse, frothy-looking, and have undigested food in them. Diarrhea is painless, but the child does have gas pains that can make them bend double. Diarrhea can be involuntary. The child is weak, irritable, nervous, oversensitive to touch and even drafts, and may have problems sleeping.

This remedy is for a child weakened from loss of fluids from diarrhea and vomiting. They have much sweating, and may feel faint or have ringing in the ears. This feeling persists after the child is no longer vomiting or passing diarrhea, because they are so dehydrated. Give the remedy every 2 hours until improvement. If there is no improvement in twenty-four hours, call your healthcare practitioner. Rehydrate them as soon as possible.

Worse from: Drafts, noise, impure water, nighttime, and after eating. **Better from:** Much quiet rest, firm pressure, bending double, warmth, and gently moving the limbs.

Zingiber

Nausea: The stomach feels heavy and empty, rumbling, and full of gas and acidity. The taste of any food remains for a long time after ingesting. They have a dry mouth, with much thirst.

Diarrhea: Extremely loos diarrhea, with lots of gas and belching. The pains are cutting. There is a feeling that the anus is loose, and it feels hot, with much soreness. The child will feel exhausted and weak. The face is red and hot. They may feel hot and chilly at the same time. They are confused, nervous, and fidgety, and become irritable in the evening.

Worse from: Eating, especially bread, touch, lying down, impure water, evening, around 3 AM, and cold damp air. **Better from:** Sitting, standing, and being uncovered.

Persistent Diarrhea

A watery diarrhea that persists more than fourteen days may indicate a parasitical infection. It can seem like a mild gastric virus that is not clearing or responding to the remedies. This is the case with *Giardia lamblia,* a protozoan intestinal parasite found in impure water or food that has been washed in impure water. The stools become extremely foul-smelling, pale, and fatty. A stool sample may be required to determine whether there is a parasite. *This condition must be treated by a professional, because parasites can cause dehydration and malnutrition from malabsorption.* A baby can become listless, weak, and pale, with sunken-looking eyes. The fontanel (soft spot on top of the head) is sunken. The urine has a strong smell, and the skin has no rebound (if you press the shinbone, the skin does not spring back quickly).

Children are particularly affected by parasites because their systems can be depleted so quickly. The main remedy is **Arsenicum**, but this is often inadequate on its own. You need to consult a healthcare professional who can work on a natural biochemical level alongside the remedies. Parasites can also spread quickly within families, so it is important to deal with them as soon as possible.

Also see "Diarrhea, Nausea, and Vomiting" (page 30).

Dosage: Give 2 pellets every 15 minutes, for four doses, then hourly until improvement. If there has been no improvement after six doses, choose a new remedy. As soon as there is improvement, repeat the remedy only if there is a return of any symptoms.

Supportive Measures:

It is imperative that the child is kept hydrated with pure or filtered water. You can make a homemade fluid replacement with a fifty-fifty mix of apple (or any clear, pulp-free) juice and water. Fresh, pulp-free watermelon juice and water is one of the most quick and natural ways to replenish electrolytes. Even if the child is vomiting, encourage them to drink small sips frequently. Giving a child bananas, applesauce, white toast, and white rice will give binding power to the intestines and slow the diarrhea.

Supportive Measures (cont):

These foods can also be reintroduced after vomiting. It is better for the child to eat small amounts frequently. Cut out all dairy products, and any fruit besides bananas or applesauce. Use organic foods when possible. Miso soup is very nourishing to the gut after an episode like this.

Have the child get plenty of rest. After a heavy loss of fluids from vomiting and diarrhea, improvement is gradual. Do no overtax the system by reintroducing rich or fatty foods too quickly. If the child has no appetite, encourage them to eat just a little. Some young children want to stop eating for fear of vomiting, if the symptoms have been severe. **Cinchona** (China Officinalis) is often needed if the child is weak, exhausted, and can't seem to get their energy back.

Call your healthcare practitioner if:

- Your child is lacking in social skills for maintaining good relationships.
- Your child develops a phobia about going to school.
- There has been no response in twenty-four hours.
- The skin has no rebound effect (if you press the shin-bone, the skin does not spring back quickly).
- There is *severe* abdominal pain that worsens, or has not responded to remedies.
- Your baby is under three months old and has any rise in temperature.
- Your child is over three months old and has a temperature over 103 degrees.

Call your healthcare practitioner if (cont):

- Your child is under two years of age and has had a fever for more than twenty-four hours.
- Your child is over two years of age and has had a fever for more than three days.
- Blood repeatedly appears in the stools or vomit.
- Your child cannot stop vomiting.
- There is vomiting after a head injury or a severe blow to the abdominal area.
- There is unexplained vomiting with severe pain around the navel, or in the extreme lower-right abdominal area, as this can indicate appendicitis in an older child.
- Your baby is refusing to drink. In a baby or toddler, dehydration can set in quite quickly. You must get to an urgent-care facility or emergency room. Shock and collapse with dehydration can cause severe damage to brain cells.
- You suspect that your child has a parasite.
- Your child is depleted, in pain, or becoming dehydrated—go to an urgent-care facility or emergency room. Then follow up with your homeopath.

Handy Tips for Travel in Developing and Tropical Countries

- When your family brushes their teeth, do not rinse the mouth with tap water.
- Do not take ice in your drinks unless they can assure you it has been made with filtered water.
- Never, ever eat food from a street vendor.
- Be careful to not overexert in a hot climate. If your child does get overheated, sponge them down

with cool water—cold drinks or a cold shower will be too much of a shock on their system.

- Rabies runs rampant in some countries. If your child is bitten by an animal, seek immediate medical advice.

- It is sensible in hot climates to avoid drinking any water other than bottled water, and it is necessary to avoid any dairy products, including ice cream, that does not come with a sealed wrapper out of a freezer. Do not eat salads or any fresh fruit without a peel, as it may have been washed in unfiltered water.

- For snake and suspected poisonous insect or spider bites, if possible, capture the animal or write down the details of what it looked like. Stay calm, and try to keep the child calm, keep the bitten part below the level of the heart, and apply an ice pack to minimize spreading of venom. Seek medical help immediately.

- If you are near the ocean, inform your children not to swim alone (especially at night), how to look for riptides, how to swim parallel to shore to escape a riptide, and how to test the depth and temperature before swimming out. Make sure they stay out of the water after eating for twenty minutes, to prevent cramping. Make sure they are drinking plenty of fluids. Use natural sunscreen or wear a coverup to avoid sunburn.

WINTER FIRST AID

Frostbite

Frostbite occurs when a part of the body becomes frozen after being exposed to cold for too long. This can happen especially at the tip of the nose, fingers, and toes. The area becomes white and hard. As the area starts to warm back up again, the child will experience throbbing pain and redness. The skin may itch and form blisters. If your child has experienced frostbite, they may be sensitive to it again in the future. If any area remains red long after it has been frostbitten, you can give a dose of **Zincum Metal**. (This is not included in the Childhood First-Aid Kit available at www.hchild.com, but it is in the general Childhood Kit.)

The most common remedies for frostbite:

Agaricus: For frostbite of feet, toes, or hands. There is burning, much itching, swelling, and inflammation. Blisters may develop later. The legs feel heavy and stiff. There will be pain before the skin is warmed back up again, and sensations as if they are being pierced by needles of ice. The child will be clumsy and appear almost drunk.

Worse from: Cold and touch. **Better from:** Warmth and moving about slowly.

Hepar Sulph: The skin is very sensitive to touch, with splinter-like pains. The child will want to be warmly wrapped up because they are very chilly. However, because the area is so sensitive, they may not want anything touching it. You can try using a blowdryer set on low on the affected area; or put the affected area next to a mild heat source to gradually warm the area. The child is very weak. They are ill-humored, low-spirited, indifferent, and lazy.

Worse from: Cold, touch, and the least draft. **Better from:** Warmth, being wrapped up, and eating warm food.

Petroleum: The skin is moist, itches, burns, and becomes purple; it may also become raw and cracked, and bleed easily, which makes it hard to heal, especially in the folds. The child is extremely irritable, both physically and mentally. They have anxiety with fear. They are angry and excitable.

Worse from: Cold fresh air, dampness, wintertime, eating cabbage, and touch. **Better from:** Warm air, dry air, and lying down.

Pulsatilla: The skin of the frostbitten area is very itchy, swollen, inflamed, and purplish. The pains are intense, with burning and pricking. The area feels hot to the touch, and lacks sensation. If the toes are frostbitten, there is intense, burning pain. The child is clingy, whimpering, whiny, weepy, and fretful, but affectionate. Your older son may feel sorry for himself. This child needs attention and gentleness.

Worse from: Heat or warmth of any kind, and warm stuffy rooms. **Better from:** Resting, fresh air, and cool drinks.

Rhus Tox: The skin is red, hot, swollen with intense itching, and very sensitive to cold air. Dark-red blisters may form. The pains are burning, tearing, shooting, and needle-like. There can also be numbness. The child is anxious, weepy, helpless, mildly delirious, and extremely restless.

Worse from: Cold damp, cold food or drinks, being uncovered, drafts, lying still, the first movement after resting, and nighttime. **Better from:** Warm drinks and food, constant gentle movement, gentle stretching, warmth, changing positions, and gentle massage.

Dosage: Give 2 pellets every 15 minutes for four doses, then hourly until improvement.

Supportive Measures:

Warm the affected area as soon as possible with warm water, a warm compress, or warm air, but not anything that is excessively hot. Do not expose the affected area to unnecessary cold or chill. Keep the frostbitten area clean, warm, and dry. Gently move the affected area around to encourage circulation.

Call your healthcare practitioner if:

- Your child is in extreme pain, and none of the remedies are working.
- The skin turns black. This may happen if the frostbite is severe. Seek immediate medical attention, because gangrene can set in and may make amputation necessary.
- Frostbitten skin breaks open.

Hypothermia

This is a condition where the body has been exposed to the cold for so long that it can no longer warm itself. The child will become drowsy, confused, disoriented, and delirious. Give 2 pellets of **Aconitum,** and repeat if there is a return of symptoms. Once in a warm setting, remove any wet clothing, and wrap the child in a warm blanket. Give them very warm (not boiling hot) drinks. Call your healthcare practitioner.

If the child is unconscious, call 911. To administer a remedy if a child's breathing is severely compromised, or if they are unconscious, put the remedy into a half-glass of water and dab it with your finger onto the child's lips or onto the wrist where the pulse is beating (just above the thumb).

Overexertion or Strains

Arnica: Give *at the end of a day of winter sports,* to prevent soreness the next day. Also use for exhaustion. This remedy prevents a buildup of lactic acid in the muscles, which is what makes you sore. If you wait until the next day, it will be too late because the lactic acid has already accumulated in the muscles.

Rhus Tox: Use this remedy if there is stiffness the next day that feels better with heat. With soreness indicating this remedy, the first movements are achy and stiff. The child feels better as they move about and limber up.

Ruta Grav: If there are sensations of lameness, heaviness, and weariness, especially in the limbs.

Dosage: Give 2 pellets. Repeat only if there is a return of symptoms.

Snow Blindness

This can occur from the glare of the sun reflected off of snow. Give 2 pellets of **Aconitum**. Repeat only if there is a return of symptoms.

Snow Headaches

Glonoinum: This remedy is for a headache from snow blindness, with throbbing as if the head is going to burst open.

Better from: Pressure and cold applications. Give 2 pellets every 15 minutes, for four doses. Repeat only if there is a return of symptoms. Do not exceed six doses.

Handy Tips for Winter Fun

- Do not allow your child to ski alone in the backcountry. Keep within the marked trail boundaries, and follow the instructions on signs.
- Most accidents happen at the end of the day when you are tired. Stop if you or the child feels tired or weak.
- Wear layers.
- Remember to apply natural sunscreen.
- Protect the eyes from UV rays and snow blindness by wearing good-quality goggles or sunglasses.
- Unless the family skis on a regular basis and ev-

eryone is in tiptop shape, take **Arnica** immediately after coming off the slopes. The next morning will be too late, as the lactic acid will have settled in the muscles, causing soreness.

- If skiing in whiteout conditions and the terrain is particularly uneven or rolling, an older child may experience motion sickness. Giving 2 pellets of **Zingiber** will be very helpful at the bottom of the slope.
- Make sure your child has well-insulated gloves and socks to prevent frostbite.

WOUNDS

If your child is in shock, refer to the "Shock" section.

Never put **Arnica** cream, gel, or tincture on an open wound.

How to Care for a Wound:

- Allow a shallow wound to bleed for a short time. This is very cleansing for the wound, and activates the lymphocytes (immune cells that produce antibodies).
- Wash the wound well with warm, mild-soapy water.
- Directly apply a solution of Calendula Tincture: Put 5 drops of the tincture into a quarter-cup of bottled spring water, or fresh water that has been boiled and cooled. Anything stronger can cause initial painful stinging.
- Apply a sterile piece of gauze or a Band-Aid® dampened with Calendula Tincture solution (above). It is important to keep the gauze moist to prevent it from sticking to the wound. The dressing should be changed once a day. Calendula Tincture helps to prevent scarring, and keeps pus from forming. It prohibits germs from thriving, but does not kill them. That is why *it is important to clean the wound first.*

Even with great care, some wounds may become slightly inflamed, swollen, and there may be redness evenly distributed around the wound. If this is the case, you can give **Hepar Sulph** 3 times a day for 3–5 days.

Wounds that become severely infected will exhibit pus filled pockets, extreme redness, swelling, and tenderness. In a case of severe infection, there will be red streaks running toward the heart, and there may or may not be a fever present. *If this is the case, do not delay. Take your child to the nearest urgent-care facility or emergency room.*

Abrasion of the Eye or Scratched Cornea

Give 2 pellets of **Calendula** internally. **Calendula** has an affinity for the cornea of the eye. Repeat **Calendula** up to three times per day as needed till all the soreness and inflammation is gone. You can use **Hypericum** as well, if there is a feeling of sharp nerve pain in the eye after the injury. These two remedies may be alternated. If the pain is severe, you can give them at two-hour intervals—first giving **Calendula** and then **Hypericum**—until the symptoms are gone.

Bleeding

The following remedies can help bleeding to slow:

Carbo Veg: Steady flow of dark-colored blood that puts the child on the verge of collapsing. Breath, hands, and feet are cold. May gasp for air. Clammy, cold sweat on hands and feet. Anxious, confused, irritable, and sluggish.

Cinchona (China Officinalis): The child is faint, **weak, and dizzy from loss of blood.** Ringing in the ears. Vision is dim. The child is thirsty, pale, cold, and shivering. May gasp for air. Nervous, anxious, sensitive to light, and noise.

Crotalus: Slow, oozing, dark, thin blood. Either no clots or very few of them. Skin feels cold and dry. Weakness with trembling. Helpful for absorption after eye bleeds. Child is weepy and spacey. Older child may feel they are going to die.

Ipecacuanha: **Gushes of bright-red blood.** Severe nausea with possible vomiting. Increased salivation, weak pulse, very pale, and clammy cold sweat. Gasping for breath. May have blue circles under the eyes. Irritable and whiny.

Hamamelis: **Dark-red blood.** Great exhaustion. The area that is bleeding feels very sore, painful, and bruised. There can be a backup of blood, which causes venous congestion and gives the area a bluish tint. Child may have throbbing headache. Their temperament while bleeding is calm. Afterwards, they are irritable.

Lachesis: **Thin, dark, almost black blood.** Great exhaustion. Much bleeding from small wounds. May feel constriction in the throat. Cold, clammy skin. They are tense and nervous, both physically and mentally. They may talk a lot.

Millefolium: **Profuse bright-red blood. Blood is very thin.** Wound feels bruised, but not much pain. Keep the child resting, because the bleeding will start again upon exertion. Especially helpful *after a tonsillectomy or nosebleed.* The child will be moaning and spacey.

Phosphorus: **Bright-red, thin, constant, slow-streaming blood.** Persistent bleeding of even small wounds. The wound tends to break open and bleed again. The child is pale and weak. This remedy is helpful *after tooth extractions.* The child will be anxious and fearful, with a large thirst for ice-cold drinks.

Dosage: Give every 15 minutes until the bleeding stops; repeat only if bleeding begins again.

Bleeding from the Mouth

After getting the bleeding to stop, you can spray on diluted Calendula Tincture. This solution can be used for three times a day until the wound is healed. See third bullet in "How to Care for a Wound" section, above.

Bleeding from the Nose

After getting the bleeding to stop, the blood vessels in the nose are in a delicate state. Your child may keep having bloody noses. Put a small dab of calendula cream on a cotton swab, and apply to the septum of the nose three times a day. The septum of the nose is the bone and cartilage that divide the nasal cavity of the nose in half. You can purchase calendula cream at a health-food store or natural pharmacy. Consult your healthcare practitioner, if there is no improvement.

Minor Cuts, Abrasions, and Lacerations

A **minor cut** is a straight cut into the skin.
An **abrasion** is when the top layer of the skin has been scraped off.
A **laceration** is a jagged or torn cut into the skin.
Note: Use these remedies even if stitches are required.

Calendula pellets can be given internally for lacerations, especially of the **lips or scalp, or for deep wounds.** It discourages infection in the incision, promotes skin repair, and reduces scarring. Give 2 pellets 2 times a day until there is improvement.

Hypericum can be used if the wound is inflamed, with severe pains that shoot upwards. This remedy is for cuts of the **lips, fingers, toes, or any other areas of the body that are rich in nerves.** Give 2 pellets internally. Repeat only if the symptoms return. If the pain is intense, you can give this remedy hourly, and then as needed.

Hamamelis can be used if the wound and the surrounding area feel painful, sore, and bruised. Give 2 pellets internally. Repeat only if the symptoms return.

Staphysagria can be used for **knife wounds.** The wound becomes dark-red, or sometimes bluish. There is usually swelling. The wound is very sensitive and tender. In many cases it bleeds more than it seems it should for its size. Give 2 pellets every 4 hours for three doses. If there is still pain in the cut area after it has healed, give 2 pellets once. Consult your healthcare practitioner if there is no improvement.

Minor Puncture Wounds

A puncture wound is penetration of the skin by a pointed object such as a nail, ice pick, needle, pitchfork, splinter, or shard of glass. Puncture wounds tend to have less swelling. It is important to encourage this wound to bleed a little, so any offending bacteria can be flushed out.

Aconitum is used for an injury from a sharp object penetrating the **eye.** Give 2 pellets and wait for 15 minutes. Repeat if the pain or discomfort returns.

Ledum: The pains are shooting and pricking. The child may say the wound feels cold, and it feels cold to the touch. But cool applications will feel best. Use **Ledum** up to three times a day for two days. Repeat whenever the pains return.

Ledum can be alternated with **Hypericum** if the child stepped on a nail, or if there is a puncture in any nerve-rich area like lips, fingers, or toes. The **Hypericum** pains will be sharp and shooting upwards. **Hypericum** will help deal with severe nerve pain, and **Ledum** will help with any muscle pain. Give 2 pellets every 4 hours—first **Ledum** and then **Hypericum**—until the symptoms are gone. If the pain is severe, you can alternate them every hour.

Silicea (also known as **Silica Terra**): Encourages the gradual and safe elimination of any foreign objects that may have penetrated the skin, but especially the **eye.** However small or deeply buried a foreign object might be, **Silicea** will gently ooze it out. *However, it will still be necessary to go to the emergency room with such an eye injury.* You can use **Silicea** with confidence that it will expel any foreign objects. Use three times a day, unless otherwise directed by your homeopath.

Road Rash

Evaluate for shock, and treat if necessary. (See "Shock," page 304.) If there is debris in the skin, it is important to get it washed out. Not an easy task with a screaming child! At first, you can give Hypericum every 15 minutes until you can get the area washed and covered with sterile gauze. Then you can give it on an as-needed basis.

If the road rash is deep and/or covering a large area, you can give **Silicea** (also known as **Silica Terra**) once a day to encourage the body to expel any foreign objects. Discontinue when everything has finished oozing and the scab is well formed. If there is redness evenly distributed around the wound, with some heat, you can give **Hepar Sulph** 3 times a day for three to five days. Wounds that become infected will exhibit pus-filled pockets, extreme redness, swelling, and tenderness. In a case of severe infection, there will be red streaks running toward the heart and there may or may not be a fever present. *If this is the case, do not delay. Take your child to the nearest urgent-care facility or emergency room.*

Note: *Do not use calendula spray for road rash.* Calendula helps to form a scab quite quickly on a wound, and this is a wound that needs to be free to drain itself rather than scabbing over.

Supportive Measures:

Always make sure your hands are clean when washing out or dressing a wound. If available, use surgical gloves. If bleeding is profuse, apply sterile gauze with gentle pressure on the wound, and hold it under cold water. This will slow down the bleeding. Once the bleeding has slowed down, wash the wound with warm, mild-soapy water. Then dab on a solution of Calendula Tincture made by putting 5 drops of the tincture in a quarter-cup of bottled spring water, or fresh water that has been boiled and

Supportive Measures (cont):

cooled, and dry the wound with sterile gauze or fabric. Assess whether stitches are needed.

If you cannot slow down the bleeding, keep applying pressure and *take the child to the emergency room.* If possible, avoid using a waterproof or plastic Band-Aid®, because they prevent air reaching the wound. For a speedy, healthy repair, the wound should be kept clean, with a good flow of air. The worse the cut, the longer it needs to be kept covered. Re-dress a minor wound at least once a day. A deeper wound should be re-dressed according to the advice of your healthcare practitioner. The sight of blood can be quite disturbing to a child. *Remind them to take slow, deep, and rhythmical breaths.*

X-RAYS, SCANS, AND ULTRASOUND

Contact your homeopath if anyone in your family is going in for an x-ray or a CAT, PET, or MRI scan, so they can prescribe a remedy to provide as much protection as possible. If any of these procedures were performed in an emergency situation, you should still contact your homeopath. These tests can be life-saving procedures, or may be needed for diagnostic reasons, but should not be performed frivolously, as they can have side effects. This is true of x-rays and CAT or PET scans because of the radiation they emit. Excessive exposure to radiation has long-term negative effects on the body. Because of this concern, there are now programs being purchased by healthcare providers that keep track of how many rads of radiation a person has received from birth.

X-rays emit radiation. We are told that we are only receiving small amounts or acceptable doses of radiation. As with everything, some people will have no reaction. However, there are some people who are ill affected. Unfortunately, there are no tests to tell whether one of these diagnostic tools has had a negative side effect. If you cannot reach your homeopath, give **Arnica** to assist in clearing radioactivity from the child's body. X-ray radiation, even in small quantities, can attach itself to the electrodynamic field of the body. One x-ray may be negligible, but dozens are not. Dental x-rays emit lower radiation levels and are taken at separate times over several years. However, radiation does not diminish over time. Each new x-ray adds to the effects of all the previous ones. For radiation burns, see the above sections on "Burns," or consult your homeopath.

CAT and PET scans are a form of x-ray, but they are more powerful and emit higher doses of radiation. One side effect is that after the procedure there may be an "energy leak" of sorts, and the child will feel constantly tired and drained. This kind of radiation poisoning can easily be missed, or dismissed as a cause. Consult your healthcare practitioner if this occurs.

MRI (magnetic resonance imaging) scans record images through the use of a giant ring magnet inside which the patient is placed. Within the cell's nucleus there is a positive charge, so when the magnet is turned on, the nucleus is pulled against the side of the cell wall. A picture is then taken of the tissue to be analyzed. When the scanner is turned off, the nucleus of the cell goes back to its original position. The result is mild trauma, and a disruption of each cell's nucleic energy. Children and adults who are sensitive can feel its effects for hours afterward.

Take **Arnica** before and after an MRI. You can call your homeopath and get a **Magnetis Pol-Ambo 30C** (homeopathic magnet) to help undo any ill effects from the MRI. This is not available in any kit. You can also order this remedy from Natural Health Supply. (See "Resources" section at the end of the book.)

Ultrasound is a completely different procedure. Cells of the tissue being analyzed are subjected to a bombardment of sound waves, above the upper limit of the normal range of what a human can hear, which are reflected back to a machine that reads them. Although this procedure is considered noninvasive, the local cells are mildly traumatized. Give **Arnica** before and after.

If an ultrasound is taken of the abdomen, give **Bellis Perennis** before and after. This is even more important for pregnant women, because ultrasound affects the developing cells of the fetus. It is not uncommon for babies who have been subjected to multiple ultrasounds to be born with hematomas (areas of bruising). Mothers report that when ultrasound starts, the fetus moves in the womb. There are pictures of a fetus *in utero* holding their hands over their ears during the procedure; this is because the amniotic fluid amplifies sound. If at all possible, do not subject the fetus to this. Try to avoid any ultrasound performed before twenty-four weeks. However, *you must always use prudent judgment and carefully weigh all options.* In an emergency, do not take a chance with the health of the fetus, or your own.

PART FOUR

Sports On and Off the Field
(including Dance and Gymnastics)

ATHLETE'S FOOT

Wash feet daily with a natural, mild soap. Lavender or calendula is best. Spray on diluted Calendula Tincture, which may be obtained at a health-food store or natural pharmacy: Put one full dropper of tincture into one half-cup of bottled spring water, or fresh water that has been boiled and cooled. Calendula has antifungal properties, as does lavender. Keep the feet exposed to air, and as dry as possible. Only wear cotton, wool, hemp, or other natural-fiber socks. If the feet are dry, you can use virgin organic coconut oil, which has antifungal properties. As much as possible, wear leather or canvas shoes so that the feet can breathe.

BLISTERS

Wash the area well and apply a few drops of diluted Calendula Tincture, which may be obtained at a health-food store or natural pharmacy. Add 5 drops of the tincture to a quarter-cup of bottled spring water, or fresh water that has been boiled and cooled.

CHARLEY HORSE

Give 2 pellets of **Arnica** every 15 minutes until relieved.

CRAMPS IN THE CALVES FROM RUNNING

Give 2 pellets of **Ledum;** repeat if necessary.

CUTS

Wash the cut. Put a few drops of diluted Calendula Tincture on the cut, which may be obtained at a health-food store or natural pharmacy. Use 5 drops of the tincture to a quarter-cup of bottled spring water, or fresh water that has been boiled and cooled. This will help stop the bleeding, and discourage bacterial growth. Apply a sterile dressing. When a child sees blood, it can be quite disturbing; remind them to take slow, deep, and rhythmical breaths. Assess whether there is shock, and give the appropriate remedy. (See the section on "Shock," page 304; also see "Wounds," page 347, if you have any concerns about the cut.)

DISLOCATIONS

Give 2 pellets of **Arnica** hourly as needed for pain, while waiting to get x-rays. Once the reduction of the dislocation is complete, give 2 pellets of **Arnica** in the morning and 2 pellets of **Rhus Tox** in the afternoon for three days. Give Rhus Tox for **lower-jaw dislocations** every 4 hours, and then once a day for three days. If the pain is severe, you can alternate the remedies every hour, or give them hourly, for severe pain from jaw dislocation.

FATIGUE

If there is severe fatigue, give 2 pellets of **Arnica**, which will improve stamina.

JOCK ITCH

Keep the groin area dry. You can spray it with diluted Calendula Tincture from a health-food store or natural pharmacy. Use one full dropper of tincture to one half-cup of bottled spring water, or fresh water that has been boiled and cooled. Calendula has antifungal properties. After the area has dried, dust it with organic cornstarch to keep it dry.

NOSEBLEEDS

Give 2 pellets of **Arnica**. Repeat if there is swelling, or the child complains of a bruised feeling.

After the bleeding stops, the blood vessels in the nose are in a delicate state. Your child may keep having bloody noses. Put a small dab of calendula cream on a cotton swab and gently apply to the septum of the nose (the bone and cartilage that divide the nasal cavity in half). Apply three times a day. You can purchase calendula cream at a health-food store or natural pharmacy. Consult your healthcare practitioner if there is no improvement.

OVEREXERTION

Arnica will help if the child feels bruised, sore, and beat-up from aching muscles and joints, with great fatigue and exhaustion. Give 2 pellets every 4 hours until improvement. Repeat only as needed. On the first few days of practice in a new season, give the child a dose of **Arnica** after each practice, to keep the lactic acid from accumulating in the muscles, which is what makes them sore the next day.

Rhus Tox: Use this if there is stiffness the next day that is relieved by heat. If the soreness subsides as the child moves about and limbers up, this remedy is indicated. Give 2 pellets. Repeat only if there is a return of symptoms.

Ruta Grav: If there are sensations of lameness, heaviness, and weariness, especially in the limbs, this is the indicated remedy. Give 2 pellets. Repeat only if there is a return of symptoms.

PERFORMANCE ANXIETY

Gelsemium can be given for fear of public performance, or fear of crowds. Even though they are anxious and afraid, the child's reactions become slow, with great weakness, confusion, exhaustion, and trembling. They become dull, heavy, sluggish, and sometimes dizzy. They may stutter. A younger child may want to be held.

This state can also occur if the child has become overexcited. They may get diarrhea. The head may ache at the forehead and/or the back of the head. The eyelids are droopy, and the child looks drowsy. It is helpful to have them bend forward while sitting, or to lie down with their head slightly elevated. They need fresh air. The older child may completely freeze up mentally and physically in a public performance situation. Give 2 pellets every 15 minutes until they calm down, then use on an as-needed basis.

SHIN SPLINTS

Arnica: Give three times a week until there is improvement. After improvement, give 2 pellets of **Calc Phos** once a week for three weeks. This remedy is derived from phosphorous and calcium, the cellular building blocks for bone repair from structural stress and injury.

Note: It is important that young athletes do not run up and down concrete stairs for training purposes. Some coaches or trainers are not aware that this can cause shin splints and, in some cases, permanent damage.

SMASHED OR CRUSHED FINGERS OR TOES

Hypericum: Give 2 pellets every 15 minutes until pain is relieved.

STITCHES IN THE SIDE

Bryonia: Give 2 pellets, and repeat if necessary.

TENNIS ELBOW

Ruta Grav: Give 2 pellets daily for five days.

VOICE LOSS FROM YELLING

Arnica: Give 2 pellets every 4 hours until relieved. Do not exceed six doses.

WHIPLASH

Assess for shock first. (See the "Shock" section, page 304.) Give 2 pellets of **Rhus Tox** every 4 hours for the first twenty-four hours, then once a day for three days. Also see "Whiplash" (page 288) in the "First Aid" section.

WIND KNOCKED OUT

Give 2 pellets of **Arnica** immediately. Repeat only if necessary.

Other sections in this book to familiarize yourself with are:

Bites and Stings, Fainting and Collapse, Heat Exhaustion and Sunstroke, Injuries, Shock, and Wounds—all found under "First Aid and Travel" (page 227).

First-Aid Remedy Kits:

You may purchase a Soccer Mom's Homeopathic Kit from my website, www.hchild.com. It includes an *On the Field Remedy Guide,* and ten remedies in a compact case.

You may also make your own first-aid kit that includes the following remedies: **Aconitum Napellus, Arnica Montana (200C potency), Bellis Perennis, Bryonia Alba, Gelsemium Sempervirens, Glonoinum, Hypericum Perforatum, Ledum Palustre, Rhus Toxicodendron,** and **Ruta Graveolens.** Use 30C potencies for all of these except the **Arnica**—this is best in a 200C potency, which you can get from Natural Health Supply. (See "Resources," below.)

THE TEN MOST COMMON REMEDIES FOR PROBLEMS ON THE SPORTS FIELD

	Aconitum	Arnica	Bellis	Bryonia	Gelsemium	Glonoinum	Hypericum	Ledum	Rhus Tox	Ruta Grav
Anxiety or Fear	Fear of crowds, anxiety, faintness, hyperventilation, heart palpitations, restlessness, and impatience.	Nightmares about an injury that occurred, or flashbacks of the injury.			Paralyzing fear of losing control, and fear of public performance. Dizziness, heavy limbs, diarrhea, and trembling.					
Blows to Muscles		Muscle feels sore, bruised, and beat-up. This remedy reduces pain and swelling.	For deeper trauma with more severe swelling and bruising than for Arnica. Sore, achy, and throbbing pain.	Tearing and needle-like pain. Child does not want to move. This remedy reduces swelling and inflammation.					Tearing pains, inflammation, and stiffness.	
Blows to the Back or Tailbone		Give this remedy first for tailbone injury, then Hypericum. Back feels sore, tender, beat up, and bruised.					For tailbone injury, or a back injury with intense pressure and shooting pains. Child is tender, sore, weak, and trembling.			
Injuries to the Eye	For splinters or sharp objects that penetrate the eye. Red and inflamed eye.	Eye socket and surrounding soft tissue feels bruised and very sore. There is swelling.					Intense, severe, and shooting pain. Also for pain after removal of a foreign object.	Severe black eye. Area around eye usually feels cold. Eye is swollen, tender, and purple.		
Blows to the Head		Give 2 pellets right away. Reduces swelling of bumps on head. Put 2 pellets inside of cheek if they are knocked out.					Bursting headache, dizzy, shooting pains or heavy feeling.			

	Aconitum	Arnica	Bellis	Bryonia	Gelsemium	Glonoinum	Hypericum	Ledum	Rhus Tox	Ruta Grav
Blows to the Lips, Mouth, or Teeth		Soreness, swelling, or bruising to teeth or mouth.					Area is extremely tender and sensitive. This remedy relieves nerve pain that shoots up.			
Heat Exhaustion or Sunstroke				Severe, splitting, and bursting headache. Does not want to move.	Drowsy, with droopy eyes, flushed face, cold hands and feet, and dry, hot skin.	Sunstroke (flushed, hot face, throbbing headache, sweaty).				
Injuries to Bones		Give 2 pellets first. Helps with shock, swelling, and bruising.								For injury to shin or collar bone. Intense soreness and achy pains. Reduces bruises and inflammation. Weariness.
Injuries to Soft Tissue			Injuries to soft tissue of breasts, abdomen, and pelvic area. Bruised, swollen, sore, and achy.							
Puncture Wounds							For insect bites that are very painful. Shooting pain in nerve-rich areas such as fingers, toes, or lips.	Wounds to palm of hand or sole of foot. Insect bites or splinters. Affected area feels cold and numb. Pains are shooting, pricking.		

THE TEN MOST COMMON REMEDIES FOR PROBLEMS ON THE SPORTS FIELD (CONT)

	Aconitum	Arnica	Bellis	Bryonia	Gelse-mium	Glonoi-num	Hyper-icum	Ledum	Rhus Tox	Ruta Grav
Shock	Child is fearful, anxious, very re-active to pain, in-consolable. Glassy eyes or dilated pupils. Screaming and crying out in terror.	Child is stunned, exhausted, and irritable when offered help. Anxious because they do not want to be touched.								
Sprains and Strains		Muscle feels sore, bruised and beat-up. Over-stretching of a joint. This remedy re-duces pain and swelling.	Deeper trauma with more severe swelling and bruising than Arnica. Sore, achy, and throbbing.	Tearing and needle-like pains. Reduces swelling and inflammation. Red around joint. Good for knees. Does not want to move.				Injured joint is very swol-len, cold, and numb.	Tearing and shooting pains. Hot, swollen joint. Much inflamma-tion and stiffness on first movement after being still.	Intense, sore, deep, achy pains. Reduces bruises, weariness, and heat. Good for wrists and ankles, and torn tendons.

Resources

Books

Homeopathic Educational Services is a comprehensive homeopathic bookstore with great pricing. They have user-friendly search options to help you find what you want, and a great selection of beginner books on homeopathy: www.homeopathic.com

Clothing for children that is "green"

Consult the "Clothing" and "Fair Trade" categories in the National Green Pages at www.greenpages.org

Consultations

You can log onto www.homeopathic.org/resources/practitioners to find qualified and reputable homeopathic practitioners in your area.

Education

The National Center for Homeopathy is a good resource to help you find a reputable homeopathic school in your area: www.homeopathic.org

Homeopathic kits

You can order homeopathic kits from my website, Homeopathy for the Child: www.hchild.com

Homeopathic pharmacy

Natural Health Supply: Call 1-888-689-1608, email nhs@a2zHomeopathy.com, or go to: www.a2zHomeopathy.com.

Hahnemann Labs: Call 1-888-427-6422, or go to: www.hahnemann labs.com

Natural art supplies

Eco-kids® is a line of art supplies that gives children the tools to create using nontoxic, natural ingredients and environmentally friendly packaging. All products are made in the USA: www.ecokidsusa.com

Natural toys

Organic and natural toys for babies and toddlers: www.hazelnutkids.com

Organizations

Holistic Moms Network is a nonprofit organization connecting parents who are passionate about holistic health and green living: www.holisticmoms.org

Skincare

Lovely lines of products for children and parents that are organic, natural, cruelty-free, and gluten-free: www.aubrey-organics.com or www.weleda.com

Websites

- Information on natural alternatives to be used for various conditions, including herbal and nutritional support: www.alternativemedicine.com
- Information about diseases, diagnoses, medical terms, and drugs: www.webmd.com and www.medlineplus.gov
- Information about drug interactions and side effects: www.rxlist.com

Remedies with Latin and English Names

Aconitum Napellus (monkshood)

Aethusa Cynapium (fool's parsley)

Agaricus Muscarius (amanita mushroom)

Allium Cepa (red onion)

Alumina (aluminum)

Antimonium Crudum (antimony sulphide)

Antimonium Tartaricum (tartar emetic)

Apis Mellifica (honeybee)

Argentum Nitricum (silver nitrate)

Arnica Montana (leopard's bane)

Arsenicum Album (oxide of arsenic)

Baptisia Tinctoria (wild indigo)

Baryta Carbonica (carbonate of barium)

Belladonna (nightshade)

Bellis Perennis (daisy)

Borax (sodium borate)

Bryonia Alba (white bryony)

Calcarea Carbonica (oyster shell)

Calcarea Fluorica (fluoride of lime)

Calcarea Phosphorica (calcium phosphate)

Calcarea Sulphurica (calcium sulphate)

Calendula Officinalis (pot marigold)

Cantharis (Spanish fly)

Carbo Vegetabilis (vegetable charcoal)

Carbolicum Acidum (phenol)

Causticum (potassium hydrate)

Chamomilla (German chamomile)

Cinchona Officinalis or **China Officinalis** (Peruvian bark)

Cocculus Indicus (Indian cockle)

Coccus Cacti (cochineal)

Coffea Cruda (unroasted coffee)

Colocynthis (bitter cucumber)

Crotalus Horridus (from the North American rattlesnake)

Cuprum Metallicum (copper)

Dioscorea Villosa (wild yam)

Drosera Rotundifolia (sundew)

Dulcamara (woody nightshade)

Echinacea Angustifolia (purple coneflower)

Eupatorium Perfoliatum (boneset)

Euphrasia Officinalis (eyebright)

Ferrum Phosphoricum (iron phosphate)

Gelsemium Sempervirens (yellow jasmine)

Glonoinum (nitroglycerin)

Graphites (black pencil lead)

Guaiacum (lignum vitae)

Hamamelis Virginiana (witch hazel)

Hepar Sulphuris (calcium sulphate)

Hypericum Perforatum (St. John's wort)

Ignatia Amara (St. Ignatius bean)

Iodium (iodine)

Ipecacuanha (ipecac root)

Kali Bichromicum (potassium bichromate)

Kali Muriaticum (potassium chloride)

Kali Sulphuricum (potassium sulphate)

Kreosotum (wood tar)

Lachesis Mutus (from the bushmaster snake)

Lathyrus Sativus (chickpea)

Ledum Palustre (wild rosemary)

Lycopodium Clavatum (club moss)

Magnesia Muriatica (chloride of magnesia)

Magnesia Phosphorica (phosphate of magnesia)

Medusa (jellyfish)

Mercurius Dulcis (mercurius chloride)

Mercurius Iodatus Flavus (proto-iodide of mercury)

Mercurius Iodatus Ruber (bin-iodide of mercury)

Mercurius Vivus or **Mercurius Sol** (quicksilver)

Millefolium Achillea (yarrow)

Natrum Muriaticum (sodium chloride, common salt)

Natrum Sulphuricum (sodium sulphate)

Nitricum Acidum (nitric acid)

Nux Moschata (nutmeg)

Nux Vomica (Quaker buttons)

Petroleum (rock oil)

Phosphoricum Acidum (phosphoric acid)

Phosphorus (phosphorus)

Phytolacca Decandra (poke root)

Podophyllum Peltatum (May apple)

Pulsatilla Nigricans (windflower)

Pyrogenium (decomposed beef)

Rheum Officinale (rhubarb)

Rhus Toxicodendron (poison ivy)

Rumex Crispus (yellow dock)

Ruta Graveolens (garden rue)

Sabidilla (cevadilla seed)

Sambucus Nigra (black elderberry)

Sepia (cuttlefish ink)

Silicea or **Silica Terra** (pure flint)

Spongia Tosta (roasted sea sponge)

Staphysagria (delphinium)

Sticta Pulmonaria (lungwort)

Stramonium (jimson weed)

Strontium Carbonicum (carbonate of strontia)

Sulphur (sulphur)

Symphytum Officinale (comfrey)

Tabacum (tobacco)

Thuja Occidentalis (white cedar)

Urtica Urens (stinging nettle)

Veratrum Album (white hellebore)

Zincum Metallicum (the metal zinc)

Zingiber Officinale (ginger)

Bibliography

Birch, Kate, RSHom. *Vaccine Free Prevention and Treatment of Infectious Contagious Disease with Homeopathy.* Victoria, BC: Trafford Publishing, 2007.

Boericke, William, MD. *Pocket Manual of Homoeopathic Materia Medica and Repertory.* New Delhi, India: B. Jain Publishers Pvt. Ltd., 1993.

Castro, Miranda, FSHom. *The Complete Homeopathy Handbook.* New York: St. Martin's Press, 1990.

Cave, Stephanie, MD, FAAFP, with Deborah Mitchell. *What Your Doctor May Not Tell You about Children's Vaccinations.* New York: Grand Central Publishing, 2004.

Curtis, Susan, RSHom. *Homeopathic Alternatives to Immunisation: A guide for travellers and parents looking for an alternative to being immunised.* Kent, UK: Winter Press, 2002.

Griffith, Colin, MCH, RSHom. *The Practical Handbook of Homeopathy.* London, UK: Watkins Publishing, 2006.

———. *The Companion to Homeopathy.* London, UK: Watkins Publishing, 2005.

Hershoff, Asa, ND, DC. *Homeopathic Remedies.* Garden City Park, New York: Avery Publishing Group, 2000.

Lessell, Colin, MB, BS, BDS, MRCS, LRCP. *The Dental Prescriber.* Devon, UK: Abbot Litho Press Limited, 1983.

———. *The World Travellers' Manual of Homeopathy.* UK: Random House, 2004.

Marieb, Elaine, RN, PhD. *Essentials of Human Anatomy and Physiology.* Redwood City, California: The Benjamin/Cummings Publishing Company, Inc., 1994.

Mendelsohn, Robert S., MD. *How to Raise a Healthy Child ... In Spite of Your Doctor.* New York: Random House, 1987.

Miller, Neil Z. *Vaccines: Are They Really Safe and Effective?* Santa Fe, NM: New Atlantean Press, 2002.

Murphy, Robin, ND. *Homeopathic Remedy Guide.* Blacksburg, Virginia: H.A.N.A. Press, 2000.

Panos, Maesimund, MD and Jane Heimlich. *Homeopathic Medicine at Home.* New York: Penguin Group (USA), 1980.

Phatak, S.R., Dr. *Materia Medica of Homeopathic Medicines.* Bombay, India: B. Jain Publishers Pvt Ltd, 1977.

Rose, Barry, MD. *The Family Health Guide to Homeopathy.* Berkeley: Celestial Arts, 1992.

Speight, Leslie J. *Sports Injuries: Their Treatment by Homoeopathy and Acupressure.* Saffron Walden, Essex, UK: The C. W. Daniel Company Limited, 1992.

Ullman, Robert, ND and Judyth Reichenberg-Ullman, ND. *Homeopathic Self-Care.* Rocklin, California: Prima Publishing, 1997.

Index

Charts are indicated with "c."

dry, 145, 150, 151–155, 158,
159, 160–164, 168c
homemade treatments for, 166
moist, 145, 150–151, 157, 159,
160, 169c
observations, 149
overview and descriptions,
144–145
spasmodic, 145, 152–158, 170c
supportive measures, 165
symptoms of concern, 166–167
whooping, 147–149, 151–159, 162
CPR (cardio-pulmonary
resuscitation), 229, 320
cradle cap, 61
cramping
menstrual, 87–94
pap tests causing, 102
running causing calf, 359
stitches in the side, 362
swimming causing, 342
Crotalus Horridus, 240, 348
croup, 146–147, 150, 153, 157,
158, 159, 160, 161
Cuprum Metallicum, 34, 69,
155–156, 170c
cuts, 350–351, 359–360

D

dehydration
diarrhea and/or vomiting
causing, 30–31, 302–303, 339
fainting due to, 269
fevers and, 193, 194
headaches due to, 77
heat exhaustion and, 271
influenza, 205
dental procedures, 313, 318,
326–327, 354
dentists, fear of, 259, 263,
322–323
depression
from grief, 260
headaches with, 80
from influenza, 198
insect bite infection causing,
242

postoperative, 318
from vaccinations, 117, 118
diaper rash, 61–62
diarrhea
contaminated drinking water
causing, 337–341
continued weakness due to, 40
diet causing, 37
emotional stress causing, 34–35
exhausting and bloody, 36
fainting due to, 268
food poisoning causing, 32–34,
35–36, 38, 297–303
overview, 30–31
parasitical infections causing,
338–340
performance anxiety causing,
34–35, 361
remedies, overview, 32–39, 42c
shock from, 306–307
supportive measures, 39
symptoms of concern, 40–41
teething causing, 34
Dioscorea Villosa, 16, 69
dislocations, 284, 292, 360, 367c
diving in cold water, 320
doctors, fear of, 259, 262, 263
dog bites, 237, 239
driving, 329–330, 331–334
drooling on pillow, 127, 167
Drosera Rotundifolia, 156–157,
170c
drowning, near-, 320–321
drug poisoning, 105–106, 296–297
DTaP vaccines, 117, 148
Dulcamara, 10, 34, 64, 125, 131
dust allergies, 230, 231–232
dysmenorrhea, 87–94

E

ear, swimmer's, 321
earaches (otitis media)
antibiotics and misdiagnoses
of, 123
dosage, 178
overview and observations,
171–172

Index

R